Smart Materials for DRUG DELIVERY

Smart Materials for DRUG DELIVERY

– Author –

Biju Chillara

Mallesh Bhattiprolu

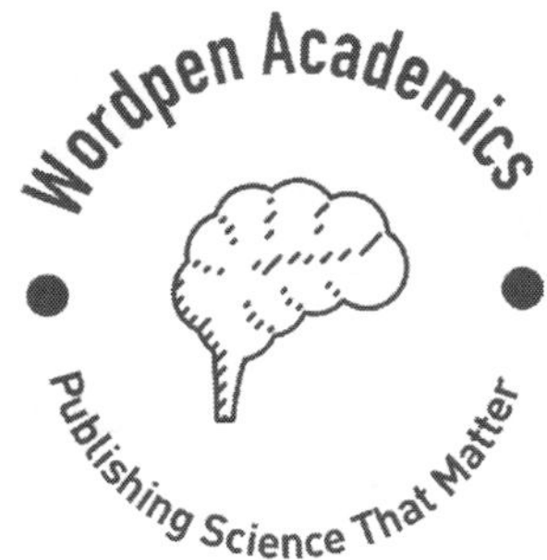

ISBN: 978-81-19283-07-1 (Hardback)

Published by : **WORDPEN ACADEMICS**
4736/23, Ansari Road, Darya Ganj,
New Delhi – 110 002
Phone: +91-011-35004336
E-mail: info@wordpenacademics.com

Printed at **:** **Replika Press Pvt. Ltd.**

Exclusive Distributor: ***Bio-Green Books, New Delhi***

Preface

Smart materials are materials that have the ability to sense changes in their environment and respond accordingly. They can be used in a variety of applications, including drug delivery. Smart materials for drug delivery refer to materials that can release drugs in a controlled manner, based on various stimuli such as pH, temperature, light, magnetic or electric fields, or specific biomolecules. These materials can be used to design drug delivery systems that are more efficient, effective, and targeted than traditional drug delivery methods. For example, a smart material-based drug delivery system could release a drug at a specific site in the body, reducing the risk of side effects and improving the drug's therapeutic effect. There are many different types of smart materials that can be used for drug delivery, including polymers, hydrogels, liposomes, and dendrimers. Researchers are actively exploring new materials and methods for drug delivery to improve the efficiency and effectiveness of drug treatments.

Smart materials for drug delivery have several applications in the field of medicine. Smart materials can be designed to release drugs only in the targeted area of the body. This can improve the efficacy of drugs and reduce side effects.Smart materials can be programmed to release drugs over a specific period, which can help maintain a consistent drug concentration in the body.Smart materials can be designed to release drugs in response to specific stimuli such as temperature, pH, or the presence of particular biomolecules. Smart materials can be used to deliver drugs directly to a localized site of infection or injury, reducing the need for systemic drug administration.Smart materials can be used to create implantable drug delivery systems that can release drugs over an extended period. These systems can reduce the need for repeated drug administration. Smart materials for drug delivery have the potential to revolutionize the way drugs are administered, improving their efficacy and reducing side effects. Researchers are actively exploring new materials and applications for smart materials in drug delivery to improve patient outcomes.

It focuses on a specific aspect of smart materials for drug delivery and discusses the properties of liposomes and how they can be used to improve drug delivery. It explains the protein and peptide drug delivery and discusses the different types of protein and peptide drugs and how they can be delivered using smart materials. It describes the the use of smart drug-delivery systems in the treatment of rheumatoid arthritis, phospholipid-based nano drug delivery systems of phytoconstituents and discusses how these compounds can be delivered using smart materials. It discusses strategies to develop cyclodextrin-based nanosponges for smart drug delivery, targeted nano-drug delivery systems to colon cancer and explains the use of smart materials to target drugs to specific areas of the body. It also explores the use of artificial intelligence in healthcare and discusses the potential applications of AI in drug delivery and other aspects of healthcare. It discusses the applications of statistical tools for optimization and development of smart drug delivery systems and also explores the use of statistical tools to improve drug delivery and optimize the use of smart materials. The book is an essential resource for researchers and professionals working in the field of drug delivery and nanotechnology.

We are grateful to all those persons as well as various books, manuals, periodicals, magazines, journals etc. that helped in the preparation of this book. In spite of the best efforts, it is possible that some errors may have occurred into the compilation and editing of the book. Further queries, constructive suggestions and criticisms for the improvement of the book are always welcomed and shall be thankfully acknowledged.

Biju Chillara
Mallesh Bhattiprolu

Contents

SECTION-II

NOVEL TOOLS AND TECHNIQUES IN DRUG DELIVERY SYSTEM

Section 1

Drug Delivery System

Chapter 1

Drug Delivery through Liposomes

Abstract

Several efforts have been focused on targeted drug delivery systems for delivering a drug to a particular region of the body for better control of systemic as well as local action. Liposomes have proven their efficiency as a choice of carrier for targeting the drugs to the site of action. The main reason for continuous research on liposomes drug delivery is they largely attributed to the fact that they can mimic biological cells. This also means that liposomes are highly biocompatible, making them an ideal candidate for a drug delivery system. The uses found for liposomes have been wide-spread and even include drug delivery systems for cosmetics. Several reports have shown the applicability of liposomal drug delivery systems for their safe and effective administration of different classes of drugs like anti tubercular, anti cancer, antifungal, antiviral, antimicrobial, antisense, lung therapeutics, skin care, vaccines and gene therapy. Liposomes are proven to be effective in active or passive targeting. Modification of the bilayer further found to increase the circulation time, improve elasticity, Trigger sensitive release such as pH, ultrasound, heat or light with appropriate lipid compositions. The present chapter focuses on the fundamental aspects of liposomes, their structural components, preparation, characterization and applications.

Keywords: liposomes, phoipsholipids, cholesterol, stealth liposomal technology, vaccines, doxorubicin

1. Introduction

Liposomes are microscopic vesicles containing aqueous volume enclosed by lipid bilayer membrane [1]. A.D. Bangham and R.W. Thorne first described about liposomes in 1964 when observed under electron microscope while analyzing phospholipids dispersion in aqueous environment [2]. They observed spontaneous arrangement of phospholipids into "bag-like" circular structures. Gerald Weissman, one of the colleagues of Bangham suggested the structures as liposomes [3]. This discovery helped as a multipurpose tool in several fields like biology, biochemistry and medicine. Liposomes gained popularity in vesicular research due their attributes of biocompatibility and similar structural features of biological cells (See **Figure 1**). The amount of drug loaded into the liposomes and the size of the liposomes play pivotal roles in the pharmacokinetic and pharmacodynamic parameters of the drug. The size scale of liposomes varies with typical a mean size of 100 nm. Due to their size and hydrophobic and hydrophilic character liposomes are promising systems for drug delivery.

Several reports showed the applicability of liposomes for the safe and effective administration of therapeutic molecules of different classes like antitubercular, anticancer, antifungal, antiviral, antimicrobial, antisense, lung therapeutics, skin

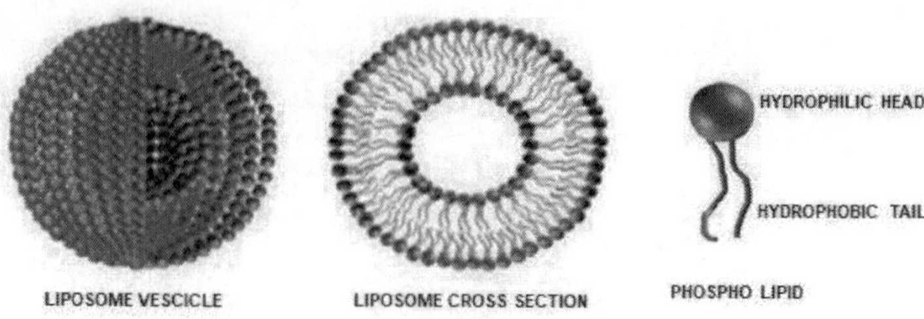

Figure 1.
Structure of liposomes.

care, vaccines, genes etc. [4]. Liposomes have proven their commercial importance from the first product 'Doxil', a PEGylated doxorubicin liposomal formulation [5, 6] to the latest 'Marqibo', vincristine sulfate liposomal formulation [7, 8]. Liposome properties differ considerably with lipid composition, surface charge, size, and the method of preparation. The nature of phospholipid bilayer determines the 'rigidity' or 'fluidity' and the charge of the vesicles. Further modifications of bilayer help in modulation of circulation time, permeability, stimuli response drug release from the liposomes.

2. Structural components present in liposomes

Liposome vesicles are composed of phospholipids as an important structural component of the bilayered membrane and cholesterol is the other component mostly stabilizes the membrane. The properties of liposomes depend on the nature of phospholipids that are being used [9].

2.1 Phospholipids

Phospholipids are amphipathic [10, 11] molecules present in membrane. They contain hydrophilic head and hydrophobic tail. The hydrophilic head has phosphorus molecule as phosphoric acid group, and two hydrophobic tails have long hydrocarbon chain groups (See **Figure 2**). Phosphoglycerides, phosphoinositides and phosphosphingosides are three classes of phospholipids [12].

2.1.1 Phosphoglycerides

Phosphoglycerides are the mostly used phospholipids which contain three OH groups in glycerol moiety and among them two OH groups are linked to two fatty acids and phosphoric acid linked with one OH group. Phosphoglycerides are differed with their attached 'polar head alcohol group' esterified with phosphoric acid. All phosphoglycerides will have two nonpolar "tails" of fatty acid (C16 or C18) and among them one is saturated and other is unsaturated which always attaches to middle or β-hydroxyl group.

a. **Lecithins (Phosphatidyl Cholines):** Lecithin is synonym for phosphotidylcholine which is a phospholipid containing phosphate obtained either from yolk of egg or from soya beans. Lecithin contains unsaturated non polar fatty acids, glycerol and phosphoric acid attached to nitrogen base choline (See **Figure 3**).

b. **Cephalins:** Cephalins have similar basic structure to that of lecithins. The choline present in lecithin is replaced with ethanolamine or serine and examples are phosphatidyl ethanolamine (See **Figure** 4) and phosphatidyl serine (See **Figure** 5). Cephalin exists in α and β forms based on position of two attached fatty acids. The primary amino group present in ethanolamine is weak base compared to quaternary ammonium group of choline. Hence, cephalins are more acidic and less soluble in alcohol than lecithins.

c. **Plasmalogens (Phosphoglyceracetals):** Plasmalogens contains only 10% of phospholipids and are structurally same like other two phosphoglycerides with change of one fatty acid replaced with unsaturated ether. The nitrogen base attached to phosphoric acid of plasmalogens can be choline, ethanolamine or serine and hence, names are phosphatidal choline (See **Figure 6**), phosphatidal ethanolamine (See **Figure** 7) and phosphatidal serine (See **Figure 8**).

2.1.2 Phosphoinositides (phosphatidyl inositols)

Phosphoinositides are phospholipids which have cyclic hexahydroxy alcohol called inositol attached to phosphoric acid. The phosphoinositides on hydrolysis

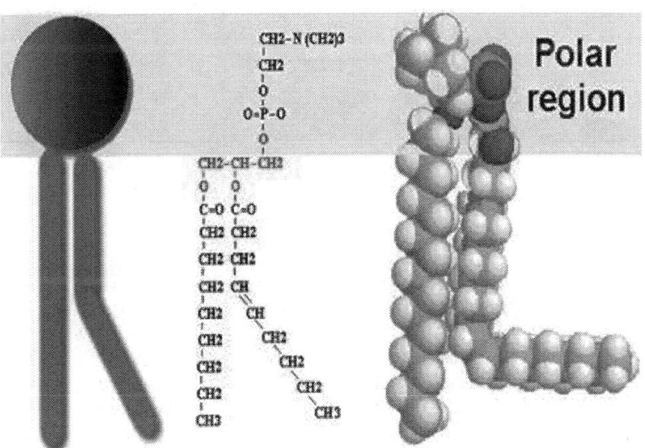

Figure 2.
Structure of phospholipid molecule.

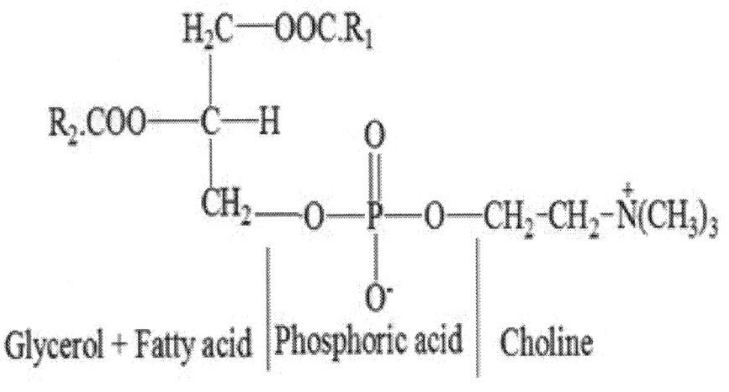

$$
\begin{array}{l}
H_2C-OOC.R_1 \\
R_2.COO-C-H \\
CH_2-O-\overset{O}{\overset{\|}{P}}(O^-)-O-CH_2\text{-}CH_2\text{-}\overset{+}{N}(CH_3)_3
\end{array}
$$

Glycerol + Fatty acid | Phosphoric acid | Choline

Figure 3.
Structure of lecithin.

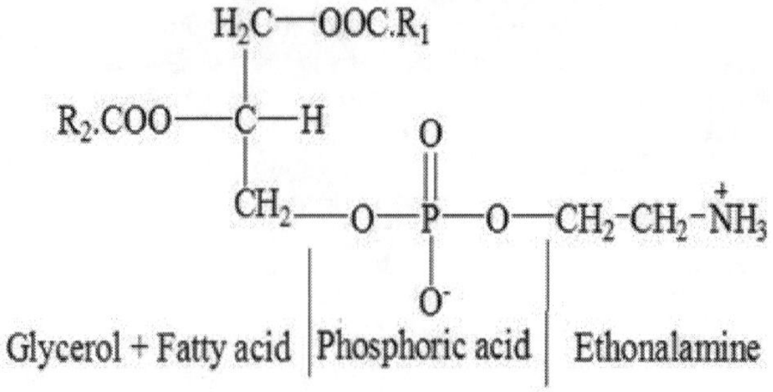

$H_2C—OOC.R_1$

$R_2.COO—C—H$ O

$CH_2—O—P—O—CH_2\text{-}CH_2\text{-}\overset{+}{N}H_3$

O^-

Glycerol + Fatty acid | Phosphoric acid | Ethonalamine

Figure 4.
Structure of Phosphatidyl Ethanolamaine.

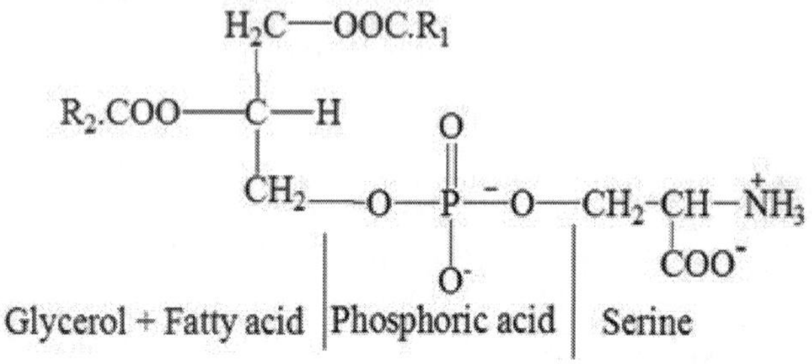

$H_2C—OOC.R_1$

$R_2.COO—C—H$ O

$CH_2—O—P—O—CH_2\text{-}CH—\overset{+}{N}H_3$

O^- COO^-

Glycerol + Fatty acid | Phosphoric acid | Serine

Figure 5.
Structure of Phosphatidyl serine.

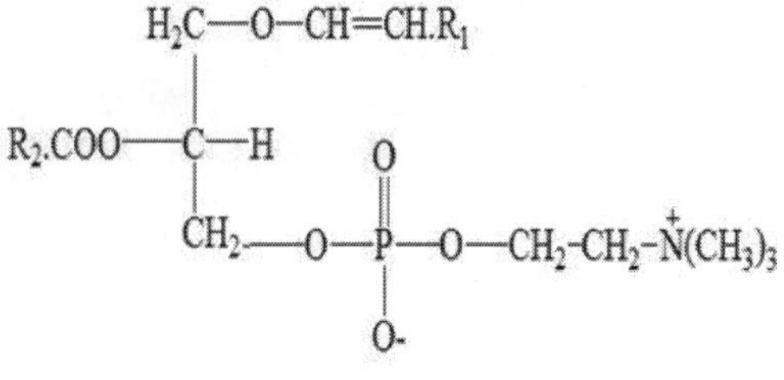

$H_2C—O—CH=CH.R_1$

$R_2.COO—C—H$ O

$CH_2—O—P—O—CH_2\text{-}CH_2\text{-}\overset{+}{N}(CH_3)_3$

O-

Figure 6.
Structure of Phosphatidal choline.

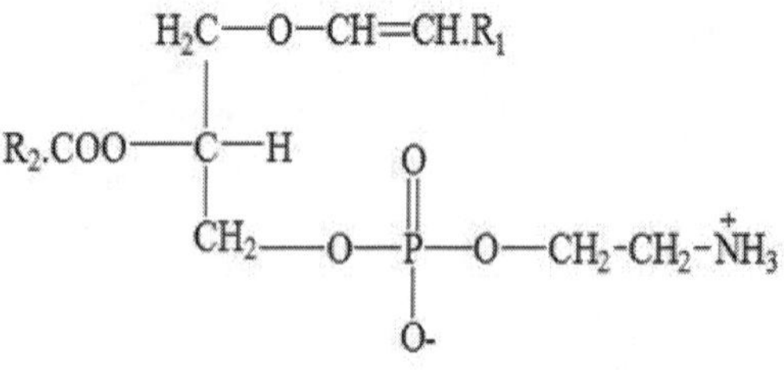

$H_2C—O—CH=CH.R_1$

$R_2.COO—C—H$ O

$CH_2—O—P—O—CH_2\text{-}CH_2\text{-}\overset{+}{N}H_3$

O-

Figure 7.
Structure of Phosphatidal ethanolamine.

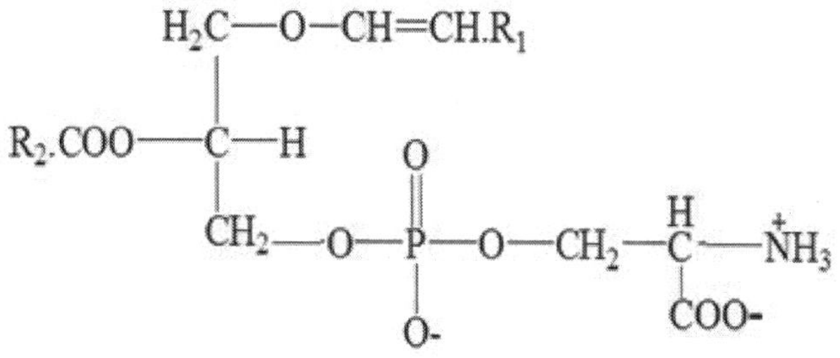

$$\begin{array}{l} H_2C-O-CH=CH.R_1 \\ R_2.COO-C-H \\ CH_2-O-P(=O)(O^-)-O-CH_2-CH(COO^-)-\overset{+}{N}H_3 \end{array}$$

Figure 8.
Structure of Phosphatidal serine.

gives glycerol, fatty acids, inositol and phosphoric acid with 1 or 2 or 3 moles. Because of this monophosphoinositide (See **Figure 9**), diphosphoinositide and triphosphoinositide (See **Figure 10**) are found. Phosphoinositides are glycolipids which contains carbohydrate residue.

2.1.3 Phosphosphingosides (=sphingomyelins)

Sphingomyelins are structurally different from that of other phospholipids by lacking glycerol moiety and presence of nitrogeneous sphingosine or dihydrosphingosine along with choline. These are electrically charged molecules with polar head phosphocholine.

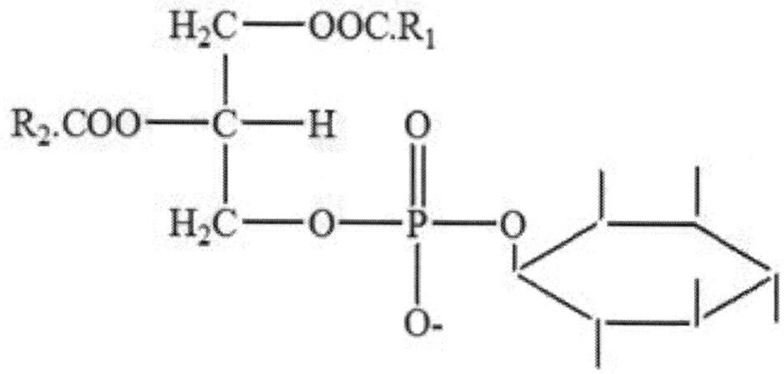

$$\begin{array}{l} H_2C-OOC.R_1 \\ R_2.COO-C-H \\ H_2C-O-P(=O)(O^-)-O-\text{(inositol ring)} \end{array}$$

Figure 9.
Structure of Monophosphoinositide.

$$\begin{array}{l} H_2C-OOC.R_1 \\ R_2.COO-C-H \\ H_2C-O-P(=O)(O^-)-O-\text{(inositol ring with (P)O)}-O-P(=O)(OH)-O^- \end{array}$$

(P) = phosphate

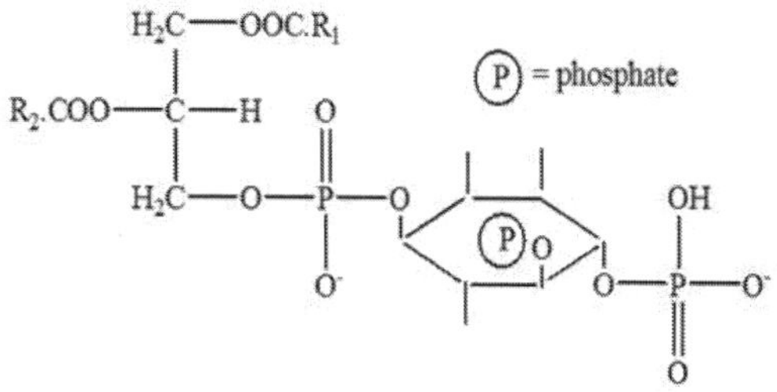

Figure 10.
Structure of Triphosphoinositide.

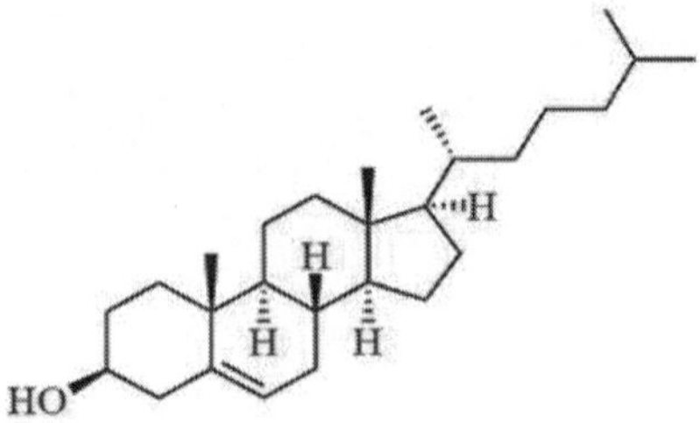

Figure 11.
Structure of cholesterol.

2.2 Cholesterol

Cholesterol is lipid containing steroidal ring with attached hydroxyl group (See **Figure 11**). The OH group present in cholesterol is united with phosphate head group of the phospholipids on biological cell membrane to keep them firm and fluid [13]. Cholesterol has a molecular formula, $C_{27}H_{45}OH$. It is a white crystalline solid and is optically active.

3. Advantages of liposomes

1. Reported methods showed liposomes are non-toxic, biocompatible and completely biodegradable.

2. Liposomes increases therapeutic index and efficacy of drugs.

3. Drug molecules will be stable inside liposomes.

4. Drug toxicity can be decreased when formulated into liposomes.

5. Liposome reduces exposure to sensitive tissues with toxic drugs.

6. Binds to specific site to achieve targeted drug delivery.

7. Liposomes are suitable in delivering aqueous as well as lipid soluble molecules.

4. Disadvantages of liposomes

1. Phospholipids undergo hydrolysis and oxidation.

2. Leakage of loaded drug molecules.

3. Short shelf life and stability.

4. Liposomes production is of very high cost.

5. Liposomes classification

Liposomes are classified [14] mainly by structure, method of preparation, composition with application, conventional liposomes and specialty liposomes (See **Figure 12**).

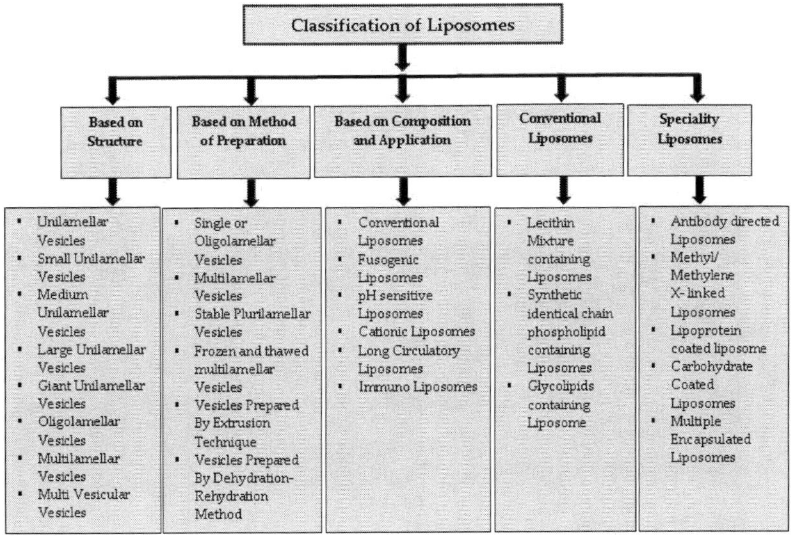

Figure 12.
Classification of liposomes.

6. Methods for liposomes preparation

Liposomes are prepared by using different methods (See **Figure 13**) in which the drug is entrapped by either passive or active loading [15, 16].

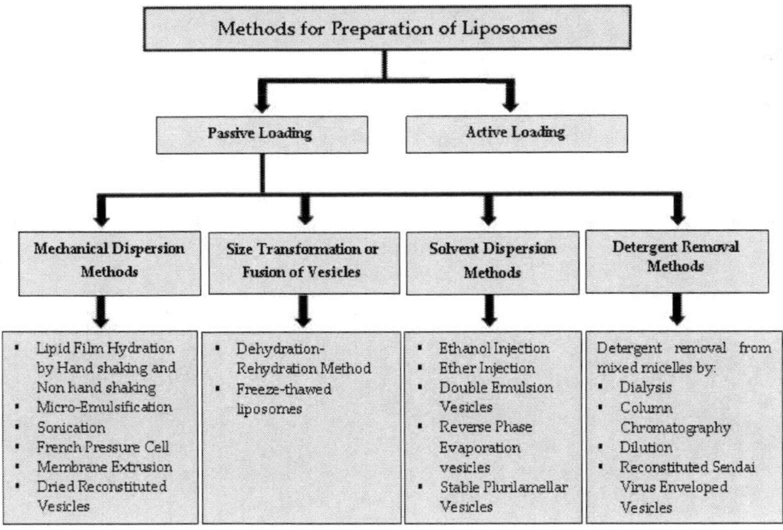

Figure 13.
Methods used for the preparation of liposomes.

6.1 Passive loading methods

This loading technique is to load or encapsulate drug molecules before forming or during preparing liposomes [9]. During liposomes preparation when the lipid film dissolved in drug containing aqueous buffer then that hydrophilic or water soluble drugs is loaded at the centre of liposome vesicle. When lipophilic drugs added to lipid phase of liposome components then that lipophilic drug will load in between lipid bilayers. The unentrapped drug is removed using gel-filtration chromatography or dialysis for liposomal dispersion [17]. The drug loading is low for hydrophillic compounds and high for lipophilic compounds in passive loading method. Liposomal vesicles with large size will have superior drug loading than small sized vesicles [18]. Lipid composition always influence for better drug loading by passive loading method [19].

Passive loading includes four types of methods namely,

1. Mechanical Dispersion.

2. Based on replacing organic solvent (Solvent Dispersion Method).

3. Based on size change or combination vesicle.

4. Detergent removal methods

6.2 Active loading methods

Certain compounds which have both aqueous and lipid solubility and having ionisable groups can be loaded after formation of vesicles [20]. This type of method is called remote or active loading of drug molecules. In this remote or active loading several methods exist in preparing of liposomes. Doxil™ is one of the liposomal products prepared by this method [21, 22].

6.3 Mechanical dispersion methods

6.3.1 Hand shaking or non hand shaking of lipid based film by hydration

This method was first described by [1] and which is simple for liposomes formation with one limitation of having low drug loading. Phospholipids and cholesterol are to be dispersed in organic solvent and then evaporated by using rotary evaporator at low pressure and vacuum. When solvent is evaporated then a dry film will be formed on the wall of rota flask and that should be hydrated by using aqueous phase buffer. The lipids in film spontaneously gets swell when hydrated to form heterogeneous multilamellar liposomes (MLVs).

6.3.2 Micro-emulsification

Micro fluidizer helps in preparing small MLVs from liposomal dispersion [23]. Micro fluidizer pumps liposomal fluid at pressure of 10,000 psi through 5 μm orifice and by micro channels that directs two pathways of dispersion to colloid with high velocity. The large MLVs liposomal dispersion or organic medium containing lipids can also be passed through fluidizer. The dispersion collected is replaced through the micro fluidizer until vesicles with spherical dimensions obtained.

6.3.3 Sonication method

When the liposomal vesicles sizes are above 1 μm then sonication is done to reduce size to form SUVs or extrusion done with polycarbonate filters for producing smaller and uniform sized vesicles. Size reduction by ultrasonication for aqueous dispersion can be done mainly by bath or probe sonicators [24].

6.3.4 French pressure cell

The French pressure press breaks cells with appropriate conditions compared with ultrasound techniques [25]. French pressure press is advantage because sonication procedure degrades lipids, proteins and sensitive compounds. This cell can be used for dispersions with low volume of less than 40 ml and not applicable for high volume production batches. Hence, a scale-up-based strategy was established by using micro fluidization technique.

6.3.5 Membrane extrusion

Another method for liposomes downsizing is extrusion. The vesicles with force are passed through membranes with a lower pressure than french press. Extrusion studies using polycarbonate filters were done and performed on extrusion behavior and membrane properties [26, 27]. Lipex Biomembranes Inc., now called Northern Lipids Inc., invented extrusion vessel from milliliter to several liters. This Lipex extruder allows higher temperatures with jacketed mode. An alternative to this lipex extruder is Maximator device, which is continuous pumping system which was introduced by Schneider et al., 1994. The Maximator has glass vessel which is thermostable and connected directly to pneumatic piston pump. This method consists of preparing liposomes followed by freeze–thaw and finally extrusion. This long process and disadvantage because of high product loss.

6.4 Methods on fusion of preformed vesicle

6.4.1 Dried and reconstituted vesicles (DRVs)

This method follows freeze drying for empty SUVs to form powder (See **Figure 14**). Then that freeze dried powder is rehydrated with aqueous phase media containing materials that are to be entrapped. This dispersion contains solid lipids which are in subdivided form. Freeze drying organizes membrane structure when rehydrated with water to fuse and reseal vesicles. For preparing uni or olio lamellar vesicles of 1.0 μm or less in diameterthis method is used [28].

6.4.2 Extrusion method by freeze thaw

This is extension to above DRV method and lipid film formed by film hydration is mixed with solute containing entrapped materials to form vesicles. The obtained dispersion extruded for three times after two freeze thaws, vortexed and again freeze thawed 6 times followed by 8 extrusions. Then liposomes get fused and forms large unilamellar vesicles, and this method mostly used for proteins encapsulation [29].

6.5 Solvent dispersion methods

In these methods the lipids and non-aqueous soluble drug are added in organic phase and then that lipid phase injected into aqueous phase.

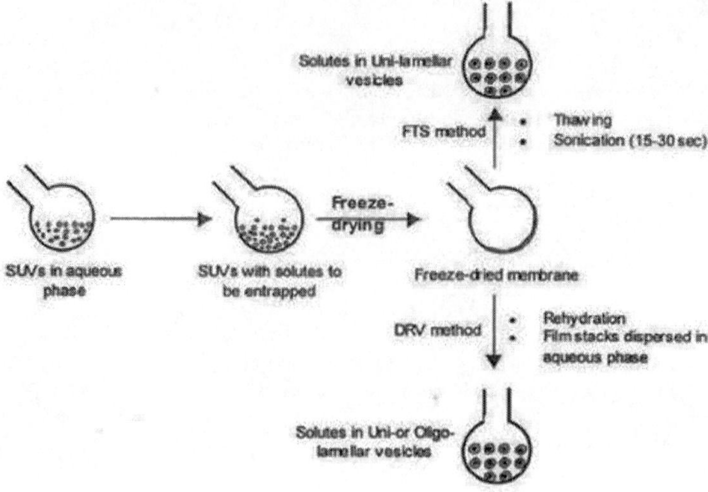

Figure 14.
Preparation of dried reconstituted liposomal vesicles.

6.5.1 Solvent injection method

In this solvent injection method (See **Figure 15**) lipids are added into organic phase (ethanol or ether or chloroform) and that lipid phase is injected into aqueous phase to obtain liposomes [30]. This method again sub divided two methods depending on solvent used.

6.5.1.1 Ethanol injection method

A lipid solution of ethanol is rapidly injected to a large quantity of aqueous buffer. This ethanol injection method gives small liposomes without any extrusion or sonication [31, 32]. This method has some disadvantages that the liposomes formed are very dilute, difficulty of ethanol removal from azeotropic mixture and possible inactivation of various biologically active macromolecules in the presence ethanol.

6.5.1.2 Ether injection method

This ether injection method is different to ethanol injection. Ether is aqueously insoluble and requires hot condition to remove solvent from liposomal dispersion. This method involves single jet injecting lipid phase containing ether into heated aqueous phase. A solution of lipids dissolved in diethyl ether or ether-methanol mixture is gradually injected to an aqueous solution of the material to be encapsulated at 55–65°C or under reduced pressure. The ether vaporizes and the dispersed lipid forms primarily unilamellar liposomes [33]. Ether injection method has advantage over ethanol injection method because the used ether is removed to obtain a concentrated liposomal dispersion and high entrapment efficiency.

6.5.2 Double emulsion vesicles

The double emulsions are prepared by controlling flow rates at three different phases (i.e. 2 aqueous phases and 1 oil/lipid phase) to form single drop of aqueous

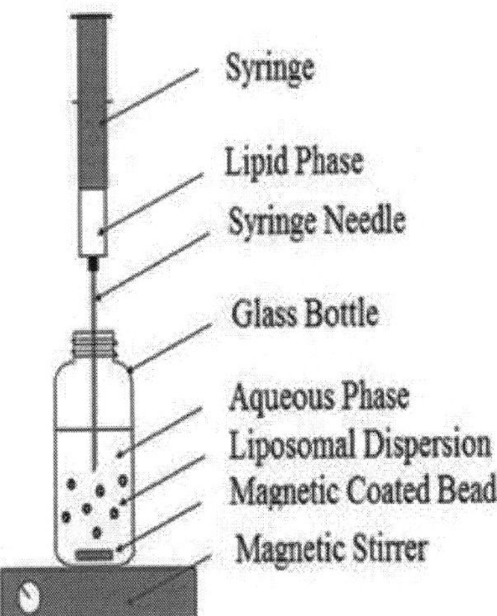

Figure 15.
Solvent injection method.

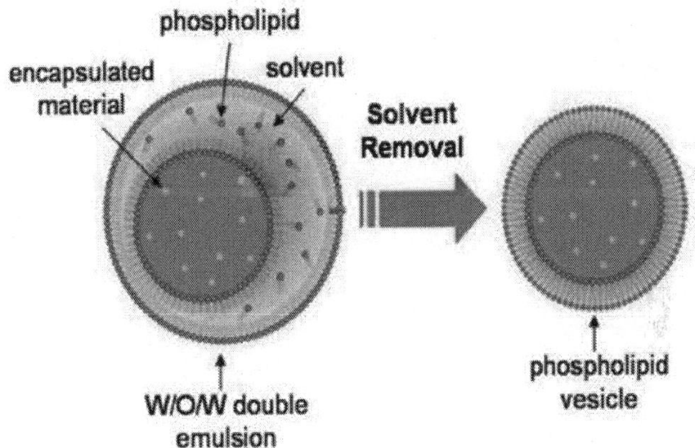

Figure 16.
Double emulsion liposomal vesicles.

solution within a single drop of oil in a continuous aqueous phase (See **Figure 16**). A method by using glass capillary micro fluidic device was fabricated from double emulsion containing phospholipid vesicles [34].

6.5.3 Reverse phase evaporation

The solvent containing lipid is taken in rota flask and evaporated by rotary evaporator kept under low pressure. The formed lipid film was nitrogen purged and then dissolved again in diethyl ether or isopropyl ether containing organic phase to form vesicles. This forms an emulsion and that formed emulsion is again evaporated at low pressure and forms semisolid gel. These obtained liposomal vesicles are called reverse phase evaporation vesicles (REV) [35, 36].

6.5.4 Stable plurilamellar vesicles

Stable plurilamellar vesicles (SPLVs) are prepared using method described by [37]. The phospholipid suspension is to be taken in round bottom flask and evaporated using rotary evaporator to form dried film. To the dried phospholipid suspension an aqueous phase (HEPES [N-2-hydroxyethylpiperazine-N9–2-ethanesulfonic acid] buffer) was added and mixed. The mixture is to be shaken in mechanical shaker and placed in bath sonicator with a nitrogen gas passed through it to facilitate evaporation during the sonication. The liposomes are to be suspended again in the HEPES buffer. The elimination of the nonencapsulated material was done by column filtration and three washes needed in HEPES buffer.

6.6 Detergent removal methods

6.6.1 Detergent dialysis

In liposomal preparations some bile salts and alkyl glycosides are used as detergents for solubilization of lipids in micellar systems. The shape, size of liposomal vesicles always depends on used detergent chemical nature, concentration and lipids [38–40]. The common procedures for removing detergent from micelles are by dilution method [41, 42], gel chromatography [43] and dialysis by hollow fibers [44] or membrane filters [45, 46]. By combining ethanol injection and cross flow injection a new technique was developed to form proteo liposomes [47]. Liposomes of size range 40–180 nm is seen when detergent solubilises lipids to yield micelles [48]. Other methods like calcium induced fusion [49], nanoprecipitation [50] and emulsion techniques [51, 52] are used for liposomes preparation. These classical methods need more solvents and very harmful to human health, also require complete removal of organic solvent.

7. Large-scale liposomes production

The liposomes production extended by techniques such as heating method, super critical reverse phase evaporation, spray drying, freeze drying and modified ethanol injection technique.

7.1 Heating method

A new heating method was available for production of liposomes [53]. All materials are to be mixed in aqueous phase and then to it glycerol (3% v/v) is to be added which will increase the stability for lipid vesicles. The glycerol containing lipid mixture will be heated up to 120° C to form vesicles. The studies on TLC of lipids showed that there is no degradation at mentioned temperature [54].

7.2 Spray-drying

Spray-drying of lipid mixture and drug is one of the methods for large scale industry production. The lecithin and mannitol are to be dissolved in chloroform, sonicated in bath sonicator and spray dried using mini spray dryer to form dried liposomal vesicles. Spray-drying conditions of temperatures 120° C for inlet and 80°C for outlet and 1000 ml/hr. of air flow rate are to be maintained. The obtained spray dried product is to be rehydrated using aqueous phase [55]. The liposomes size depends on used aqueous phase volume for rehydration [55].

7.3 Freeze drying

Freeze drying is a new method for preparation of submicron sized liposomes which are sterile and pyrogen-free [56]. Freeze drying method depends on dispersion having lipids with water-soluble carriers like sucrose and mannitol. Sucrose and mannitol are dissolved in cosolvent system containing tert-butyl alcohol and water. Lyophilizer can be used for freeze drying. The conditions for freeze drying are first freezing to be maintained at −40° C for eight hours followed by 1° drying maintained at −40°C for 48 hours and then secondary drying maintained at 25°C for 10 hours. Mainly 20 pascal pressure is to be maintained in freeze drying chamber at drying process. After reconstitution with aqueous phase the prepared freeze dried product forms liposomal dispersion. The lipid/carrier ratio plays vital role in size and polydispersity of the liposomal dispersion [56].

7.4 Super critical reverse phase evaporation (SCRPE)

This is single step process for preparation of liposomes under supercritical carbon dioxide condition [57]. Liposomal dispersion is formed by emulsion formation with water mixed in ethanol, LR-dipalmitoylphosphatidylcholine, and supercritical carbon dioxide at stirring condition with required pressure. Transmission electron microscopy (TEM) results showed large unilamellar vesicles formed at size range 0.1 to 0.2 μm [57]. The entrapment efficiency results also showed that five times more drug was entrapped by this method compared with Bangham method [57]. Results showed SCRPE is one best technique with single step for large single lamellar vesicles with good entrapment efficiency [58, 59].

7.5 Modified ethanol injection method

Novel approaches are available for liposomes production with principle of ethanol injection which are namely cross flow-injection technique [60–63], microfluidic channel method [64–66] and membrane contactor method [67].

7.5.1 Cross flow injection method

This cross flow is one of large scalable liposome preparation technique with a module with two tubes welded crossly [60–63]. To the cross connecting point, one injection hole is adapted. The used concentration of lipid, injecting hole diameter, injection pressure, flowing rate of buffer and performance of system are important parameters to be considered in preparation of liposomes [62]. A minimum amount of buffer flow rate and lipid concentration with higher injection pressures is needed for batch homogeneity. Reproducibility and scale up data of prepared liposomes with this method showed good results on vesicle size, size distribution, stability and robustness [60].

7.5.1.1 *Microfluidization*

Liposomes are prepared by injecting lipid and water phases with microfluidic hydrodynamic focusing (MHF) into a microchannel [64]. Microfluidic flow is a low rate laminar flow with. Uniform mixing is observed when multi flow steams injected into microchannel [64].

7.5.2 Membrane contactor

In recent studies ethanol injection method was used along with membrane contractor for large production of liposomes [67]. The lipid phase contains cholesterol and phospholipid mixed in ethanol. That mixture has to be pressed through membrane using nitrogen gas with pressure below 5 bars. Tangentially aqueous phase was passed through the same membrane into organic phase to form liposomal dispersion. This new process has advantages with simple design, control of liposome size and scale up batch abilities [67].

8. Recent technologies for preparation of liposomes

Different liposome technologies developed for preparation of liposome formulations. All these technologies have their unique characteristics with unique properties for drug delivery.

8.1 Stealth liposomal technology

In stealth liposomal technology method some strands of polymer are attached to drug molecule for safety to that therapeutic agents. In PEGylation process polyethylene glycol is used. Linkage of PEG to liposomes protects drug molecules in physiochemical properties along with changes in hydrodynamic size and prolongs circulatory time. PEGylation reduces frequency of dosage and provides hydrophilic nature for hydrophobic drugs. Drug efficacy will not be changed by this method and also shows reduced toxicity [68]. With the help of this technology a liposome-based formulation Doxil® which is intravenous injection was prepared for ovarian cancer, multiple myeloma, and Kaposi's sarcoma associated with HIV.

8.2 Non-PEGylated liposomal technology

Non-PEGylated liposome technology (NPLT) is another technology for liposomes delivery in cancer treatment which has more benefits compared to PEGylation process. This technology eliminates PEG side effects and hand foot syndrome (HFS) in chemotherapy treatment. Non-PEGylated liposome Doxorubicin (NPLD) decreases cardiac toxicity related with DOX and dose limiting toxicity with Doxil® like painful HFS [69]. Myocet® is another NPLD used in advanced stage IV breast cancer which was manufactured by company Elan Pharmaceuticals.

8.3 DepoFoam™ liposome technology

This technology was invented by Pacira Pharmaceuticals for preparation of multivesicular liposomes without changing molecular structure of encapsulated drug and releases drug for long period (1 to 30 days). DepoFoam® is a core technology for liposomal marketed products in names Depocyt(e)® containing cytarabine, DepoDur® contains morphine sulfate and Exparel® contains bupivacaine. These formed vesicles are microscopic spheroids with 3–30 μm in size having granular structure with single layered lipid molecules composed like honeycomb and drug molecules are loaded in central aqueous core [70].

8.4 Lysolipid thermally sensitive liposomal (LTSL) technology

Thermally sensitive liposomes release drug from sites which have elevated temperature in our body. Phospholipids like DPPC and MSPC are generally used for preparing these types of liposomes. They are called temperature dependent liposomes. Lipid components present in these thermosensitive liposomes first forms gel to liquid during higher temperature which will be more permeable for drug release. ThermoDox® liposomal formulation prepared with LTSL technology by Celsion Corporation contains doxorubicin drug and present in clinical phase III trials. ThermoDox® has more drug concentration compared to intravenous doxorubicin and present in clinical studies (phase II) used in breast cancer associated to chest wall [71].

9. Characterization of liposomes

Liposomes are mainly characterized physically, chemically and biologically.

9.1 Physical characterization

The physical characterization of liposomes will be known by evaluating their shape, size, morphology, lamellarity behavior and drug release.

9.1.1 Vesicle shape, size and morphology

The liposomes physical stability depends on their size and polydispersibility index [72]. The size is important in parenteral formulations [73]. Electron microscopy is used for measurement of liposome vesicle size and determining their morphology and lamellarity [74–76]. Transmission electron microscopy (TEM) is mostly used in measurement of size distribution. Cryo transmission electron microscopy helps in visualizing liposomes that are in frozen state [77]. This is advantageous because analysis is done at their storage environment and prevents disruption of vesicles [78]. Liposomes are applied in a thin film form to a grid and that grid is to be kept in cooling medium (mostly liquid nitrogen) and viewed under microscope and imaged [79, 80]. This microscopy method is advantageous because vesicles can be measured individually which gives detailed information in size and matrix [81, 82].

9.1.2 Surface charge

The surface charge of liposomes in dispersion can be known by zeta potential [82]. The zeta potential is the total charge obtained by liposomes in liposomal dispersion [83]. The liposomes stability always depends on zeta potential [84]. The liposomal dispersion is always stable when vesicles remain separate without any aggregation. When vesicles have charge then repulsion is seen between vesicles in dispersion with repulsive forces and become stable. For stable liposomal dispersion there will be maximum vesicle charge. Liposomal dispersion with zeta potential of greater that 30 mV or lesser than −30 mV are considered to be more stable.

9.1.3 Lamellarity

The lipid bilayers present in liposomal vesicles represents the lamellarity. This lamellarity of liposomes is mostly applicable in encapsulation efficiency, drug release, fate of drug, and applications [85]. Lamellarity is identified using nuclear magnetic resonance (NMR) spectroscopy. In this ^{31}P NMR method, paramagnetic ion Mn^{2+} or Co^{2+} or Pr^{3+} are added into liposomal dispersion [86, 87]. These ions quenches ^{31}P signal from outer part of phospholipids on reaction with negative phosphate groups. This causes disturbance in spin relaxation and decreases ^{31}P resonance signal. The lamellarity is calculated from comparing signal before and after addition of reagent.

9.1.4 Liposomal dispersion phase behavior

Liposomal dispersion phase behavior can be identified by using differential scanning calorimetry (DSC) [88]. Differential scanning calorimetry method depends on temperature measurement at excess heat capacity of liposomes [89].

9.1.5 Encapsulation efficiency

Percentage encapsulation efficiency (% EE) can be determined by ultracentrifugation method [90, 91]. To find out the entrapment efficiency the liposomal dispersions are to be centrifuged at 5° C at 18,000 rpm for 1 h. The sediment portion of the mixture containing liposomes will be separated and lysised using methanol. Then the concentration of drug from lysised liposomes after suitable dilution was estimated by using UV Visible Spectrophotometer at respective wave length. The entrapment efficiency can be calculated by using following formula.

$$\text{Entrapped Efficiency} = \frac{\text{Entrapped Drug Content}}{\text{Total Drug Content}} \times 100 \qquad (1)$$

9.2 Chemical characterization

Chemical characterization studies gives results for identification of purity in liposomal constituents.

9.2.1 Phospholipids concentration

Phospholipids concentration can be known by using barrlet assay and its principal depends on colorimetric method by inorganic phosphate measurement. The concentration of phospholipid in liposomes is identified by addition of perchloric acid and that gives inorganic phosphate. On adding ammonium molybdate, inorganic phosphate will be converted into phospho-molybdic acid. On adding 4-amino-2-napthyl-4-sulfonic acid to phospho-molybdic acid under hot condition its gives blue color complex which can be determined calorimetrically at 830 nm.

9.2.2 Cholesterol concentration

The adequate separation of cholesterol and its oxidation products in liposomal dispersion can be analyzed by HPLC method. This is mainly studied in stability tests for liposomal formulations.

9.2.3 Fatty acid composition in phospholipids

The fatty acid composition in phospholipid or liposomal dispersion is analyzed by gas chromatography. This method is suitable in estimation of fatty acids oxidation. Two types of column are used in gas chromatography. One is packed column in which liquid phase is coated on granular support and packed into a coiled tube of glass or stainless steel. Other is capillary column which is much narrower in bore, longer and made of glass or fused silica capillary and contains no packing but the liquid phase is coated directly on to inner capillary wall.

9.2.4 Phospholipids per-oxidation

Most oxidation products are further subjected to degradation and at least two separate tests should be performed for estimation of oxidation. Gas liquid chromatography (GLC) and UV absorbance are most quantitative methods to estimate oxidation. This UV method is based on the absorbance of conjugated dienes and trienes at 233 nm 270 nm and phospholipids do not absorb at these wave lengths. TBA (thiobarbituric acid) method is widely used lipid peroxidation assay. In this method the samples are heated with an aqueous TBA solution. Under these conditions the lipid oxidation product malondialdehyde reacts with TBA gives a pink chromophore and spectrophotometrically quantified at 533 nm.

9.2.5 Phospholipids hydrolysis

The phospholipids in liposomes will hydrolyse to free fatty acids and 2-acyl- and 1-acyl-lysophospholipids. The lysophospholipids further hydrolysed to glycerol phosphor compounds. The hydrolysed products can be analyzed by using HPLC method or TLC method and glycerol phosphor compounds can be analyzed by total phosphate analysis of the supernatant (methanol/water phase) after lipid extraction.

9.3 Biological characterization

Biological characterization identifies safety of liposomes formulations when *in vivo* studies are done [16]. The liposomes characterization depends on selection of phospholipid, size characteristics and charge behavior [92, 93]. Sterility of liposomes can be identified by preparing aerobic or anaerobic cultures and pyrogenicity can be known by pyrogen test on rabbits.

10. Stabilization of liposome

Stability is that prescribed preparation should remain with required pre-established limits at predetermined time period. Chemical instability is physical not stability with leakage in loaded drug molecules from lipid bilayers, vesicles fusion with forming aggregation [94]. Physicochemical instability of liposome suspension like hydrolysis, aggregation, fusion and oxidation can be avoided by preparing pro-liposomes [95]. Liposomal stability will be increased when preparing efficient formulation using lyophillization or freeze drying to form powder liposomes which can be reconstituted upon usage. Selection of lipid composition, concentration of bilayers, buffers, antioxidant, chelating agents and cryo protectants play vital role in liposomes preparation. Buffer solutions having neutral pH decreases hydrolysis and antioxidant like sodium ascorbate will decrease oxidation in liposomal dispersion.

Oxygen potential is minimized with nitrogen gas purging to liposomal dispersion to obtain stable formulation [96]. Using antioxidants, buffers with neutral pH and lyo or cryo protectants in freeze drying also gives stable liposomal formulation.

11. Applications of liposomes

Liposomes with varying size, morphology, lipid composition and cholesterol are suitable for many applications to drug delivery [97]. Liposome vesicles interact with body cells for targeted drug delivery [98].

11.1 Liposome for respiratory disorders

Liposome formulations are used in lung disorders and respiratory aerosol which contains liposomes has more advantage compared to normal aerosol. Liposomal aerosols have advantages like sustained action, no local irritation, less toxicity and more stability [93]. Liposome products related to respiratory disorders available in market with brand names are ambisome, Myocet and Fungisome.

11.2 Liposome in nucleic acid therapy

The liposomes bind to nucleic acid with passive charge lipids and pH related surfactants [99, 100]. Liposomes related to gene delivery are under research [101, 102].

11.3 Liposome in eye disorders

Liposomes are used with disorders associated to front and later segments. Retinal diseases cause eye blindness in most advanced countries. Liposomal formulations related to eye disorders are approved for patents and few are in clinical trials. Verteporfin is one of the liposomal based products used in leak of blood vessels at eye caused by pathologic myopia, histoplasmosis (a fungal infection) to eye and age-related macular degeneration.

11.4 Vaccine adjuvant liposomes

Liposomes acts as immune adjuvant and has potentiating activity for cell and non cell mediated immunity [103]. Liposomes are immunological (vaccine) adjuvant, vaccines, carrier of immune modulation and tool in immune diagnostics. Liposomal immuno-adjuvant releases encapsulated antigen very slowy and passively accumulates in lymph node [104] by coupling to the liposomal membrane [105]. Liposomal vaccines can be stored in refrigerator for about 12 months.

11.5 Brain targeting liposomes

Liposomes have biocompatible and eco-friendly action which leads to exploration to brain drug delivery [106]. Liposomes with small and large size undergo easy diffusion through blood brain barrier (BBB). Small unilamelar vesicles (SUVs) coupled to brain drug transport maybe transported through blood brain barrier by receptors or transcytosis. To the liposomes preparations on addition of sulphatide will help to cross blood brain barrier [107]. Wang *et al.* reported in his studies that liposomes with mannose coated targets brain tissue by passing through blood brain barrier [108, 109].

Product Name (Approved Year)	Drug	Lipid Ratio	Route	Indication	Manufactured Company	References
Abelcet® (1995)	Amphotericin B	DMPG and DMPC of molar ratio 3:7	IV	Fungal infections	Sigma-Tau Pharmaceuticals	[120]
Ambisome® (1997)	Amphotericin B	Amphoteracin B, DSPG, HSPC and cholesterol of molar ratio 0.4:0.8:2:1	IV	Fungal infections	Astellas Pharma	[121, 122]
Amphotec® (1996)	Amphotericin B	Cholesteryl Sulfate	IV	Fungal Diseases	Ben Venue Laboratories Inc.	[123]
DaunoXome® (1996)	Daunorubicin	Cholesterol and DSPC of molar ratio 1:2	IV	Blood tumors	NeXstar Pharmaceuticals	[121, 124, 125]
Depocyt® (1999)	Cytarabine	Triolein, DPPG, DOPC and Cholesterol of molar ratio 1:1:7:11	Spinal	Neoplastic meningitis	SkyPharma Inc.	[121]
DepoDur® (2004)	Morphine sulfate	Triolein, DPPG, DOPC and Cholesterol of molar ratio 1:1:7:11	Epidural	Pain management	SkyPharma Inc.	[126]
Doxil® (1995)	Doxorubicin	PEG 2000 DSPE, cholesterol, and HSPC of molar ratio 5:39:56	IV	Breast cancer or Kaposi's sarcoma, Ovarian	Sequus Pharmaceuticals	[121, 127, 128]
Epaxal® (1993)	Inactivated hepatitis A virus	DOPE, DOPC	IM	Hepatitis A	Crucell, Berna Biotech	[129, 130]
Exparel® (2011)	Bupivacaine	Cholesterol, DPPG and DEPC	IV	Pain management	Pacira Pharmaceuticals, Inc.	—
Inflexal® V (1997)	Inactivated hemaglutinine of Influenza virus strains A and B	DOPE, DOPC	IM	Influenza	Crucell, Berna Biotech	[131]
Lipodox® (2013)	Doxorubicin	PEG 2000 DSPE, cholesterol, and HSPC of molar ratio 5:39:56	IV	Breast cancer or Kaposi's sarcoma, ovarian/	Sun Pharma Global FZE	[132]
Marqibo® (2012)	Vincristine sulfate	Egg sphingomyelin and cholesterol	IV	Acute lymphoblastic leukemia	Talon Therapeutics, Inc	[133, 134]

Product Name (Approved Year)	Drug	Lipid Ratio	Route	Indication	Manufactured Company	References
Mepact® (2004)	Mifamurtide	POPC:DOPS of molar ratio 7:3	IV	Non-metastatic osteosarcoma	Takeda Pharmaceutical Limited	—
Myocet® (2000)	Doxorubicin	Cholesterol and EPC of molar ratio 45:55	IV	Breast cancer	Elan Pharmaceuticals	[121, 127, 135]
Onivyde™ (2015)	Irinotecan	DSPE, DSPC, MPEG-2000 of molar ratio 0.015:3:2	IV	Metastatic adenocarcinoma of the pancreas	Merrimack Pharmaceuticals Inc.	—
Visudyne® (2000)	Verteporfin	DMPC, EPG of molar ratio 5:3	IV	Ocular histoplasmosis	Novartis	[11, 136]

Table 1.
Commercial liposome products.

Product name	Drug	Lipid	Indication	Route	Clinical phase	References
Arikace	Amikacin	Cholesterol, DPPC	Lung infection	Aerosol	III	[137, 138]
Aroplatin	L NDDP Cisplatin analog	DMPG, DMPC	Metastatic colorectal carcinoma	Intrapleural	II	[139]
Atragen	Tretinoin	Soybean oil, DMPC	Acute promyelocytic leukemia, hormone -refractory prostate cancer	IV	III	[140]
CPX-1	Floxuridine, Irinotecan HCL	Cholesterol, DSPG, DSPC	Colorectal cancer	IV	II	[141]
CPX-351	Daunorubicin, Cytarabine	Cholesterol, DSPG, DSPC	Acute myeloid leukemia	IV	II	[142]
EndoTAG1	Paclitaxel	Paclitaxel, DOPC, DOTAP in molar ratio 3: 47:50	Anti angiogenic properties, breast cancer	IV	II	[143–145]
INX0076	Topotecan	Egg sphingomyelin, Cholesterol in molar ratio 55: 45	Advanced solid tumors	IV	I	[121]
INX0125	Vinorelbine	Egg sphingomyelin, Cholesterol in molar ratio 55:45	Advanced solid tumors	IV	I	[121, 146]
LE SN38	irinotecan active metabolite SN38	Cardiolipin, cholesterol, DOPC	Metastatic colorectal cancer	IV	I/II	[121, 147]
LEM ETU	Mitoxantrone	Cardiolipin, cholesterol, DOPC in molar ratio 5:5:90	Leukemia, breast, stomach, liver, ovarian cancers	IV	I	[121, 148]
LEP ETU	Paclitaxel	Cardiolipin, cholesterol, DOPC in molar ratio 5:5:90	Ovarian, breast, and lung cancers	IV	I/II	[121, 149]
Lipoplatin	Cisplatin	mPEG 2000, SPE, PPG,SPC, cholesterol	Pancreatic, head and neck cancer, mesothelioma, breast and gastric cancer, non squamous	IV	III	[121, 150]
Liposomal Grb2	Antisense oligodeoxynucleotide Grb2	—	Acute myeloid leukemia, chronic myelogenous leukemia, acute lymphoblastic leukemia	IV	I	[151]
Liposome annamycin	Annamycin	Tween, DSPG, DSPC	Acute lymphocytic leukemia	IV	I/II	[121]
Liprostin	Prostaglandin E1	Unknown	Peripheral vascular disease	IV	II/ III	—

Product name	Drug	Lipid	Indication	Route	Clinical phase	References
Nyotran	Nystatin	Cholesterol, DMPG, DMPC	Systemic fungal infections	IV	I/II	[121]
OSI211	Lurtotecan	Cholesterol, HSPC in molar ratio 2:1	Ovarian cancer, head, and neck cancer	IV	II	[125, 152]
S CKD602	Camptothecin analog	PEG, DSPE and DPSC in molar ratio 5:95	Recurrent or progressive carcinoma of the uterine cervix	IV	I/II	[153, 154]
SPI077	Cisplatin	DSPE PEG, cholesterol, SHPC	Head and neck cancer, lung cancer	IV	I/II	[121]
Stimuvax	MUC1 targeted peptide BLP25 lipopeptide	Cholesterol,, DMPG, Monophosphoryl lipid A, DPPC	Cancer vaccine for multiple myeloma developed encephalitis	Subcutaneous	III	[155, 156]
T4N5 liposome lotion	Endonuclease 5 Bacteriophage T4	Unknown	Xeroderma pigmentosum	Topical	III	[140]
ThermoDox	Doxorubicin	PEG 2000 DSPE, MSPC, DPPC	Non resectable hepatocellular carcinoma	IV	III	[157, 158]

Table 2.
Liposomal products under clinical trails.

11.6 Liposome as anti-infective agents

Amphotericin B (ambisome) is now available in liposome based formulation has passed all the clinical trials. Liposomal Amphotericin B targets liver and spleen by passively and reduces renal toxicity at normal dose and toxicity appears back when given at higher dose [110, 111].

11.7 Liposome in tumor therapy

Long therapy treatment with anticancer drugs gives several toxic effects but liposomal for tumor cells showed less side effects. Reported methods showed liposomes targets to tumor cells and circulate for longer time period with enhanced vascular permeability [112, 113]. In the year 1995, Doxil which is Doxorubicin PEGylated liposomes, for intravenous administration prepared by stealth technology was approved for hematological tumors [5, 6]. Caelyx and myocet are other liposome preparations for same doxorubicin used for advanced breast cancer [114–116].

12. Commercially and clinically available liposomal based products

Various attempts have been made in research to develop novel liposomal formulations for commercial importance and some are under clinical trials. Liposomes have gained their commercial importance with Intravenous formulations. However some recently developed liposomal formulations which are under clinical trials is Arikace (Amikacin for lung infections) [117, 118] which can be given as subcutaneous injection or inhaled as aerosols. Apart from intravenous route and nasal route, the research is being focused and investigated on liposomal formulations for topical route by applying new strategies in the preparation of cosmetics such as skin creams, anti-aging creams, after shave, lipstic, sun screen and make-up [119]. The liposomal-based drugs that are available in market and are under clinical trials are shown in **Tables 1** and **2** respectively.

13. Conclusion

In the last decade, liposomes have become much popular due to research and commercial importance. They offer several advantages for the delivery of different molecules in various routes of administration. Hence the regulatory agencies through the globe is also implemented the subject of liposome into their guidelines. In conclusion, continuous efforts are going in the area of liposome technology to make them better for drug delivery.

Acknowledgements

The authors are thankful to University Grants Commission (UGC, New Delhi, India) for providing financial assistance for carrying the research work. The authors would like to acknowledge M/s. GITAM Institute of Pharmacy, Gandhi Institute of Technology and Management (GITAM) Deemed to be University, Rushikonda, Visakhapatnam, Andhra Pradesh, India for providing facilities and giving support to conduct this work.

Conflict of interest

There is no conflict of interest.

References

[1] Bangham AD, Standish MM, Watkens JC. Diffusion of Univalent Ions Across the Lamellae of Swollen Phospholipids. Journal of Molecular Biology. 1965;13(1): 238-252.

[2] Betageri GV, Jenkins SA, Parsons DL. Liposome Drug Delivery Systems. Technomic Publishing Co., Pennsylvania; 1993. p. 109–125.

[3] Deamer DW. From "Banghasomes" to Liposomes: A Memoir of Alec Bangham 1921–2010. The FASEB Journal. 2010;24(5):1308-1310.

[4] Abdus S, Sultana Y, Aqil M. Liposomal Drug Delivery Systems: An Update Review. Current Drug Delivery. 2007;4(4):297-305.

[5] Barenholz Y. Doxil® the First FDA-Approved Nano-Drug: Lessons Learned. Journal of Controlled Release. 2012;160: 117-134.

[6] Fassas A, Anagnostopoulos A. The Use of Liposomal Daunorubicin (Daunoxome) In Acute Myeloid Leukemia. Leukemia & Lymphoma. 2005;46:795-802.

[7] Sarris AH, Hagemeister F, Romaguera J, Rodriguez MA, McLaughlin P, Tsimberidou AM, Medeiros LJ, Samuels B, Pate O, Oholendt M, Kantarjian H, Burge C, Cabanillas F. Liposomal Vincristine in Relapsed Non-Hodgkin's Lymphomas: Early Results of an Ongoing Phase II Trial. Annals of Oncology. 2000;11(1):69-72.

[8] Rodriguez MA, Pytlik R, Kozak T, Chhanabhai M, Gascoyne R, Lu B, Deitcher SR, Winter JN. Vincristine Sulfate Liposomes Injection (Marqibo) In Heavily Pretreated Patients with Refractory Aggressive Non-Hodgkin Lymphoma: Report of the Pivotal Phase 2 Study. Cancer. 2009;115(15): 3475-3482.

[9] New Roger RC. Liposomes: A Practical Approach, Oxford University Press; Oxford; 1990.

[10] Federico P, Vladimir PT. Recent Trends in Multifunctional Liposomal Nanocarriers for Enhanced Tumor Targeting. Journal of Drug Delivery. 2013;1-32.

[11] Fahr A, Van Hoogevest P, May S. Bergstrand, N., Leigh, M.L.S., Transfer of Lipophilic Drugs Between Liposomal Membranes and Biological Interfaces: Consequences for Drug Delivery. European Journal of Pharmaceutical Sciences. 2005;26(3-4):251-265.

[12] Jain JL, Sunjay J, Nitin J. Fundamentals of Biochemistry. S. Chand & Company Ltd. Ram Nagar, New Delhi; 2005. P. 245-268.

[13] Alberts B, Johnson A, Lewis J, Raff M, Roberts K, Walter P. Molecular Biology of the Cell. Fourth Edition, New York: Garland Science; 2002. 588 p.

[14] Hope MJ, Bally MB, Mayer LD, Janoff AS, Cullisa PR. Generation of Multilamellar and Unilamellar Phospholipid Vesicles. Chemistry and Physics of Lipids. 1986;40(2-4):89-107.

[15] Ostro MJ. Liposomes: From Biophysics to Therapeutics. Marcel Dekker, New York; 1987.

[16] Talsma H, Crommelin DJA. Liposomes as Drug Delivery Systems, Part I: Preparation, Pharmaceutical Technology. 1992;16: 96-102.

[17] Tyagi N, Rathore SS, Ghosh PC. Efficacy of Liposomal Monensin on the Enhancement of the Antitumour Activity of Liposomal Ricin in Human Epidermoid Carcinoma (KB) Cells. Indian Journal of Pharmaceutical Sciences. 2013;75(1):16-22.

[18] Akbarzadeh A, Rezaei-Sadabady R, Davaran S, Joo SW, Zarghami N, Hanifehpour Y. Liposome: Classification, Preparation, and Applications. Nanoscale Research Letters. 2013;8(1):102-108.

[19] Bozzuto G, Molinari A. Liposomes as Nanomedical Devices. International Journal of Nanomedicine. 2015;10: 975-999.

[20] Lasic DD, Ceh D, Stuart MCA, Guo L, Frederik PM, Barenholz Y. Transmembrane Gradient Driven Phase Transitions within Vesicles: Lesson for Drug Delivery. Biochimica et Biophysica Acta (BBA)-Molecular and Cell Biology of Lipids. 1995;1239(2):145-156.

[21] Lasic DD, Frederik PM, Stuart MC, Barenholz Y, McIntosh TJ. Gelation of Liposome Interior. A Novel Method for Drug Encapsulation. FEBS Letters. 1992; 312(2-3):255-258.

[22] Haran G, Cohen R, Bar LK, Barenholz Y. Transmembrane Ammonium Sulfate Gradients in Liposomes Produce Efficient and Stable Entrapment of Amphipathic Weak Bases. Biochimica et Biophysica Acta (BBA)-Molecular and Cell Biology of Lipids. 1993;1151(2):201-215.

[23] Mayhew E, Lazo R, Vail WJ, King J, Green AM. Characterization of Liposomes Prepared Using A Microemulsifier. Biochimica et Biophysica Acta (BBA)-Molecular and Cell Biology of Lipids. 1984;775(2): 169-74.

[24] Hwang KJ, Padki MM, Chow DD, Essien HE, Lai JY, Beaumier PL. Uptake of Small Liposomes by Non-Reticuloendothelial Tissues. Biochimica et Biophysica Acta (BBA)-Molecular and Cell Biology of Lipids. 1987;901(1): 88-96.

[25] Barenholzt Y, Amselem S, Lichtenberg D. A New Method for Preparation of Phospholipid Vesicles (Liposomes). FEBS Letters. 1979;99(1): 210–214.

[26] Olson F, Hunt CA, Szoka FC. Preparation of Liposomes of Defined Size Distribution by Extrusion through Polycarbonatemembranes. Biochimica et Biophysica Acta (BBA)-Molecular and Cell Biology of Lipids. 1979;557(1): 9–23.

[27] Mayer LD, Hope MJ, Cullis PR. Vesicles of Variable Sizes Produced by A Rapid Extrusion Procedure. Biochimica et Biophysica Acta (BBA)-Molecular and Cell Biology of Lipids. 1986;858(1): 161–168.

[28] Gregoriadis G, Leathwood PD, Ryman BE. Enzyme Entrapment in Liposomes. FEBS Letters. 1971;14(2): 95-99.

[29] Mayer LD, Hope MJ, Cullis PR, Janoff AS. Solute Distributions and Trapping Efficiencies Observed in Freeze-Thawed Multilamellar Vesicles. Biochimica et Biophysica Acta (BBA)-Molecular and Cell Biology of Lipids. 1985;817(1):193-196.

[30] Szebeni J, Breuer JH, Szelenyi JG, Bathori G, Lelkes G, Hollan SR. Oxidation and Denaturation of Hemoglobin Encapsulated in Liposomes. Biochimica et Biophysica Acta (BBA)-Molecular and Cell Biology of Lipids. 1984;798(1):60-67.

[31] Batzri S, Korn ED. Single Bilayer Liposomes Prepared without Sonication. Biochimica et Biophysica Acta (BBA)-Molecular and Cell Biology of Lipids. 1973;298(4):1015-1019.

[32] Stano P, Bufali S, Pisano C, Bucci F, Barbarino M, Santaniello M, Carminati P, Luisi PL. Novel Camptothecin Analogue (Gimatecan)-Containing Liposomes Prepared by the Ethanol Injection Method. Journal of

Liposome Research. 2004;14(1-2): 87-109.

[33] Deamer DW. Preparation and Properties of Ether-Injection Liposomes. Annals of the New York Academy of Sciences. 1978;308:250-258.

[34] Shum HC, Lee D, Yoon I, Kodger T, Weitz DA. Double Emulsion Templated Monodisperse Phospholipid Vesicles. La ngmuir. 2008;24(15):7651-7653.

[35] Papahadjopoulos D, Vali WJ, Jacobson K, Poste G. Cochleate Lipid Cylinders: Formation by Fusion of Unilamellar Lipid Vesicles. Biochimica et Biophysica Acta (BBA)-Molecular and Cell Biology of Lipids. 1975;394(3): 483-491.

[36] Szoka FJ, Papahadjopoulos D. Procedure for Preparation of Liposomes with Large Internal Aqueous Space and High Capture by Reverse-Phase Evaporation. Proceedings of the National Academy of Sciences of the United States of America. 1978;75(9): 4194-4198.

[37] Fountain MW, Weis SJ, Fountain AG, Shen A, Lenk RP. Treatment of Brucella Canis and Brucella Abortus in Vitro and in Vivo by Stable Plurilamellar Vesicle-Encapsulated Aminoglycosides. The Journal of Infectious Diseases. 1985;152: 529- 535.

[38] Frokjaer S. Double Emulsion Vesicles, in Liposomes. A Practical Approach, R. R. C. New, Ed., IRLPress, Oxford, UK; 1989.

[39] Anholt RRH. Solubilization and Reassembly of the Mitochondrial Benzodiazepine Receptor. Biochemistry. 1986;25(8):2120–2125.

[40] Jackson ML, Litman BJ. Rhodopsin-Phospholipid Reconstitution by Dialysis Removal of Octyl Glucoside. Biochemistry. 1982;21(22):5601–5608.

[41] Driessen AJM, Wickner W. Solubilization and Functional Reconstitution of the Protein-Translocation Enzymes of Escherichia Coli. Proceedings of the National Academy of Sciences of the United States of America. 1990;87(8):3107–3111.

[42] Kagawa Y, Racker E. Partial Resolution of the Enzymes Catalysing Oxidative Phosphorylation, Reconstitution of Vesicles Catalysing $^{32}P_i$ Adenosinetriphosphate Exchange. The Journal of Biological Chemistry. 1971;246:5477–5487.

[43] Schurtenberger P, Mazer N, Waldvogel S, Kanzig W. Preparation of Monodisperse Vesicles with Variable Size by Dilution of Mixed Micellar Solutions of Bile Salt and Phosphatidylcholine. Biochimica et Biophysica Acta (BBA)-Molecular and Cell Biology of Lipids. 1984;775(1):111–114.

[44] Brunner J, Skrabal P, Hauser H. Single Bilayer Vesicles Prepared without Sonication: Physico Chemical Properties. Biochimica et Biophysica Acta (BBA)-Molecular and Cell Biology of Lipids. 1976;455(2):322–331.

[45] Goldin SM. Formation of Unilamellar Lipid Vesicles of Controllable Dimensions by Detergent Dialysis. Biochemistry. 1979;18(9): 4173–4176.

[46] Milsmann MHW, Schwendener RA, Weder HG. The Preparation of Large Single Bilayer Liposomes by A Fast and Controlled Dialysis. Biochimica et Biophysica Acta (BBA)-Molecular and Cell Biology of Lipids. 1978;512(1): 147–155.

[47] Wagner A, Stiegler G, Vorauer-Uhl K, Katinger H, Quendler H, Hinz A, Weissenhorn W. One Step Membrane Incorporation of Viral Antigens as A Vaccine Candidate Against HIV. Journal

of Liposome Research. 2007;17(3-4): 139–154.

[48] Zumbuehl O, Weder HG. Liposomes of controllable size in the range of 40 to 180 nm by defined dialysis of lipid/detergent mixed micelles. Biochim Biophys Acta. 1981; 640(1):252-262.

[49] Papahadjopoulos D, Nir S, Düzgünes N, Bioenerg J. Molecular Mechanisms of Calcium-Induced Membrane Fusion. Journal of Bioenergetics and Biomembranes. 1990; 22(2):157-179.

[50] Cauchetier E, Fessi H, Boulard Y, Deniau M, Astier A, Paul M. Preparation and Physicochemical Characterization of Atovaquone-Containing Liposomes. Drug Development Research. 1999;47 (4):155-161.

[51] Nii T, Ishii F. Encapsulation Efficiency of Water-Soluble and Insoluble Drugs in Liposomes Prepared by the Microencapsulation Vesicle Method. International Journal of Pharmaceutics. 2005;298(1):198-205.

[52] Cheung Shum H, Lee D, Yoon I, Kodger T, Weitz DA. Double Emulsion Templated Monodisperse Phospholipid Vesicles. Langmuir. 2008;24(15): 7651-7653.

[53] Mozafari MR. Liposomes: An Overview of Manufacturing Techniques. Cellular & Molecular Biology Letters. 2005;10(4):711-719.

[54] Mozafari, MR, Omri A. Importance of Divalent Cations in Nanolipoplex Gene Delivery. Journal of Pharmaceutical Sciences. 2007;96(8): 1955-1966.

[55] Skalko-Basnet N, Pavelic Z, Becirevic-Lacan M. Liposomes Containing Drug and Cyclodextrin Prepared by the One-Step Spray-Drying Method. Drug Development and Industrial Pharmacy. 2000;26(12): 1279-1284.

[56] Li C, Deng Y. A Novel Method for the Preparation of Liposomes: Freeze Drying of Monophase Solutions. Journal of Pharmaceutical Sciences. 2004;93(6): 1403-1414.

[57] Otake K, Imura T, Sakai H, Abe M. Development of a New Preparation Method of Liposomes Using Supercritical Carbon Dioxide. Langmuir. 2001;17(13):3898-3901.

[58] Otake K, Shimomura T, Goto T, Imura T, Furuya T, Yoda S, Takebayashi Y, Sakai H, Abe M. Preparation of Liposomes Using an Improved Supercritical Reverse Phase Evaporation Method. Langmuir. 2006; 22(6):2543-2550.

[59] Imura T, Otake K, Hashimoto S, Gotoh T, Yuasa, M, Yokoyama S, Sakai H, Rathman JF, Abe M. Preparation and Physicochemical Properties of Various Soybean Lecithin Liposomes Using Supercritical Reverse Phase Evaporation Method. Colloid Surface B. 2002;27(2–3):133–140.

[60] Wagner A, Vorauer-Uhl K, Kreismayr G, Katinger H. The Crossflow Injection Technique: An Improvement of the Ethanol Injection Method. Journal of Liposome Research. 2002a;12(3):259–270.

[61] Wagner A, Vorauer-Uhl K, Kreismayr G, Katinger H. Enhanced Protein Loading into Liposomes by the Multiple Crossflow Injection Technique. Journal of Liposome Research. 2002b;12 (3):271–283.

[62] Wagner A, Vorauer-Uhl K, Katinger H. Liposomes Produced in A Pilot Scale: Production, Purification and Efficiency Aspects. European Journal of Pharmaceutics and Biopharmaceutics. 2002c;54(2):213-219.

[63] Wagner A, Platzgummer M, Kreismayr G, Quendler H, Stiegler G, Ferko B, Vecera G, Vorauer-Uhl K, Katinger H. GMP Production of Liposomes–A New Industrial Approach. Journal of Liposome Research. 2006;16 (3):11-319.

[64] Jahn A, Vreeland WN, DeVoe DL, Locascio LE, Gaitan M. Microfluidic Directed Formation of Liposomes of Controlled Size. Langmuir. 2007;23(11): 6289-6293.

[65] Jahn A, Vreeland WN, Gaitan M, Locascio LE. Controlled Vesicle Self-Assembly in Microfluidic Channels with Hydrodynamic Focusing. Journal of the American Chemical Society. 2004;126 (9):2674-2675.

[66] Pradhan P, Guan J, Lu D, Wang PG, Lee LJ, Lee RJ. A Facile Microfluidic Method for Production of Liposomes. Anticancer Research. 2008;28(2A): 943-947.

[67] Jaafar-Maalej C, Charcosset C, Fessi H. A New Method for Liposome Preparation Using a Membrane Contactor. Journal of Liposome Research. 2011;21(3):213-220.

[68] Veronese FM, Harris JM. Introduction and Overview of Peptide and Protein Pegylation. Advanced Drug Delivery Reviews. 2002;54(4):453-456.

[69] Leonard RCF, Williams S, Tulpule A, Levine AM, Oliveros S. Improving the Therapeutic Index of Anthracycline Chemotherapy: Focus On Liposomal Doxorubicin (Myocet™). The Breast. 2009;18(4):218–224.

[70] Murry DJ, Blaney SM. Clinical Pharmacology of Encapsulated Sustained-Release Cytarabine. Annals of Pharmacotherapy. 2000;34(10):1173–1178.

[71] Slingerland M, Guchelaar HJ, Gelderblom H. Liposomal Drug Formulations in Cancer Therapy: 15 Years Along the Road. Drug Discovery Today. 2012;17(3-4):160–166.

[72] Armengol X, Estelrich J. Physical Stability of Different Liposome Compositions Obtained by Extrusion Method. Journal of Microencapsulation. 1995;12(5):525.

[73] Pattni BS, Chupin VV, Torchilin VP. New Developments in Liposomal Drug Delivery. Chemical Reviews. 2015;115 (19):10938-10966.

[74] Akashi K, Miyata H, Itoh H, Kinosita K. Preparation of Giant Liposomes in Physiological Conditions And Their Characterization Under An Optical Microscope. Biophysical Journal. 1996;71:3242-3250.

[75] Jiskoot W, Teerlink ET, Beuvery C, Crommelin DJA. Preparation of Liposomes Via Detergent Removal from Mixed Micelles By Dilution. Pharmaceutisch Weekblad. 1986;8(5): 259-265.

[76] Egerdie B, Singer M. Morphology of Gel State Phosphatidylethanolamine and Phosphatidylcholine Liposomes: A Negative Stain Electron Microscopic Study. Chemistry and Physics of Lipids. 1982;31(1):75-85.

[77] Kuntsche J, Horst JC, Bunjes H. Cryogenic Transmission Electron Microscopy (Cryo-TEM) For Studying the Morphology of Colloidal Drug Delivery Systems. International Journal of Pharmaceutics. 2011;417(1-2): 120-137.

[78] Gustafsson J, Arvidson G, Karlsson G, Almgren M. Complexes Between Cationic Liposomes and DNA Visualized by Crio-TEM. Biochemica et Biophysica Acta. 1995;1235(2):305-311.

[79] Almgren M, Edwards K, Gustafsson J. Cryotransmission Electron Microscopy of Thin Vitrified Samples.

Current Opinion in Colloid and Interface Science. 1996;1(2):270-278.

[80] Almgren M, Edwards K, Karlsson G. Cryo Transmission Electron Microscopy of Liposomes and Related Structures. Colloids and Surface A. 2000;174(1-2): 3-21.

[81] Blochliger E, Blocher M, Walde P, Luisi PL. Matrix Effect in the Size Distribution of Fatty Acid Vesicles. Journal of Physical Chemistry B. 1998; 102(50):10383-10390.

[82] Hunter RJ, Midmore BR, Zhang HC. Zeta Potential of Highly Charged Thin Double-Layer Systems. Journal of Colloid and Interface Science. 2001;237 (1):147-149.

[83] Lyklema J, Fleer G.J. Electrical Contributions to the Effect of Macromolecules on Colloid Stability. Colloids and Surface A. 1987;25(2-4): 357-368.

[84] Du Plessis J, Ramachandran C, Weiner N, Muller DG. The Influence of Particle Size of Liposomes On the Deposition of Drug into Skin. International Journal of Pharmaceutics. 1994;103(3):277-282.

[85] Frohlich M, Brecht V, Peschka-Suss R. Parameters Influencing the Determination of Liposome Lamellarity by 31P-NMR. Chemistry and Physics of Lipids.2001;109(1):103-112.

[86] Baeza I, Wong C, Mondragon R, Gonzalez S, Ibanez M, Farfan N, Arguello C. Transbilayer Diffusion of Divalent Cations into Liposomes Mediated by Lipidic Particles of Phosphatidate. Journal of Molecular Evolution. 1994;39(6):560-568.

[87] Stampoulis P, Ueda T, Matsumoto M, Terasawa H, Miyano K, Sumimoto H, Shimada I. Atypical Membrane-embedded Phosphatidylinositol 3,4-Bisphosphate (PI (3,4) P2)-binding Site on p47phox Phox Homology (PX) Domain Revealed by NMR. Journal of Biological Chemistry. 2012;287:17848-17859.

[88] Jousma H, Talsma H, Spied F, Joosten JGH, Junginger HE, Crommelin DJA. Characterization of Liposomes, the Influence of Extrusion of Multilamellar Vesicles Through Polycarbonate Membranes on Particle Size, Particle Size Distribution and Number of Bilayers. International Journal of Pharmaceutics.1987;35(3): 263-274.

[89] Biltonen RL, Lichtenberg D. The Use of Differential Scanning Calorimetry as a tool to Characterize Liposome Preparations. Chemistry and Physics of Lipids.1993;64(1-3):129–142.

[90] Sudhakar B, Ravi Varma JN, Ramana Murthy KV. Formulation, Characterization and Ex vivo Studies of Terbinafine HCl Liposomes for Cutaneous Delivery. Current Drug Delivery.2014;11(3):1-9.

[91] Demel RA, Geurts VanKessel WS, Mand Van Deenen LLM. The Properties of Polyunsaturated Lecithins in Monolayers and Liposomes and the Interactions of These Lecithins with Cholesterol. Biochimica et Biophysica Acta- Biomembranes.1972;266(1): 26-40.

[92] Abra RM, Hunt CA. Liposome Disposition in Vivo. III. Dose and Vesicle-Size Effects. Biochimica et Biophysica Acta. 1981;666(3):493-503.

[93] Jaroni HW, Schubert RE, Schmidt KH. Liposomes as Drug Carries. Georg thieme Verlag: Stutgart; 1986.

[94] Grit M, Zuidam NJ, Underberg WJ, Crommelin DJ. Hydrolysis of Partially Saturated Egg Phosphatidylcholine in Aqueous Liposome Dispersions and the Effect of Cholesterol Incorporation on

Hydrolysis Kinetics. Journal of Pharmacy and Pharmacology.1993;45 (6):490–495.

[95] Chen CM, Alli D. Use of Fluidized Bed In Proliposome Manufacturing. Journal of Pharmaceutical Sciences.1987;76(5):419-419.

[96] Uster PS, Deamer DW. Fusion Competence of Phosphatidylserine-Containing Liposomes Quantitatively Measured by A Fluorescence Resonance Energy Transfer Assay. Archives of Biochemistry and Biophysics.1981;209 (2):385-395.

[97] Mayer LD, Cullis PR, Balley MB. Medical Application of Liposome. Elsevier Science BV: New York; 1998.

[98] Dunnick JK, Rooke JD, Aragon S, Kriss JP. Alteration of Mammalian Cells by Interaction with Artificial Lipid Vesicles. Cancer Research.1976;36 (7 PT 1):2385-2389.

[99] Fidler IJ, Therapy of Spontaneous Metastases by Intravenous Injection of Liposomes Containing Lymphokines. Science. 1980;208(4451):1469-1471.

[100] Fidler IJ, Sone S, Fogler WE, Barnes ZL. Eradication of Spontaneous Metastases and Activation of Alveolar Macrophages by Intravenous Injection of Liposomes Containing Muramyl Dipeptide. Proceedings of the National Academy of Sciences of the United States of America.1981;78(3):1680-1684.

[101] Deodhar SD, James K, Chiang T, Edinger M, Barna BP. Inhibition of Lung Metastases in Mice Bearing A Malignant Fibrosarcoma by Treatment with Liposomes Containing Human C-Reactive Protein. Cancer Research. 1982; 42(12):5084-5088.

[102] Thombre PS, Deodhar SD. Inhibition of Liver Metastases in Murine Colon Adenocarcinoma by Liposomes Containing Human C-Reactive Protein or Crude Lymphokine. Cancer Immunology Immunotherapy. 1984;16 (3):145-150.

[103] Gluck R, Mischelar R, Brantschen S, Just M, Althaus B, Cryz SJJ. Immunopotentiating Reconstituted Influenza Virus Virosome Vaccine Delivery System for Immunization Against Hepatitis A. Journal of Clinical Investigation. 1992; 90(6):2491-2495.

[104] Dehaan A, Tomee JFC, Huchshorn JP, Wilschut J. Liposomes as an Immunoadjuvant System for Stimulation of Mucosal and Systemic Antibody-Responses Against Inactivated Measles-Virus Administered Intranasally to Mice. Vaccine. 1995;13 (14):1320-1324.

[105] Wassef NM, Alving CR, Richards RL. Liposomes as Carriers for Vaccines. Immunomethods. 1994;4(3): 217-222.

[106] Mc Cauley JA, Flory's Book, Mc Comb TG. Biochimica et Biophysica Acta.1992;30(112).

[107] Rose JK, Buoncore L, Whitt MA. A New Cationic Liposome Reagent Mediating Nearly Quantitative Transfection of Animal Cells. Biotechniques.1991;10(4):520-525.

[108] Prathyusha K, Muthukumaran M, Krishnamoorthy B. Liposomes as Targetted Drug Delivery Systems Present And Future Prospectives: A Review. Journal of Drug Delivery & Therapeutics. 2013;3(4):195-201.

[109] Schroeder U, Sommerfeld P, Ulrich S, Sabel BA. Nanoparticle Technology for Delivery of Drugs Across the Blood-Brain Barrier. Journal of Pharmaceutical Sciences.1998;87(11): 1305-1307.

[110] Black CDV, Watson GJ, Ward RJ. The Use of Pentostam Liposomes in the

Chemotherapy of Experimental Leishmaniasis. Transactions of the Royal Society of Tropical Medicine and Hygiene.1977;71(6):550-552.

[111] Desiderio JV, Campbell SG. Liposome-Encapsulated Cephalothin in the Treatment of Experimental Murine Salmonellosis. Journal of the Reticuloendothelial Society.1983;34(4): 279–287.

[112] Gabizon AA. Selective Tumor Localization and Improved Therapeutic Index of Anthracyclines Encapsulated In Long-Circulating Liposomes. Cancer Research. 1992;52(4):891-896.

[113] Lawrence DM, Jennifer R, Marcel BB. Intravenous Pretreatment with Empty Ph Gradient Liposomes Alters the Pharmacokinetics and Toxicity of Doxorubicin Through in Vivo Active Drug Encapsulation. Journal of Pharmaceutical Science. 1999; 88(1):96-102.

[114] Dinesh T, Namdeo A, Mishra PR, Khopade AJ, Jain NK. High-Entrapment Liposomes for 6-Mercaptopurine—A Prodrug Approach. Drug Development and Industrial Pharmacy. 2000;26(12): 1315-1319.

[115] Tashuhiro I, Yoshihiro T, Hisako D, Isao Y, Hiroshi K. Encapsulation of an Antivasospastic Drug, Fasudil, into Liposomes, and in Vitro Stability of the Fasudil-Loaded Liposomes. International Journal of Pharmaceutics. 2002;232(1):59-67.

[116] Moustapha H, Zuzana H, Christina N, Mohamed AR, Susanne K, Birgitta E, Nils K. Pharmacokinetics and Distribution of Liposomal Busulfan in the Rat: A New Formulation for Intravenous Administration. Cancer Chemotherapy and Pharmacology. 1998; 42(6):471-478.

[117] Li Z, Zhang Y, Wurtz W, Lee JK, Malinin VS, Krishnan SD, Meers P, Perkins WR. Characterization of Nebulized Liposomal Amikacin (Arikace) as a Function of Droplet Size. Journal of Aerosol Medicine and Pulmonary Drug Delivery. 2008;21(3): 245-254.

[118] Okusanya OO, Bhavnani SM, Hammel J, Minic P, Dupont LJ, Forrest A, Mulder GJ, Mackinson C, Ambrose PG, Gupta R. Pharmacokinetic and Pharmacodynamic Evaluation of Liposomal Amikacin for Inhalation In Cystic Fibrosis Patients with Chronic Pseudomonal Infection. Antimicrobial Agents and Chemotherapy. 2009;53(9): 3847-3854.

[119] Lasic DD. Applications of Liposomes, Handbook of Biological Physics, (Editors, Lipowsky, R., Sackmann, E.,) Liposome Technology, Inc., Chapter 10, Hamilton Court, Menlo Park, California, USA 94025, 1995;1: p. 491-519.

[120] Wasan KM, Lopez-Berestein G. Characteristics of Lipid-Based Formulations that Influence their Biological Behavior in the Plasma of Patients. Clinical Infectious Diseases. 1996;23(5):1126–1138.

[121] Immordino ML, Dosio F, Cattel L. Stealth Liposomes: Review of the Basic Science, Rationale, and Clinical Applications, Existing and Potential. International Journal of Nanomedicine. 2006;1(3):297–315.

[122] Meunier F, Prentice HG, Ringdén O. Liposomal Amphotericin B (Ambisome): Safety Data from a Phase II/III Clinical Trial. Journal of Antimicrobial Chemotherapy. 1991;28 (Suppl B):83–91.

[123] Denning DW, Lee JY, Hostetler JS, Pappas P, Kauffman CA, Dewsnup DH, Galgiani JN, Graybill JR, Sugar AM, Catanzaro A. NIAID Mycoses Study Group Multicenter Trial of Oral Itraconazole Therapy for Invasive

Aspergillosis. The American Journal of Medicine. 1994;97(2):135–144.

[124] Rivera E. Liposomal Anthracyclines in Metastatic Breast Cancer: Clinical Update. Oncologist. 2003;8(Suppl 2):3-9.

[125] Tomkinson B, Bendele R, Giles FJ, Brown E, Gray A, Hart K, LeRay JD, Meyer D, Pelanne M, Emerson DL. OSI-211, A Novel Liposomal Topoisomerase I Inhibitor, is Active in SCID Mouse Models of Human AML and ALL. Leukemia Research. 2003;27(11):1039–1050.

[126] Patil SD, Burgess DJ. Liposomes, Design and Manufacturing, In: Burgess DJ, editor. Injectable Dispersed Systems: Formulation, Processing and Performance (Drugs and the Pharmaceutical Sciences Series). New York: Marcel Dekker; 2005; p. 249–303.

[127] Park JW. Liposome-Based Drug Delivery in Breast Cancer Treatment. Breast Cancer Research.2002;4(3):95–99.

[128] Hoarau D, Delmas P, David S, Roux E, Leroux JC. Novel Long-Circulating Lipid Nanocapsules. Pharmaceutical Research. 2004;21(10): 1783–1789.

[129] Usonis V, Bakasénas V, Valentelis R, Katiliene G, Vidzeniene D, Herzog C. Antibody Titres After Primary and Booster Vaccination of Infants and Young Children with A Virosomal Hepatitis a Vaccine (Epaxal). Vaccine. 21(31):4588–4592.

[130] D'Acremont V, Herzog C, Genton B. Immunogenicity and Safety of a Virosomal Hepatitis a Vaccine (Epaxal) In the Elderly. Journal of Travel Medicine. 13(2):78–83.

[131] Herzog C, Hartmann K, Künzi V, Kürsteiner O, Mischler R, Lazar H, Glück R. Eleven Years of Inflexal V-A Virosomal Adjuvanted Influenza Vaccine. Vaccine. 2009;27(33):4381–4387.

[132] Hong RL. Liposomal Anti-Cancer Drug Researches the Myth of Long Circulation. Journal of Chinese Oncological Society. 2004;20(2):10–21.

[133] Sarris AH, Hagemeister F, Romaguera J, Rodriguez MA, McLaughlin P, Tsimberidou AM, Medeiros LJ, Samuels B, Pate O, Oholendt M, Kantarjian H, Burge C, Cabanillas F. Liposomal Vincristine in Relapsed Non-Hodgkin's Lymphomas: Early Results of an Ongoing Phase II Trial. Annals of Oncology. 2000;11(1): 69-72.

[134] Rodriguez MA, Pytlik R, Kozak T, Chhanabhai M, Gascoyne R, Lu B, Deitcher SR, Winter JN. Vincristine Sulfate Liposomes Injection (Marqibo) In Heavily Pretreated Patients with Refractory Aggressive Non-Hodgkin Lymphoma: Report of the Pivotal Phase 2 Study. Cancer.2009;115(15): 3475-3482.

[135] Gardikis K, Tsimplouli C, Dimas K, Micha-Screttas M, Demetzos C. New Chimeric Advanced Drug Delivery Nano Systems (Chi-Addnss) as Doxorubicin Carriers. International Journal of Pharmaceutics.2010:402 (1–2):231–237.

[136] Chowdhary RK, Shariff I, Dolphin D. Drug Release Characteristics of Lipid Based Benzoporphyrin Derivative. Journal of Pharmacy & Pharmaceutical Sciences. 2003;6(1):13–19.

[137] Mossalam M, Dixon AS, Lim CS. Controlling Subcellular Delivery to Optimize Therapeutic Effect. Therapeutic Delivery. 2010;1(1): 169–193.

[138] Li Z, Zhang Y, Wurtz W, Lee JK, Malinin VS, Krishnan SD, Meers P, Perkins WR. Characterization of

Nebulized Liposomal Amikacin (Arikace) as a Function of Droplet Size. Journal of Aerosol Medicine and Pulmonary Drug Delivery.2008;21(3): 245-254.

[139] Dragovich T, Mendelson D, Kurtin S, Richardson K, Von Hoff D, Hoos A. A Phase 2 Trial of the Liposomal DACH Platinum L-NDDP in Patients with Therapy-Refractory Advanced Colorectal Cancer. Cancer Chemotherapy and Pharmacology.2006; 58(6):759–764.

[140] Zahid S, Brownell I. Repairing DNA Damage in Xeroderma Pigmentosum: T4N5 Lotion and Gene Therapy. Journal of Drugs in Dermatology.2008;7(4):405–408.

[141] Batist G, Sawyer M, Gabrail N, Christiansen N, Marshall JL, Spigel DR, Louie A. A Multicenter, Phase II Study of CPX-1 Liposome Injection in Patients (Pts) with Advanced Colorectal Cancer (CRC). Journal of Clinical Oncology.2008;26(15):4108.

[142] Feldman EJ, Lancet JE, Kolitz JE, Ritchie EK, Roboz GJ, List AF, Allen SL, Asatiani E, Mayer LD, Swenson C, Louie AC. First-in-Man Study of CPX-351: A Liposomal Carrier Containing Cytarabine and Daunorubicin in a Fixed 5:1 Molar Ratio for the Treatment of Relapsed and Refractory Acute Myeloid Leukemia. Journal of Clinical Oncology. 2011;29(8):979-985.

[143] Eichhorn ME, Becker S, Strieth S, Werner A, Sauer B, Teifel M, Ruhstorfer H, Michaelis U, Griebel J, Brix G, Jauch KW, Dellian M. Paclitaxel Encapsulated in Cationic Lipid Complexes (MBT-0206) Impairs Functional Tumor Vascular Properties as Detected by Dynamic Contrast Enhanced Magnetic Resonance Imaging. Cancer Biology Therapy.2006;5(1):89–96.

[144] Michaelis U, Haas H. Targeting of Cationic Liposomes to Endothelial Tissue. In: Gregoriadis G, editor. Liposome Technology, Volume III: Interactions of Liposomes with the Biological Milieu, London, UK: Informa Healthcare;2007. p. 151–170.

[145] Robert B, Campbell RB, Ying B, Kuesters GM, Hemphill R. Fighting Cancer: From the Bench to Bedside Using Second Generation Cationic Liposomal Therapeutics. Journal of Pharmaceutical Sciences. 2009;98(2): 411–429.

[146] Semple SC, Leone R, Wang J, Leng EC, Klimuk SK, Eisenhardt ML, Yuan ZN, Edwards K, Maurer N, Hope MJ, Cullis PR, Ahkong QF. Optimization and Characterization of a Sphingomyelin/Cholesterol Liposome Formulation of Vinorelbine with Promising Antitumor Activity. Journal of Pharmaceutical Sciences.2005;94(5): 1024–1038.

[147] Pal A, Khan S, Wang YF, Kamath N, Sarkar AK, Ahmad A, Sheikh S, Ali S, Carbonaro D, Zhang A, Ahmad I. Preclinical Safety, Pharmacokinetics and Antitumor Efficacy Profile of Liposome-Entrapped SN-38 Formulation. Anticancer Research.2005;25(1A):331–341.

[148] Cattaneo AG, Gornati R, Sabbioni E, Chiriva-Internati M., Cobos E., Jenkins MR, Bernardini G. Nanotechnology and Human Health: Risks and Benefits. Journal of Applied Toxicology.2010;30(8):730–744.

[149] Zhang JA, Anyarambhatla G, Ma L, Ugwu S, Xuan T, Sardone T, Ahmad I. Development and Characterization of a Novel Cremophor EL Free Liposome-Based Paclitaxel (LEP-ETU) Formulation. European Journal of Pharmaceutics and Biopharmaceutics. 2005;59(1):177–187.

[150] Stathopoulos GP, Boulikas T. Lipoplatin Formulation Review Article. Journal of Drug Delivery. 2012;1-10.

[151] Tari AM, Gutiérrez-Puente Y, Monaco G, Stephens C, Sun T, Rosenblum M, Belmont J, Arlinghaus R, Lopez-Berestein G. Liposome-Incorporated Grb2 Antisense Oligodeoxynucleotide Increases the Survival of Mice Bearing Bcr-Abl-Positive Leukemia Xenografts. International Journal of Oncology. 2007; 31(5):1243–1250.

[152] Duffaud F, Borner M, Chollet P, Vermorken JB, Bloch J, Degardin M, Rolland F, Dittrich C, Baron B, Lacombe D, Fumoleau P. Phase II Study of OSI-211 (Liposomal Lurtotecan) In Patients with Metastatic or Loco-Regional Recurrent Squamous Cell Carcinoma of the Head and Neck, An Eortc New Drug Development Group Study. European Journal of Cancer. 2004;40(18):2748–2752.

[153] Hwang JH, Lim MC, Seo SS, Park SY, Kang S. Phase II Study of Belotecan (CKD 602) as a Single Agent in Patients with Recurrent or Progressive Carcinoma of Uterine Cervix. Japanese Journal of Clinical Oncology. 2011; 41(5):624–629.

[154] Yu NY, Conway C, Pena RL, Chen JY. Stealth Liposomal CKD-602, a Topoisomerase I Iinhibitor, Improves the Therapeutic Index in Human Tumor Xenograft Models. Anticancer Research. 2007;27(4B):2541–2545.

[155] Ohyanagi F, Horai T, Sekine I, Yamamoto N, Nakagawa K, Nishio M, Senger S, Morsli N, Tamura T. Safety of BLP25 Liposome Vaccine (L-BLP25) In Japanese Patients with Unresectable Stage III NSCLC After Primary Chemoradiotherapy: Preliminary Results from a Phase I/II Study. Japanese Journal of Clinical Oncology.2011;41(5):718–722.

[156] Powell E, Chow LQ. BLP-25 Liposomal Vaccine: A Promising Potential Therapy in Non-Small-Cell Lung Cancer. Expert Review of Respiratory Medicine.2008;2(1):37–45.

[157] Dromi S, Frenkel V, Luk A, Traughber B, Angstadt M, Bur M, Poff J, Xie J, Libutti SK, Li KC, Wood BJ. Pulsed-High Intensity Focused Ultrasound and Low Temperature-Sensitive Liposomes for Enhanced Targeted Drug Delivery and Antitumor Effect. Clinical Cancer Research. 2007; 13(9):2722–2727.

[158] Yarmolenko PS, Zhao Y, Landon C, Spasojevic I, Yuan F, Needham D, Viglianti BL, Dewhirst MW. Comparative Effects of Thermosensitive Doxorubicin-Containing Liposomes and Hyperthermia in Human and Murine Tumours. International Journal of Hyperthermia. 2010;26(5):485–498.

Chapter 2

Protein and Peptide Drug Delivery

Abstract

Protein and peptide-based drugs have great potential applications as therapeutic agents since they have higher efficacy and lower toxicity than chemical drugs. However, difficulty with their delivery has limited their use. In particular, their oral bioavailability is very low, and the transdermal delivery faces absorption limitations. Therefore, most of the protein and peptide-based drugs are administered by the parenteral route. However, this route also has some problems, such as patient discomfort, especially for pediatric use. Extensive research has been performed over the past few decades to develop protein and peptide delivery systems that circumvent the problems mentioned above. Various strategies that have been employed during this time include nanoparticle carriers, absorption enhancers, enzyme inhibitors, mucoadhesive polymers, and chemical modification of protein or peptide structures. However, most of these strategies are focused on the delivery of proteins or peptides via the oral route since it is the most preferred route considering its high level of patient acceptance, long-term compliance, and simplicity. However, other routes of administration such as transdermal, nasal, pulmonary can also be attractive alternatives for protein and peptide delivery. This chapter will discuss the most effective approaches used to develop protein and peptide drug delivery systems.

Keywords: bioavailability, liposomes, nanoparticle carriers, absorption enhancers, enzyme inhibitors, mucoadhesive polymers, chemical modification, aquasome, iontophoresis, electroporation, sonophoresis, transfersomes

1. Introduction

Proteins and peptides play vital roles in many biological processes, including catalysis, transportation, regulation of gene expression, immunity-related functions, etc. They are also involved in many pathological conditions such as diabetes, hypertension, cancer, etc. [1]. Because of their wide range of functions and their involvement in diseases, proteins and peptides are attractive therapeutic agents for combatting many diseases. Currently, there are more than 100 approved peptide-based therapeutics on the market [2]. The market for peptide and protein drugs is growing much faster than for small molecule drugs. One reason for this is that peptides and proteins can be highly selective as they have multiple points of interaction with the target. This increased selectivity will also lead to decreased side effects and toxicity.

However, the physicochemical properties of proteins and peptides make their use as drugs difficult. Firstly, proteins and peptides are not suitable for administration via the oral route because of their instability in the gastrointestinal tract (GIT). Secondly, the size and hydrophilicity of proteins and peptides lead to their poor bioavailability [3, 4]. Other routes of delivery also have some drawbacks. For example, administration via intravenous injection may not be suitable for achieving optimal therapeutic effects since many proteins and peptides have low circulation half-life [5]. This may also lead to pain or discomfort [6], severe reaction at the injection site [7, 8], scarring [9], local allergic reactions [10], cutaneous infections [11], etc. Transdermal delivery leads to absorption limitations due to the skin barrier, which prevents the passage of drug molecules with molecular weight greater than 500 Da, especially hydrophilic molecules [12, 13].

Extensive research has been performed over the past few decades to develop protein and peptide delivery systems that circumvent the drawbacks mentioned above. Different strategies that have been employed for this purpose include nanoparticle carriers, absorption enhancers, enzyme inhibitors, mucoadhesive polymers, and chemical modification of protein or peptide structures [14, 15]. Most of these approaches aim to deliver proteins and peptides via the oral route since it is the most convenient route of drug administration. However, other routes of administration such as transdermal [16], nasal [17], buccal [18], pulmonary [19] also have some attractive features such as avoidance of harsh environment of the GIT and non-invasiveness of the nature of administration. Thus, these routes can also be excellent alternatives for protein and peptide delivery [20]. This chapter will discuss the most effective approaches to developing protein and peptide drug delivery systems.

Proteins and peptides consist of amino acids connected via peptide bonds (**Figure 1**). Protein and peptide structures can be primary structure, secondary structure, tertiary structure, and quaternary structure. The primary structure provides information about the number and types of amino acids in a protein or peptide. Secondary structure gives us information about the presence of α-helix, β-sheets, loops, and turns in the protein or peptide. For example, hemoglobin is a predominantly helical protein (**Figure 2**). The tertiary structure indicates the overall three-dimensional structure of the protein. For example, the tertiary structure of hemoglobin consists of a globin fold (**Figure 2**). The quaternary structure indicates the oligomeric state of the protein. For example, hemoglobin has a tetrameric (or dimer of dimer) quaternary structure (**Figure 2**).

Various routes for delivery of protein and peptide drug has been mentioned above. Their advantages and disadvantages have been discussed briefly. The strategies adopted for enhancing the delivery of protein and peptides via various routes is discussed below.

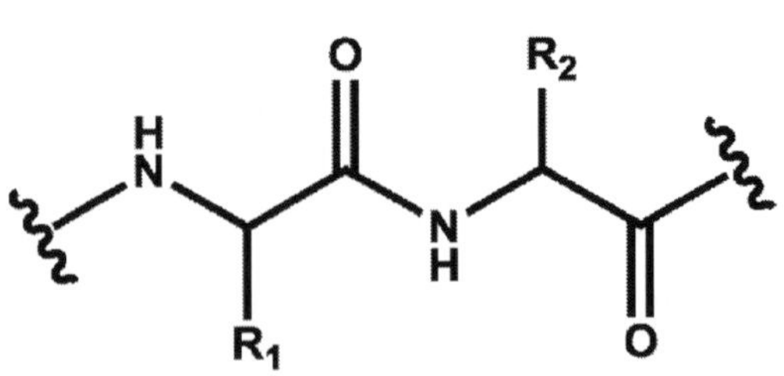

O R$_2$ H N N H R$_1$ O

Figure 1.
General structure of a peptide fragment.

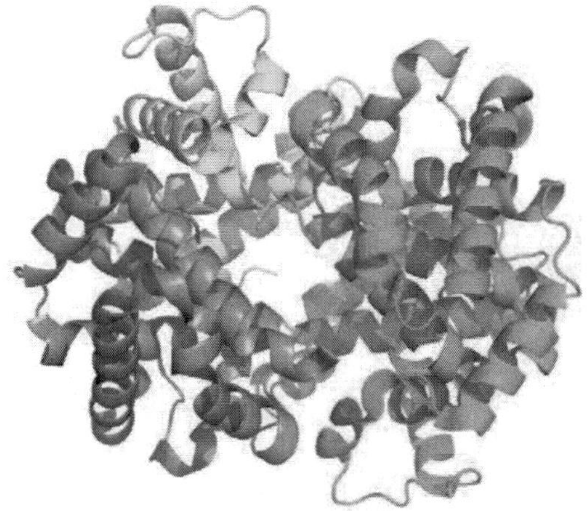

Figure 2.
Structure of hemoglobin.

2. Oral route

2.1 Chemical modification

Chemical modification of proteins and peptides is one of the strategies adopted to make these more clinically applicable [21]. This strategy eliminates some of the undesirable properties of proteins and peptides, such as susceptibility to enzyme hydrolysis, improper solubility, poor membrane permeability, etc. There are several ways of performing the chemical modification, including replacement of a specific amino acid or modification of the structure of amino acids. For example, replacement of an L-amino acid with its D-counterpart may lead to resistance to enzymatic hydrolysis, enhanced cell-membrane permeability, etc. In desmopressin (an analog of vasopressin), the C-terminal L-Arg has been replaced by D-Arg (**Figure 3**). Also, the N-terminal amino group (of cysteine) has been deaminated (**Figure 3**). These chemical modifications resulted in substantially higher oral bioavailability of desmopressin than that of vasopressin [22].

Another method of chemical modification is to incorporate a lipophilic moiety (e.g., fatty acid) in the protein or peptide. The lipophilic moiety will increase the

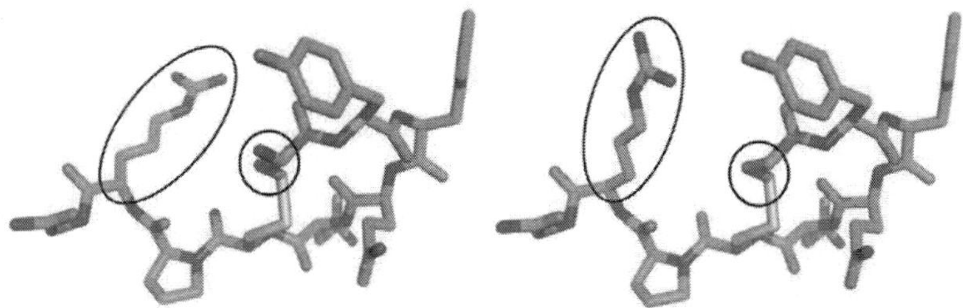

Figure 3.
Structure of vasopressin (left) and desmopressin (right).

overall hydrophobicity of the molecule, which may lead to an increase in its intestinal absorption. Increased hydrophobicity may also lead to increased stability of the protein or peptide [23]. For example, three amino acids (Gly, Phe, and Lys) in insulin were attached to 1, 3-dipalmitoyl glycerol moiety. This modification resulted in an increased hydrophobicity of insulin as well as increased intestinal absorption. The enzymatic hydrolysis of insulin was also reduced, which resulted in increased bioavailability [24].

2.1.1 PEGylation

PEGylation involves the covalent attachment of one or more polyethylene glycol (PEG) molecule(s) to a protein or peptide. PEG has some special features that make it suitable for protein and peptide delivery systems [25–28]. One important feature is that it is soluble in both organic and aqueous solvents. Another feature is that PEG can be obtained in a wide range of molecular weights. It can be obtained both as a linear or branched chain. PEG is more hydrophilic than other polymers of comparable sizes. Also, PEG is highly flexible since there is no bulky substituent around the backbone to hinder the rotation. Finally, PEG is non-toxic and non-immunogenic.

PEG improves the pharmacokinetic properties of proteins and peptides by protecting these from enzymatic hydrolysis (**Figure 4**) and by increasing solubility. PEG acts as a shield that prevents the hydrolysis of the protein or peptide by blocking its access to the proteolytic enzyme (**Figure 5**) [29]. The attachment of PEG with a protein or peptide increases its size, which increases the circulation half-life of the protein or peptide by decreasing the clearance by the renal filtration process. The attachment of PEG to a protein or peptide also reduces immunogenicity by reducing the recognition by the β-cell or antibodies. Finally, the attachment of PEG to proteins or peptides prevents their possible aggregation [30].

PEGylation process can interfere with the molecular recognition between the protein or peptide and the receptor due to the modified structure of the PEGylated protein or peptide. For example, PEGylation of a protein or peptide may cause steric hindrance, which may prevent proper binding of the protein or peptide to the target. However, this drawback is balanced by the improvements in pharmacokinetic properties, such as enhanced absorption and circulation half-life [31]. The development of Nobex Corporation's HIM2 was based on the PEGylation approach. HIM2 is hexyl insulin monoconjugate 2 that is attached to a PEG. The attachment of PEG improves the stability of the molecule and enhances bioavailability that allows oral administration [32].

2.1.2 Peptidomimetics

Peptidomimetics mimic the structure of a protein or peptide and show acceptable pharmacokinetic properties while retaining biological activity. Different modifications (N-alkylation, isosteric replacement of the amide bond, etc.) can be performed on a peptide to improve its pharmacokinetic properties [33]. Structural

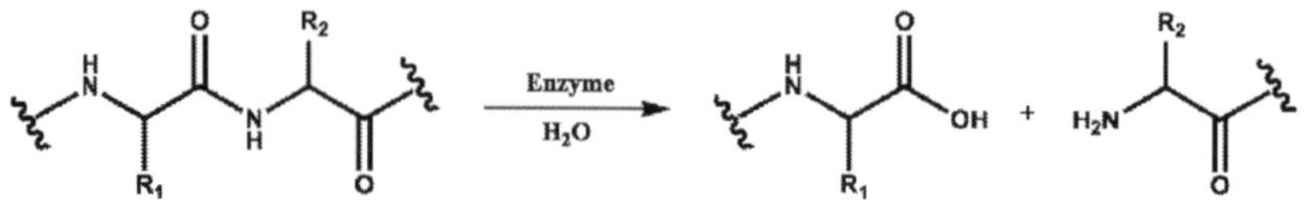

Figure 4.
Enzymatic hydrolysis of the peptide bond.

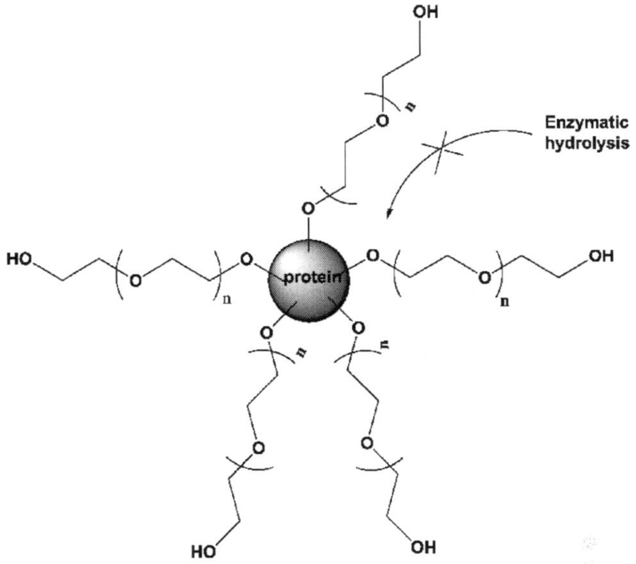

Figure 5.
PEGylaiton blocks enzymatic hydrolysis of peptides.

modifications are mainly performed to make the peptide more stable in the GIT by making it less susceptible to enzymatic degradation. Solubility, lipophilicity, and the flexibility of the peptide can also be altered to enhance stability as well as absorption. Modification of a peptide may occur at the backbone of the peptide or the side chains of amino acids, or both. The alkylation of the backbone N-atom has been shown to improve the bioavailability of peptide molecules [34].

N-alkylation, in general, leads to an increase in lipophilicity of the peptide as well as a steric hindrance. N-alkylation also leads to a reduction in H-bonding since the H-atom of the backbone amide has been replaced by an alkyl group. This decrease in H-bonding may lead to destabilization of α-helix and β-sheets, which may alter the conformation of the peptide. N-alkylation method has been used to make cyclosporine (**Figure 6**) where the N-atoms of the backbone have been alkylated by methyl groups (green spheres) [35].

Isosteric replacement of amide bond is another strategy for peptidomimetics design. This process can lead to alteration in H-bonding as well as peptide-folding. Thus, this process may affect the conformation of the peptide. For example, the replacement of a carbon-atom by an N-atom gives azapeptide class. Azapeptides can be of two types – azatides and peptoids. In azatides, all the α-carbon in the peptide backbone has been replaced by nitrogen atom. In peptoids, the α-carbon is replaced by N-atom, and the N-atom of the backbone is replaced by C-atoms. Ritonavir (**Figure 7**) is an example of a drug developed by the peptidomimetics approach [36, 37].

2.2 Enzyme inhibition

Inhibition of enzymes like proteases is a good way of improving the stability of proteins and peptides in the GIT since these enzymes hydrolyze peptide bonds in proteins and peptides administered via the oral route. Proteases can be classified into different categories depending on the catalytic amino acid residue

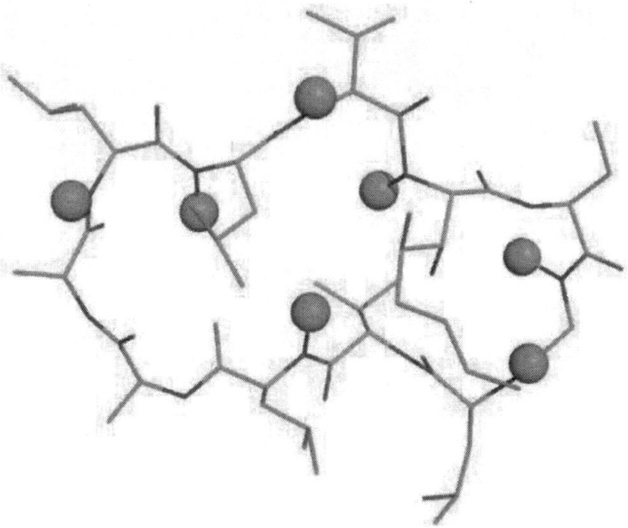

Figure 6.
Backbone N-alkylation in cyclosporine.

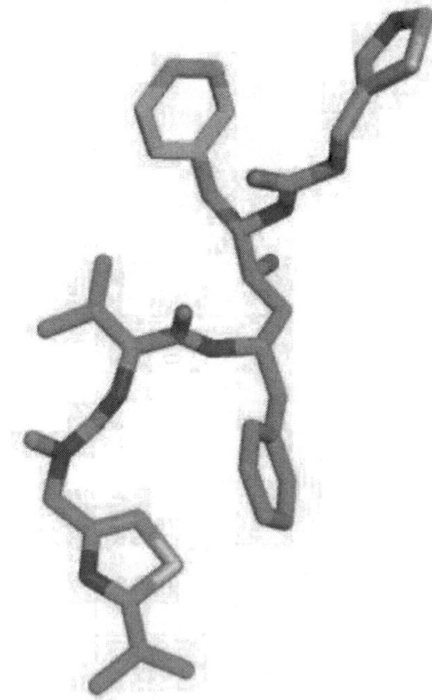

Figure 7.
Ritonavir.

(Ser, Thr, Asp, Glu, etc.) in the active site of the enzyme [38]. For example, serine proteases contain a serine residue in the active that acts as a nucleophile during the hydrolysis of the peptide bond. Another class of proteases is metalloproteases, where the water molecule used for hydrolysis is ligated to a metal ion (Zn^{2+}, Co^{2+}, Mn^{2+}, etc.) in the active site of the enzyme. Thus, one way of preventing hydrolysis of the protein or peptide drug is to co-administer protease inhibitors [39]. Insulin, for example, undergoes degradation in the GIT by different enzymes like trypsin, chymotrypsin, etc. Therefore insulin is co-administered with various synthetic (e.g., camostat mesylate) and naturally occurring inhibitors (soybean trypsin inhibitor) of trypsin and chymotrypsin. This co-administration leads to enhanced bioavailability of insulin [40]. However, the administered protein other than the therapeutic protein will not be degraded, leading to toxic side effects. Besides, the non-degraded proteins may also cause metabolic changes in the GIT [41].

Another way of protease inhibition is to alter the pH of the medium in which these enzymes work. This pH change may lead to the inactivation of the proteases. It has been reported that lowering the pH of the intestine to 4.5 or below leads to the inhibition of trypsin and chymotrypsin [23].

2.3 Absorption enhancers

Absorption enhancers are substances co-administered with protein or peptide drugs to enhance their absorption. In general, these absorption enhancers reversibly damage the physical barrier in the cell wall, which prevents a protein or peptide from crossing the intestinal wall. Thus, absorption enhancers provide a temporal path for the proteins or peptides to cross the intestinal wall and to be absorbed [42]. There are two main ways by which absorption enhancers cause the temporal opening – transcellular pathway and paracellular pathway. The transcellular mechanism involves the structural change in the cell membrane of the epithelial cells. This structural alteration leads to enhanced passive diffusion of proteins and peptides through the cell. In the paracellular pathway, the absorption enhancers facilitate the opening of tight junctions between the epithelial cells, which allows the protein and peptide to diffuse through the intercellular space present between the epithelial cells. Another absorption enhancing mechanism involves the reduction of viscosity of the mucus in the intestinal wall, which enhances the diffusion of proteins and peptides [25].

There are different types of absorption enhancers based on their molecular structure and mechanism of action. For example, ethylene diamine tetraacetic acid (EDTA) works by chelating Ca-ions, which are important in maintaining the tight junction between the cells. Therefore, when Ca-ions are complexed by EDTA, the tight junction between the cells will be opened, allowing the proteins and peptides to cross the intercellular space. However, surfactants (sodium lauryl sulfate, Tween 40, etc.) work by disrupting the intestinal membrane allowing the protein and peptide to cross the cells via the transcellular pathway [43].

It is worth mentioning that the absorption enhancers are potentially toxic since some of them disrupt the integrity of the intestinal membrane. Damage of the intestinal membrane can cause proteins or peptides other than the protein or peptide of interest to be absorbed, leading to toxicity. Besides, pathogens (virus, bacteria, etc.) may also get absorbed, which may lead to various pathological conditions. Severe damage of the intestinal membrane may also lead to inflammatory conditions and ulceration of the epithelium. Therefore, the toxicology of the absorption enhancers needs to be fully understood before their long-term applications [44].

2.4 Site specific delivery in GIT

Different regions of the GIT show differences in the absorption of proteins and peptides. These differences are due to different pH values and different distribution of proteolytic enzymes at different regions of the GIT. The pH affects both the solubility and the stability of the protein or peptide, while the proteolytic enzymes are responsible for the degradation of the protein or peptide. There is also variability in the distribution of active transporters involved in peptide transport and the efflux pumps that can lower the absorption of proteins or peptides along the GIT [45, 46].

Extensive research has been performed to locate the optimum absorption site in the GIT for proteins or peptides [47]. These results indicate that the colon region of the GIT is one of the optimum sites for protein or peptide absorption mainly due to the lower protease activity in the colon area compared to other areas in the GIT, such as the stomach and small intestine. Therefore, several strategies have been employed to deliver the therapeutic protein or peptide intact to the colon. One approach is to design a prodrug (**Figure 8**) with adequate stability in the other regions of the GIT [48]. However, it should be converted to the parent therapeutic protein or peptide in the colon. Since the microflora in the colon produces reductive enzymes, the prodrug should be designed by linking the therapeutic protein or peptide via a bond (e.g., azo bond) that can be cleaved by reductive enzymes in the colon [49]. These reducing enzymes can also be utilized to attach a polymeric carrier to the protein or peptide (**Figure 9**). This polymer will protect the therapeutic

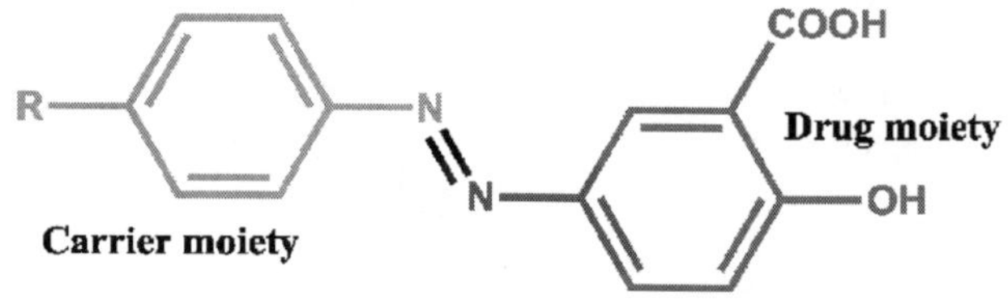

COOH
Drug moiety
R
N
N
OH
Carrier moiety

R = -CONHCH$_2$CH$_2$COONa, Balsalazine
= -CONHCH$_2$COONa, Ipsalazine
= -CH$_2$COOH, APAZA^{TM}

Figure 8.
Prodrugs with an azo bond.

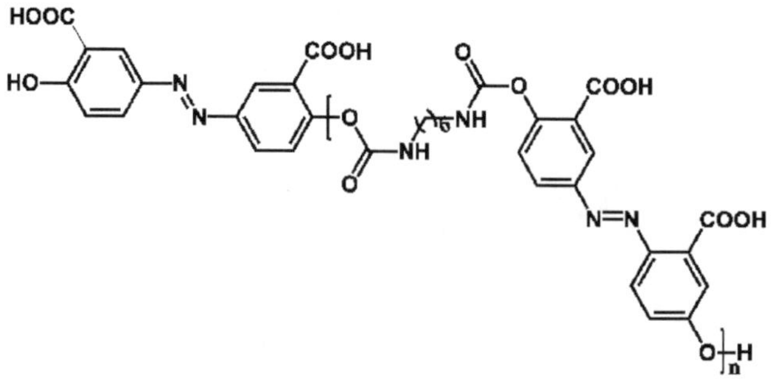

HOOC
HO
N
N
COOH
O
O
NH
NH
O
COOH
N=N
COOH
O
H
n

Figure 9.
A prodrug with a polymeric carrier.

peptide molecule along the GIT and will release the protein or peptide at the colon site, enhancing its absorption.

2.5 Membrane transporters

Epithelial cells express various amino acid and oligopeptide transporter proteins that transport various amino acids and oligopeptide found in nutrients to facilitate their absorption. Therefore, designing a therapeutic drug with structural similarity with the natural substrate of the transporter proteins will help in transporting the molecule across the epithelium to the systemic circulation. This can also be achieved by attaching a natural substrate of the transporter proteins to the bioactive molecule [50]. This linkage will allow the recognition of the attached peptide by the transporter and its binding to the transporter. However, for this process to occur, the attached peptide should be enzymatically stable in the GIT. Otherwise, hydrolysis of the peptide before reaching the transporter will prevent the recognition of the molecule by the transporter, and thus, transportation will not happen. PepT1 is a transporter protein that plays a vital role in the oral delivery of biomolecules. PepT1 can transport dipeptides and tripeptides with varying degrees of substrate specificity. PepT1 is involved in the transport of peptidomimetic drugs such as acyclovir which resembles a dipeptide [51, 52].

Generally, only small molecules can be transported by membrane transport proteins. However, molecules with relatively larger sizes are usually transported by receptor-mediated endocytosis. Endocytosis involves the binding of the large molecule to a membrane receptor, and the resulting complex gets inside the cell. In some cases, the internalized molecule can be subjected to degradation by the lysosome. In other cases, the components of the complex are kept intact following internalization and exit the cell by exocytosis. Thus, these components are transported into the systemic circulation. This kind of receptor-mediated endocytosis is called transcytosis. Epidermal growth factor, vitamin B12, and immunoglobulins are some of the substances absorbed by the transcytosis [53]. It has been reported that by attaching a therapeutic protein or peptide (e.g., erythropoietin, α-interferon, etc.) to vitamin B12, the bioavailability of the protein or peptide can be enhanced [54].

2.6 Mucoadhesive systems

Mucoadhesive systems utilize the bioadhesive phenomenon where certain components of the system (usually a polymer) form adhesion bonds with the mucosal membrane at the absorption site. This adhesion may lead to a high concentration of the therapeutic molecule, which increases absorption of the therapeutic molecule. Adhesion of the polymer in the delivery system also leads to an increase the residence time of the therapeutic molecule at the site of absorption and thus, further enhances the absorption and the bioavailability of the therapeutic agent [55].

The properties of the mucoadhesive system depends on the nature of the polymer used. The polymer should be hydrophilic enough to properly interact with the high amount of water present in the mucus layer. The polymer should be large enough (high molecular weight) to increase the possibility of interactions. The polymer should also have proper surface tension to allow the spreading of the polymer on the mucus layer. The polymer should contain functional groups (e.g., COOH, OH, etc.) to form strong H-bonds. Finally, the polymer should be non-toxic and non-immunogenic [41]. Although the main function of polymer in mucoadhesive drug delivery system is to form adhesive bonds with the mucus membrane to enhance the bioavailability of the protein or peptide, some polymers may have additional functions. For example, some polymers can act as absorption enhancers by modifying tight junctions between epithelial cells and by inhibiting proteases that hydrolyze proteins or peptides [56].

Cellulose derivatives (e.g., methylcellulose, hydroxyethyl cellulose, carboxymethyl cellulose) are used in mucoadhesive drug delivery systems. Other commonly used polymers are polyacrylic acid derivatives such as carbapol and polyacrylate. Thiol-containing polymers are also used in mucoadhesive systems. These polymers show strong adhesive binding with the mucus layer due to the formation of covalent bonds in addition to the non-covalent interactions. The thiol group in these polymers forms disulfide bonds with the cysteine residues present in the glycoproteins of the mucus. It has been reported that the increase in the thiol group in the polymer increases the strength of adhesive binding [23].

2.7 Liposomes

Liposomes are spherical microscopic vesicles containing one or more phospholipid bilayer (**Figure 10**). The inner core of the liposomes consists of hydrophilic parts of the phospholipid, while the lipophilic parts tend to remain in the lipid portion of the phospholipid bilayer. Extensive research has been carried out on the liposome-based delivery system for their application in the delivery of proteins or peptides, mainly via the oral delivery route. The advantage of liposome in oral delivery is mainly protecting the protein or peptide (e.g., insulin) from enzymatic hydrolysis in the GIT [57]. This protection is due to the encapsulation of the protein or peptide in the interior of the liposome, and thus, the protein or peptide is inaccessible to the proteolytic enzymes in the GIT. Liposomes also enhance the absorption of proteins or peptides (e.g., insulin) in the small intestine. The activity of the insulin-containing liposome depends on various factors such as the lipid components of the liposome, the charge on the surface of the liposome, etc. [58].

It is worth mentioning that the bile salts in the GIT can solvate the liposome resulting in their rupture and consequent release of the encapsulated proteins or peptides in the GIT. This solvation of liposomes is a problem with the application of liposomes as the oral delivery system. However, the problem with the *in vivo*

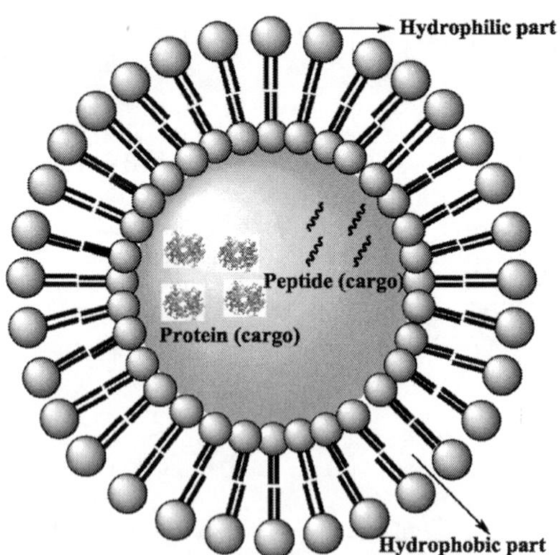

Figure 10.
General structure of liposomes.

stability of liposomes can be improved by adopting strategies like coating the liposome with a polymer or using dehydrated forms of liposomes [31].

2.8 Microspheres

Microspheres (**Figure 11**) can be prepared from polymers using various methods such as double emulsification, spray drying, complexation of macromolecules with opposite charges. Microspheres have sizes ranging from 1 μm to 1 mm. Much research has been performed on the use of microspheres for the oral delivery of protein or peptide drugs [59]. Microsphere-based delivery systems can protect the protein or peptide of interest from the harsh environment of the GIT such as enzymatic hydrolysis, acidic pH, etc. Microspheres can also enhance the absorption of the protein or peptide of interest, mainly through the paracellular pathway. The microsphere-based delivery system also allows the controlled release of the protein or peptide of interest at a specific area in the GIT by using pH-sensitive polymers. Insulin was loaded into the microsphere formed by the polymer poly (methacrylic-g-ethylene-glycol) [60]. This microsphere prevents the enzymatic degradation of insulin in the acidic environment of the stomach. However, swelling of the microsphere and consequent release of the insulin occurred in the basic environment of the intestine.

2.9 Nanoparticle-based delivery systems

Nanoparticles can be used as a delivery system to administer protein or peptide therapeutics via different routes such as oral, intravenous, subcutaneous, and transdermal. Delivery of proteins or peptides via nanoparticles can be achieved by employing different approaches such as encapsulation of the drug molecule by the nanoparticle, adsorption of the drug molecule on the surface of the nanoparticle, etc. [61]. Nanoparticle-based delivery system protects the protein or peptide of interest from enzymatic degradation in the GIT [62]. Nanoparticles can also deliver the protein or peptide to the desired location, such as tumor cell, inflammation site, etc. This site-specificity results in reduced side effects of the therapeutic agent [63, 64].

The uptake of nanoparticles by the cells usually occurs via endocytosis. This process involves phagocytosis, receptor-mediated phagocytosis, and pinocytosis.

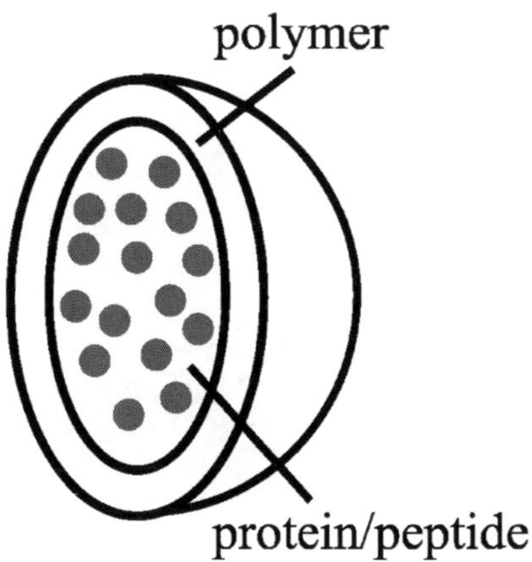

Figure 11.
General structure of microspheres.

Endocytosis starts with the association of the nanoparticle with the cell membrane to form an endosome, followed by the internalization of the endosome. Subsequent degradation of the nanoparticle by the lysosome leads to the release of the protein or peptide inside the cell [65]. Other ways of the release of drug molecules from the nanoparticle depend on factors such as the solubility of the therapeutic agent at a specific pH, polymer swelling, composition of the nanoparticle, etc. [41].

2.9.1 Solid lipid nanoparticle

Solid lipid nanoparticles (SLN, **Figure 12**) are composed of lipids that are solid at room temperature as well as body temperature and dispersed in water or an aqueous surfactant solution [66]. The lipids that can form SLN can be complex acylglycerol mixtures, highly purified triacylglycerol, or waxes. Extensive research has been performed on the solid lipid nanoparticles for their application in delivering proteins or peptides mainly due to their biocompatibility, biodegradation, and good tolerability [67]. It has been reported that SLN can enhance the bioavailability of the protein or peptide therapeutics and prolong their residence time in blood [68]. SLN can also enhance the oral absorption of many drugs [69, 70]. When SLNs are administered orally, they can be absorbed either through the M-cells (membranous epithelial cells) of the Peyer's patches in the gut-associated lymphoid tissue (GALT) or transcellularly [71].

Surface modification of nanoparticles with chitosan is an excellent way of enhancing the penetration of encapsulated proteins or peptides (e.g., insulin) through mucosal surfaces. This chitosan modified SLN has antimicrobial, mucoadhesive, absorption-enhancing properties and low toxicity in addition to good biocompatibility and biodegradation [72]. Mucoadhesive properties of chitosan may enhance drug uptake due to the longer contact period with the intestinal epithelium. This prolonged contact of the nanoparticle with the intestinal membrane leads to enhanced penetration of the protein or peptide. Also, chitosan is an effective permeability enhancer as it reversibly changes tight junctions [73, 74]. Fonte et al. showed

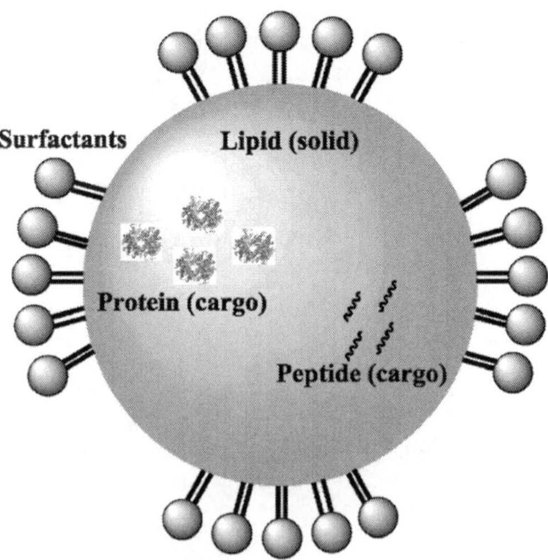

Figure 12.
General structure of solid lipid nanoparticles.

the ability of the chitosan-coated SLN to enhance the intestinal uptake of insulin by comparing with the uncoated SLN [75]. Significant improvement of hypoglycemic effect was observed for the chitosan-coated SLN compared to the uncoated SLN. Improvement of hypoglycemic effect could be due to mucoadhesive property of chitosan, which not only overcome the degradation of insulin in the GIT, but also promotes intestinal insulin uptake. However, one major limitation of the oral delivery of insulin-loaded nanoparticles is their elimination by the mononuclear phagocyte system [76, 77]. Macrophages present in various tissues such as the liver, spleen and bone marrow are also responsible for eliminating nanoparticles. The use of PEG [78] and other hydrophilic polysaccharides [79] coating to avoid phagocytosis of nanoparticles by macrophages has been reported. SLNs coated with chitosan were not internalized by the murine macrophage cell line, while the uncoated SLN were taken up by these cells [80]. Thus, chitosan was able to provide stealth properties to the SLN.

2.9.2 Chitosan based nanoparticles

Chitosan is a natural polysaccharide of glucosamine and N-acetyl glucosamine. Chitosan has some attractive features for being used in protein or peptide delivery [81]. Firstly, chitosan has high biocompatibility and low immunogenicity. Secondly, chitosan is a biodegradable polymer with high abundance. In the acidic environment, chitosan is protonated (**Figure 13**). This protonated form enhances the absorption of chitosan due to the interaction of the positively charged amino group with the cellular membrane [82–84]. This interaction leads to structural changes that opens the tight junction and allows the entry of proteins or peptides across the membrane. It is worth mentioning that chitosan exhibits absorption enhancing ability only in the acidic environment since it requires the protonated form of chitosan. Therefore, chitosan cannot act as an absorption enhancer in the neutral or basic environment [85, 86]. However, N-trimethyl chitosan (**Figure 13**) possess the absorption enhancing property over a wide range of pH, including the physiological pH. N-trimethyl chitosan-based nanoparticles loaded with insulin showed enhanced bioavailability of insulin [87]. N-trimethyl chitosan enhances the transport of proteins or peptides via both transcellular and paracellular pathways.

2.9.3 Inorganic nanoparticles

Inorganic nanoparticles are receiving more attention in the development of protein or peptide carriers due to some special properties. The protein or peptide of interest can be encapsulated inside the nanoparticle, which can provide protection against denaturation of the protein or peptide of interest. Thus, nanoparticles preserve both the structure and the biological function of the protein or peptide. Nanoparticles also prevent possible enzymatic hydrolysis and other degradation in the harsh environment of the GIT. Finally, nanoparticles improve the shelf life of the incorporated protein or peptide [88]. CaP nanoparticle has been used in

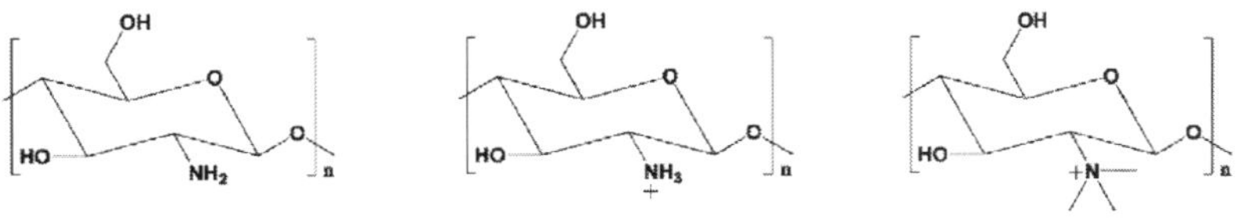

Figure 13.
Protonated (middle) and methylated (right) forms of chitosan (left).

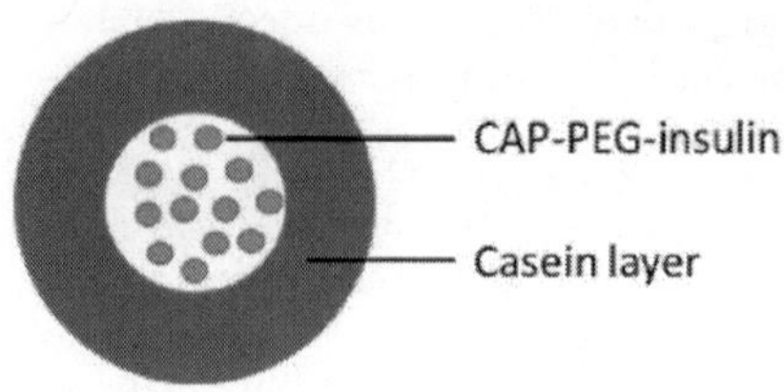

Figure 14.
Structure of a CaP-based insulin carrier.

delivering protein (e.g., insulin) via the oral route. In this formulation, PEG-insulin and casein are encapsulated in the CaP nanoparticle (**Figure 14**). This formulation was shown to increase the half-life of insulin [89].

2.9.4 Aquasomes

Aquasomes have recently emerged as solid nanoparticle drug carriers with a three-layered structure – core, coating, and drug (**Figure 15**) [90, 91]. It consists of a ceramic core coated with poly hydroxyl oligomer on which the protein or peptide of interest can be adsorbed. This polyhydroxy oligomer film protects proteins and peptides from changing shape and being damaged when they are surface-bound [92]. The layers that form aquasomes are assembled through the non-covalent bond, ionic bond, and van der Waals interactions [93].

Ceramics are mainly used as core material. These materials provide structural regularity and a high degree of order due to their crystallinity. This structure leads to efficient carbohydrate-binding on its surface resulting in the stable structure of aquasomes. Common materials used as the ceramic core in aquasomes are tin oxide, calcium phosphate, diamond nanoparticles, and hydroxyapatite. Among these, calcium phosphate and hydroxyapatite have excellent biocompatibility, biodegradability, and stability.

Carbohydrate coating provides a molecular layer capable of adsorbing therapeutic proteins or peptides without modification. Carbohydrates provide an environment that resembles water to the protein or peptide but keeps it in a dry solid-state, protecting the three-dimensional structure of the protein or peptide of interest [94, 95]. Carbohydrates commonly used for coating are trehalose,

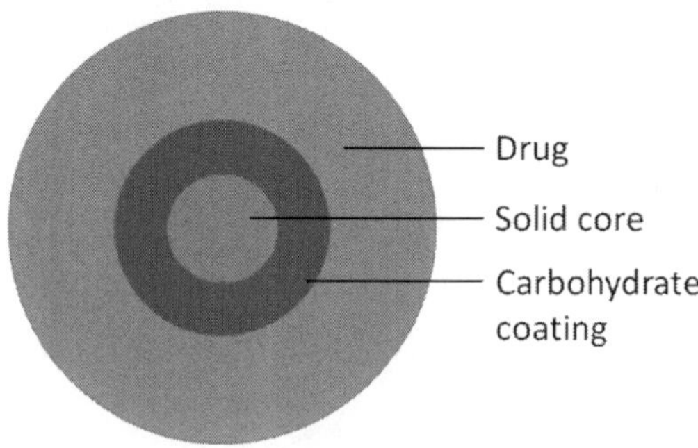

Figure 15.
General structure of aquasomes.

cellobiose, lactose and sucrose. The coating is achieved by the adsorption of the carbohydrate onto the core. The protein or peptide of interest interacts with the coating film by non-covalent or ionic interactions. Trehalose was previously reported to induce stress tolerance in bacteria, yeast, fungi, and some plants. Trehalose protects protein within the plant cell during the dehydration process and thus preserves cell structure [96]. It was observed that trehalose increased the transition temperature of proteins, resulting in increased stability [97]. Also, the hydroxyl group of carbohydrates interacts with the polar and charged group of proteins. Upon drying, the large number of hydroxyl groups of the carbohydrate replaces the water around polar groups in protein, thus maintaining their integrity [98].

A nanosized ceramic core-based drug delivery system has been developed for the oral administration of serratiopeptidase [99]. In this method, the calcium phosphate core was coated with chitosan, and the enzyme was adsorbed by the coating. The enzyme was further stabilized by encapsulating the enzyme-loaded core into alginate gel. The results indicated the ability of aquasomes to protect the structural integrity of the enzyme, resulting in a more potent therapeutic effect.

2.10 Hydrogels

Hydrogels are three-dimensional networks made of polymeric chains that are hydrophilic in nature. The polymer can be natural or synthetic and should contain a large amount of water. Although natural polymers show good biocompatibility, they are not suitable for protein or peptide delivery due to their improper mechanical strength. Natural polymers can also lead to an autoimmune response. However, hydrogels with the synthetic polymer can be designed to avoid these problems. Hydrogels can control the release of the protein or peptide of interest in response to pH [100, 101]. Hydrogels can also enhance transportation of the protein or peptide of interest. The difference of pH at different parts of the GIT has been utilized to control the release of insulin encapsulated in the hydrogels at the intestine (**Figure 16**). Hydrogels also showed rapid release of the encapsulated insulin once in the intestine. Finally, the encapsulation process of the protein (e.g., insulin) inside the hydrogel is highly efficient. These properties of the hydrogels make them promising systems for protein or peptide delivery [102].

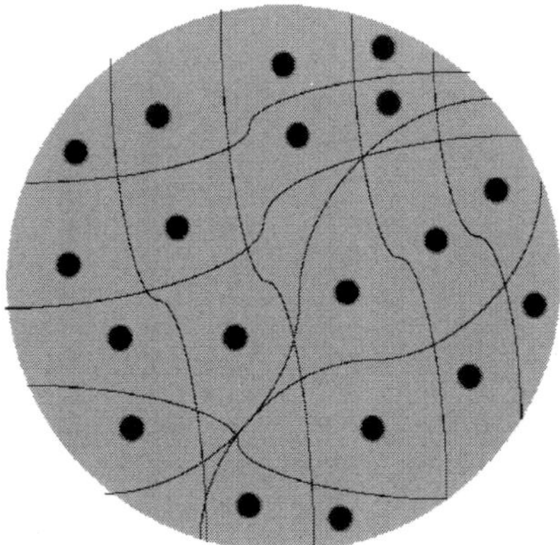

Figure 16.
Protein or peptide therapeutic (black spheres) encapsulated in a hydrogel.

2.11 Injectable nanocomposite cryogels

Although hydrogels are promising systems for protein or peptide delivery, they have some issues regarding the rapid release of the encapsulated protein or peptide of interest. This rapid release leads to a short duration of action which may not be optimal for some therapies. Another issue associated with the hydrogels is the possible denaturation of the encapsulated protein or peptide. Injectable nanocomposites have been developed to overcome some of the issues related to hydrogels. Kinetics of the release of the therapeutic protein or peptide can be controlled by using suitable components of the system [103]. This delivery system can also be used for the sustained release of various therapeutic proteins and peptides.

2.12 Cell-penetrating peptides

Cell-penetrating peptides (CPP) are capable of transporting the attached molecule across the cell membrane. Therefore, one way of enhancing the permeability of therapeutic proteins or peptides across the cell membrane is to attach them to a CPP (**Table 1**) [104]. One way CPP can penetrate the cell membrane is via endocytosis. Another way could be the perturbation of the lipid bilayer of the cell membrane by the CPP. Although minor disturbances in the membrane structure were found, toxic effects of CPP on the cell membrane have not been reported. Insulin attached to TAT (**Figure 17**) showed better permeability across the cell membrane [105].

2.13 Protein crystallization

Crystallization of therapeutic proteins offers many advantages over the traditionally used protein solution or amorphous form of the protein. The protein in the crystalline form shows significantly higher stability than the amorphous form. This higher stability is advantageous for therapeutic proteins since the high stability of the proteins maintains their biological function in different environments [106]. Crystalline form

CPP	Protein or peptide
TAT	β-galactosidase, Rnase A, Horseradish peroxidase, Domain-III of pseudomonas exotoxin A, peptides derived from VHL tumor suppressor, insulin
11-poly arginine peptide	p53
Antennapedia	p16-derived synthetic peptide
hCT (9–32)	Green fluorescence protein

Table 1.
Examples of protein and peptides delivered by CPPs.

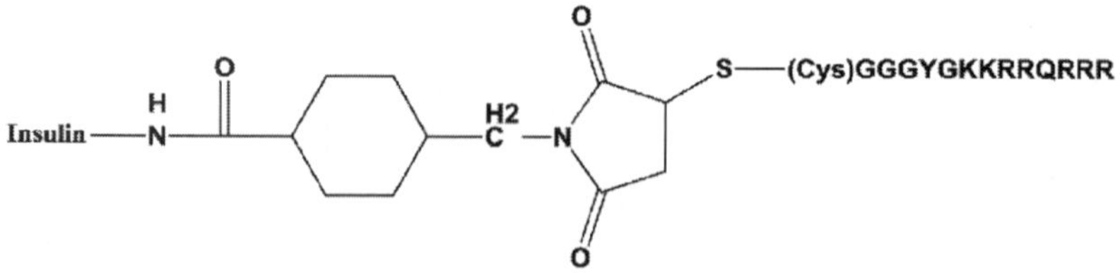

Figure 17.
Insulin attached to a CPP.

of lipase enzyme is used as a therapeutic enzyme in pathological conditions related to abnormalities in the digestion of lipid. However, a major limitation of crystallization approach is that not all proteins can be crystallized. Also, in some cases, protein crystallization is not efficient. Nevertheless, protein crystallization remains a promising approach for developing protein or peptide delivery systems [107, 108].

3. Transdermal delivery

3.1 Microneedle

Microneedle technology uses small needles, which creates small pores in the skin, allowing the protein or peptide to cross the outermost physical barrier [109]. Since one goal of transdermal delivery is to increase efficacy while still retaining an easy, non-invasive technique, microneedles are designed to breach only the stratum corneum [110]. Since the microneedles do not reach the viable dermis, both the capillaries and the nerve ends are avoided. Thus, this approach leads to painless feelings during the drug delivery. These needles have been made using various materials, including silicon, different metals, and biodegradable material such as polymers or sugars [111].

Different types of microneedles, as well as drug introduction routes, have been tested for efficient delivery of protein or peptide therapeutics [112]. In one method, needles are used to puncture the skin to create pores, followed by the drug administration. Another method involves coating the microneedle with the protein or peptide of interest. Thus, the creation of pores by the microneedles will allow the drug to enter the body. Another method involves encapsulating the drug in biodegradable microneedles. In this method, the drug will be released slowly as the microneedles degrade. Another method utilizes hollow microneedles, through which the therapeutic protein or peptide can be infused following the puncture of the skin.

3.2 Thermal ablation

Like microneedle technology, thermal ablation makes the stratum corneum more permeable [113]. Both these methods avoid the breach of deeper capillary and nerve-containing tissues. However, the difference is that short pulses of high heat (~100°C) are used (instead of needles) to create small, reversible channels in the micron range [114]. Thus, following the application of short bursts of heat, the drug can be applied to the area for entering the circulation. Multiple systems have been designed to deliver drugs via thermal ablation successfully. While these systems successfully deliver smaller drug molecules, delivery of protein or peptide via this method is a work in progress.

3.3 Iontophoresis

Iontophoresis does not require physical disruption of the skin's outer barrier. This method uses principles of electrorepulsion (for charged particles) and electroosmosis (for uncharged particles) to act on drug molecule rather than the skin [112]. During this process, a device capable of generating electric current is placed on the skin. When delivering a negatively charged peptide or protein, for example, the battery will build up a strong negative charge on the anode, which is placed in the same area of the skin as the drug molecule. Thus, the anode will drive the negatively charged protein or peptide into the skin due to charge–charge repulsion [115, 116]. It is important to note that the rate of drug release can be controlled easily by this method since the entry of the protein or peptide into the body is proportional to the current being applied to the skin [114]. Although the system successfully delivers small molecules (e.g., lidocaine), delivery of proteins or peptides via this method is still a work in progress.

3.4 Electroporation

Electroporation uses very short pulses of high voltage (10–100 V) to perforate the skin. Like microneedles and iontophoresis, this is also a non-invasive method of drug delivery since this method breaches only the stratum corneum [117]. Application of electric current disrupts the structure of the lipid-bilayer. This disruption allows the protein or peptide of interest to penetrate the skin. One advantage of this method is that the delivery of drugs can be easily changed by changing the voltage, number and duration of pulses, etc. [112].

3.5 Sonophoresis

Sonophoresis uses sound waves to increase the permeability of the skin. Similar to electroporation, sonophoresis also targets the lipid bilayer underneath the stratum corneum [112]. Sound waves (20–100 kHz) increases the pore sizes on the skin due to the increased fluidity of the lipid bilayers. Thus, sound waves allow the transcellular entry of drug molecules through the stratum corneum [114].

3.6 Biochemical enhancers

Biochemical enhancement utilizes biomolecules to enhance the permeability of the skin towards the peptide or protein of interest. This method aims to allow the entry of the drug molecule into circulation while being non-toxic, non-irritating, and non-allergenic [118]. Magainin, a 23-amino acid-containing peptide, has been reported to form pores in the bacterial cell membrane [119, 120]. Another small peptide TD1 increases the transdermal penetration capability of hEGF when fused together [121]. This system may play a vital role in delivering hydrophilic peptides transdermally.

3.7 Nanocarriers

Nanocarriers have been developed for administering protein or peptide therapeutics via the transdermal route. Nanocarriers have been found to be more effective penetration enhancers than biochemical enhancers. Nanocarriers commonly employed for delivering protein or peptide therapeutics are described below.

3.7.1 Transfersomes

Transfersomes are elastic or deformable liposomes (discussed in Section 2.7) [122]. These were developed to overcome the localization of liposomes on the skin. The membrane of transfersomes is formed by phospholipid and a single chain surfactant molecule (sodium cholate, sodium deoxycholate, Tween 20, Tween 60, dipotassium glycyrrhizinate, etc.). Transfersomes, by virtue of its tendency to avoid dry surroundings, enter into deeper layers of the skin that have higher moisture content than the surface layer. The elasticity of the membrane helps to breach the narrow gap on the surface of the skin. The enhanced drug transport by the transfersomes can be explained by its distribution on the skin surface after the adsorption on the skin [123]. The ability of transfersomes to transport protein or peptide therapeutics (e.g., insulin) has been reported [124, 125]. Encouraging results were obtained in the case of low molecular weight heparin [126].

3.7.2 Microemulsions

Water in oil microemulsions are stable dispersions consist of small water droplets dispersed within a continuous oil layer stabilized by incorporating a high concentration of surfactant/emulsifying molecules. Lipophilic surroundings of the external phase of the microemulsion resemble the environment of the upper layer of skin. This resemblance makes microemulsions ideal for application on the skin surface [127]. Also, the ease of administering microemulsions on the skin makes these ideal for passive delivery of proteins or peptides across the skin [128].

The efficacy of topically applied protein formulated with a microemulsion was investigated [129]. Rapid penetration of the molecule into the skin immediately below the application site was observed. Another study performed with desmopressin not only validated the capability of microemulsion as a transdermal carrier system but also indicated its superiority over creams and gels in delivering drugs across the skin [130]. The superior transdermal delivery of microemulsion has been attributed to the high loading capacity of the microemulsion and penetration enhancing effect of the constituents. Microemulsions have the capacity of encompassing a large amount of drugs without an increase in vehicle affinity. This capacity leads to a higher concentration gradient and higher transdermal flux from microemulsions. Also, the surfactant (e.g., isopropyl palmitate) can augment permeation by disrupting the intracellular lipid structure of stratum corneum [131, 132].

3.8 Prodrug

A prodrug is a reversible chemical modification of the drug to enhance its solubility, bioavailability, and stability without altering its pharmacological properties [133]. There are many examples where prodrug has been synthesized for proteins or peptides. For example, the thyrotropin-releasing hormone (TRH) has been successfully transported through human skin [134]. This was done by using the lipophilic prodrug of TRH, N-octyloxycarbonyl-TRH (**Figure 18**). The good skin penetration

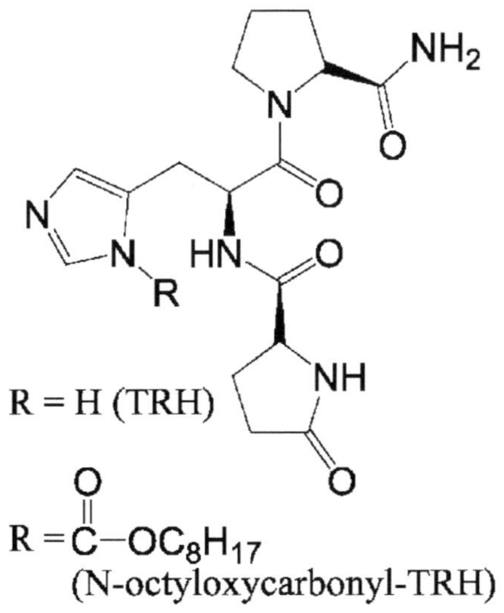

R = H (TRH)

$R = C(=O){-}OC_8H_{17}$
(N-octyloxycarbonyl-TRH)

Figure 18.
TRH and its prodrug.

behavior of this prodrug was attributed to its high water solubility and lipophilicity. Conjugation of proteins or peptides with carriers that selectively transport them across the biological membranes can be used to deliver protein or peptide therapeutics across the skin [135, 136]. For example, the toxic protein ricin is transported across the cell membrane via binding to the ricin B chain found on the surface, followed by internalization. The active component is liberated upon entering the cell, where it exerts its toxicological effects. Thus, ricin behaves essentially as a prodrug of the ricin A chain.

4. Nasal route

Delivery of protein or peptide via nasal route has been employed in delivering desmopressin, calcitonin, and seasonal influenza vaccine [137, 138]. Advantages of this method include patient convenience and comfort, elimination of needle-related injuries and infections, and decreased syringe-related medical waste. Some disadvantages of this method include nasal irritation, limitation on the amount of drug that can be delivered, peptidases, and large interpatient variability in absorption. However, highly effective and non-irritating absorption enhancers have been developed to overcome some of the limitations [139]. This route could be important for drugs used in crisis treatment (e.g., pain, sleep induction, panic attack, nausea, heart attack, etc.) due to the rapid absorption of drugs from the nasal cavity to the systemic circulation. In some of these cases, the putative pathway from nose to brain might provide a faster and more specific therapeutic effect [140]. This route is also very important for delivering drugs against respiratory infections since this route provides not only systemic immune response but also local mucosal immune response. The latter should provide a much higher immune response against these diseases. Considering the potential benefits of this route of delivery, we can expect novel nasal products in the near future. Some nasal delivery systems are described below.

4.1 Chitosan

Chitosan has attracted much attention as a nasal delivery system recently. Chitosan is produced by the deacetylation of chitin found in crustacean shells. The resulting free amino groups allow chitosan to exist in the protonated form (see Section 2.9.2) in the acidic environment. Chitosan glutamate is a pharmaceutically acceptable chitosan salt for nasal drug delivery. It has an average molecular weight of ~250 kDa and a degree of deacetylation > 80% [140]. A nasal morphine product containing chitosan as an absorption enhancer is being investigated. Morphine is a polar drug and is not readily absorbed via the nasal route using simple formulations [141]. However, the addition of chitosan to the nasal formulation leads to a remarkable increase in nasal morphine absorption. As discussed in Section 2.9.2, chitosan improves the transport of polar drugs across the epithelial membrane via the transient opening of the tight junctions in the cell membrane [142–144]. Another mechanism of improving the transport of polar drug across the epithelial membrane by chitosan is via bioadhesion. Finally, chitosan is non-toxic and non-irritant to the nasal membrane [145].

Other cationic polymers, such as poly-L-Arg and aminated gelatin has also been investigated for their application as absorption enhancers. These polymers work in a way similar to chitosan. These polymers improve the absorption of fluorescein-isothiocyanate (FITC)-dextran and insulin with negligible nasal toxicity [146–148].

4.2 Cyclodextrins

Cyclodextrins have been used as absorption enhancers in animal models [149–150]. But, their usefulness has not been confirmed in humans. However, cyclodextrin systems are in use in nasal formulations for drug stabilization.

4.3 Lipids and phospholipids

Phospholipid material didecanoyl-L-α-phosphatidyl choline was used as an absorption enhancer to develop the nasal delivery system for insulin. However, the development was halted due to low bioavailability in diabetic patients [151]. A nasal insulin formulation with a bioavailability of 35% has been reported. Irritation problems were also reported.

5. Buccal route

Delivery of proteins or peptides via buccal route involves administration of therapeutics through the mucosal membrane lining the cheeks [152]. In this process, the drug is placed in the mouth between the gum and cheek [153]. Buccal delivery has many advantages such as ease of use, bypassing the GIT, large contact surface area, etc. This method can also be employed to deliver hydrophilic macromolecules [154]. However, this method has some disadvantages such as irritation of the mucosa, low permeability of the peptide, and bitter taste of many buccal drugs. Absorption enhancers and adhesive polymers are being used to overcome some of these problems. Several drugs such as insulin, oxytocin have been successfully delivered via this route. Mucoadhesion (discussed in Section 2.6) is very important during the development of buccal drug delivery systems. Some methods employed for increased drug delivery via this route are described below.

5.1 Absorptions enhancers

Absorption enhancers are essential for delivering protein or peptide therapeutics, which generally show low buccal absorption rates. Some absorption enhancers are aprotinin, benzalkonium chloride, cyclodextrin, polyoxyethylene, sodium EDTA, etc.

5.2 pH

Permeability of acyclovir was investigated in the presence of sodium glycocholate (absorption enhancer) at a pH range of 3.3 to 8.8. The permeability of acyclovir was found to be pH dependent.

5.3 Patch design

Much research have been performed to understand the relationship between the type and amount of support materials and the drug release profile. Results indicated that these two factors are interrelated. It was also shown that single- and multi-layer patches have different drug release profiles.

6. Pulmonary route

The pulmonary route has been used to successfully deliver peptide therapeutics such as desmopressin, calcitonin, human growth hormone, parathyroid hormone, etc. [155]. There are several barriers to this route of peptide or protein delivery, such as respiratory mucus, mucociliary clearance, pulmonary enzymes, and macrophages that secrete peroxidases and proteases [156]. However, the large surface area, good vascularization, high capacity for solute exchange, and ultra-thinness are some of the attractive features of the alveolar epithelium that can facilitate systemic delivery of proteins or peptides via this route. The passage of large hydrophilic molecules through alveolar epithelium and capillary endothelium is limited. Absorption enhancers and enzyme inhibitors have been used to increase the absorption of peptide or protein therapeutics. However, these can be damaging to lung tissues. Some pulmonary delivery systems are described below.

6.1 Absorption enhancers

Cyclodextrins has been used as pulmonary absorption enhancers [157]. The relative efficiency of cyclodextrins in enhancing pulmonary insulin absorption follows the following order – dimethyl-β-cyclodextrin > α-cyclodextrins > β-cyclodextrin > γ-cyclodextrin > hydroxypropyl-β-cyclodextrin (**Figure 19**). Lanthanide ions are also effective in enhancing pulmonary insulin absorption [158].

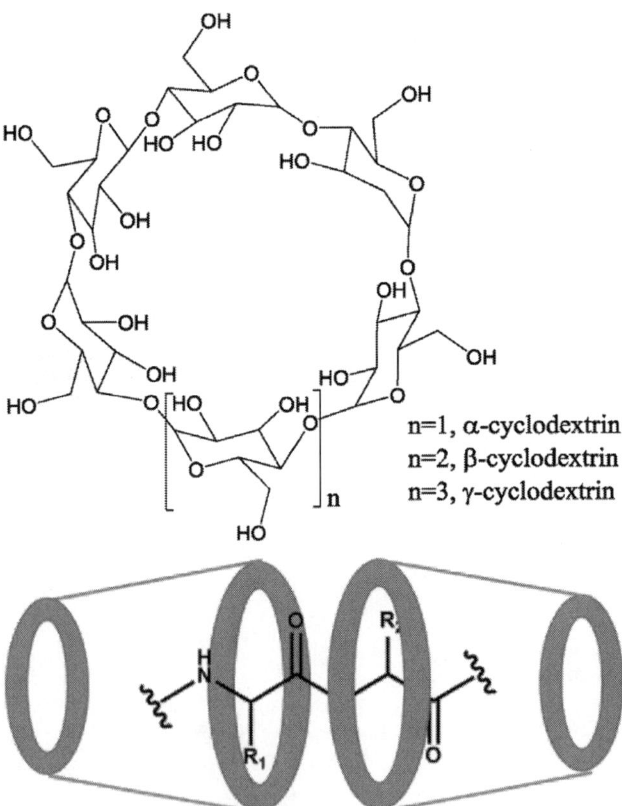

Figure 19.
Structures of cyclodextrins (top) and the cyclodextrin-drug complex (bottom).

6.2 Enzyme inhibition

Enzyme inhibitors (e.g., bacitracin, bestatin, nafamostat mesylate, soybean trypsin inhibitor, potato carboxypeptidase inhibitor, phosphoramidon) has been shown to enhance pulmonary absorption of proteins and peptides [159–161]. In addition to insulin, the absorption of calcitonin has been shown to increase [161–164].

6.3 Microparticles

The human lung is equipped with mechanisms to remove deposited particles by mucociliary clearance and phagocytosis. These clearance mechanisms should be considered while designing protein or peptide therapeutics and nanoparticles as a vehicle. The aim should be to achieve more efficient absorption and sustained therapeutic effect. It has been reported that inhalation of large porous insulin particles resulted in an elevated systemic level of insulin [165]. On the other hand, small non-porous insulin particles did not sustain therapeutic effect (4 hours vs. 96 hours for large porous particles). It has also been reported that the pulmonary delivery of insulin with nebulized DL-lactic/glycolide copolymer nanoparticle resulted in more sustained release (48 hours vs. 6 hours) compared to the nebulized aqueous solution [166].

6.4 Liposomes

Enhanced pulmonary absorption of protein or peptide therapeutics (e.g., insulin) has been shown using the Liposome (discussed in Section 2.7) as a carrier. Intratracheal administration of insulin liposomes led to increased pulmonary uptake of insulin [167]. The ability of liposome to promote pulmonary insulin absorption depends on the concentration, charge, and acyl chain length of the phospholipid [168].

6.5 PEGylation

Pulmonary absorption of protein or peptide therapeutics has been shown to increase using PEG. The pulmonary absorption of PEGylated r-huG-CSF generated a more intense response as compared to r-huG-CSF alone [169].

7. Rectal route

Rectal delivery of drugs is sometimes necessary if other routes of delivery are not applicable. This method offers some advantages such as rapid absorption of many low molecular weight drugs, partial avoidance of the first-pass metabolism, potential absorption into the lymphatic system, retention of large volumes, etc. This method is also beneficial considering the low amount of proteases compared to other parts of the GIT. This route allows both local and systemic delivery of drugs. Local delivery of drugs can be used to treat constipation, hemorrhoids, inflammation, hyperkalemia, etc. Systemic delivery of drugs can be used to treat pain, fever, nausea and vomiting, migraines, and sedation. Controlled absorption enhancement can also be achieved via this route due to the constant condition of the rectal environment. However, this method also has limitations, including limited absorption surface area, dissolution problem due to low fluid content, drug metabolism, etc. [170]. Several drugs such as insulin and pentagastrin have been successfully delivered via this route. Some rectal delivery systems are described below.

7.1 Absorption enhancers

Since the bioavailability of the peptide is low via the rectal route, various absorption enhances such as enamines, salicylate and its derivatives, surfactants, micelles, etc., have been investigated. It has been shown that enamine derivatives enhanced rectal absorption of CMZ (a hydrophilic antibiotic) [171]. Salicylate and its derivatives enhance rectal absorption of insulin, heparin, gastrin, and pentagastrin [172].

7.2 Protease inhibitors

Protease inhibitors reduce the degradation of various proteins and peptides due to the inhibition of proteases at the absorption site. Therefore, the use of protease inhibitors is one of the promising approaches for delivering protein or peptide therapeutics. Protease inhibitors (e.g., bacitracin, aprotinin, bestatin, trypsin inhibitor, puromycin, etc.) has been shown to enhance rectal absorption of protein and peptide therapeutics [173].

7.3 Chemical modification

Chemical modification of protein or peptide therapeutics is a potentially useful approach to deliver the protein or peptide of interest via the rectal route. For example, the acyl derivative of insulin improves its membrane permeability by making it more lipophilic [173]. Chemical modification may also protect the protein or peptide of interest from enzymatic degradation.

7.4 Cyclodextrins

Cyclodextrins are cyclo oligosaccharides consisting of several glucopyranose units (see Section 6.1). These act as host molecules that form inclusion complexes. Parent cyclodextrins can be modified to extend physicochemical properties and inclusion capacity. Cyclodextrins were shown to help rectal drug delivery with respect to stabilization, release, bioavailability, and alleviation of local irritation. Enhanced rectal absorption of lipophilic drugs by cyclodextrins is due to improved release from the vehicle and dissolution rate in the rectal fluid. However, the enhanced absorption of protein or peptide therapeutics is due to the action of cyclodextrins on the rectal epithelial cells [174].

8. Conclusion

Proteins and peptides are essential in various biochemical processes. These are also involved in various pathophysiological conditions. Therefore, the application of proteins and peptides to combat diseases, including cancer and diabetes, will be beneficial. However, unfavorable physicochemical properties of protein and peptides such as large size, hydrophilicity, and stability limit their use. Various approaches (discussed in this chapter) have been developed to overcome these problems. However, there is no general strategy for the delivery of protein or peptide therapeutics. One reason for the absence of a general strategy is the complex nature and variety of peptides and proteins. Thus, many strategies discussed in this chapter were focused on the delivery of the protein or peptide of interest. The long-term safety and efficacy of all these strategies should be considered. So, there are challenges to overcome in delivering the protein or peptide therapeutics. However, the future of protein and peptide delivery is bright considering the growing number of materials and combinatorial approaches. Also, emphasis is placed on developing cost-effective, tunable, biodegradable, and biocompatible materials for protein and peptide delivery. In the near future, it will be excellent to have a system that can be used for the delivery and systemic stability of different proteins and peptides.

References

[1] Voet D, Voet JG. Amino acids, Biochemistry., fourth ed. Wiley, USA; 2011. p. 67-82. https://www.wiley.com/en-us/Biochemistry%2C+4th+Edition-p-9780470570951

[2] Craik DJ, Fairlie DP, Liras S, Price D. The future of peptide-based drugs. Chem. Biol. Drug Des. 2013; 81(1): 136-147. DOI:10.1111/cbdd.12055

[3] Goldberg M, Gomez-Orellana I. Challenges for the oral delivery of macromolecules. Nat. Rev. Drug. Discov. 2003; 2(4):289-295. DOI:10.1038/nrd1067

[4] Park K, Kwon IC, Park K. Oral protein delivery: Current status and future prospect. React. Funct. Polym. 2011; 71(3):280-287. DOI:10.1016/j.reactfunctpolym.2010.10.002

[5] Werle M, Bernkop-Schnu¨rch, A. strategies to improve plasma half lifetime of peptide and protein drugs. Amino Acids 2006; 30(4): 351-367. DOI:10.1007/s00726-005-0289-3

[6] Shone A, Burnside J, Chipchase S, Game F, Jeffcoate W. Probing the validity of the probe-to-bone test in the diagnosis of osteomyelitis of the foot in diabetes. Diabetes Care 2006; 29:945-945. DOI:10.2337/diacare.29.04.06.dc05-2450

[7] Thomaidou E, Ramot Y. Injection site reactions with the use of biological agents. Dermatol. Ther. 2019; 32:e12817. DOI:10.1111/dth.12817

[8] Hilhorst N, Spanoudi-Kitrimi I, Goemans N, Morren MA. Injection site reactions after longterm subcutaneous delivery of drisapersen: A retrospective study. Eur. J. Pediatr. 2018; 178:253-258. DOI:10.1007/s00431-018-3272-1

[9] Messer LH, Berget C, Beatson C, Polsky S, Forlenza GP. Preserving skin integrity with chronic device use in diabetes. Diabetes Technol. Ther. 2018; 20:S254–S264. DOI:10.1089/dia.2018.0080

[10] Richardson T, Kerr D. Skin-related complications of insulin therapy: Epidemiology and emerging management strategies. Am. J. Clin. Dermatol. 2003; 4: 661-667. DOI:10.2165/00128071-200304100-00001

[11] Kerbleski JF, Gottlieb AB. Dermatological complications and safety of anti-TNF treatments. Gut 2009; 58:1033-1039. DOI:10.1136/gut.2008.163683

[12] Bos JD, Meinardi MM. The 500 Dalton rule for the skin penetration of chemical compounds and drugs. Exp Dermatol. 2000; 9(3):165-169. DOI:10.1034/j.1600-0625.2000.009003165.x

[13] Ruan RQ, Wang SS, Wang CL, Zhang L, Zhang YJ, Zhou W, et al. Transdermal delivery of human epidermal growth factor facilitated by a peptide chaperon. Eur J Med Chem. 2013; 62:405-409. DOI:10.1016/j.ejmech.2012.12.054

[14] Morishita M, Peppas NA. Is the oral route possible for peptide and protein drug delivery? Drug Discov. Today 2006; 11(19-20): 905-910. DOI:10.1016/j.drudis.2006.08.005

[15] Shantanu B, Nabamita B, Pran Kishore D, Chhater S, Rakesh KT. Chapter-12: Pre-formulation studies of drug substances, protein and peptides: Role in drug discovery and pharmaceutical product development. In: Tekade, R.K. (Ed.), Dosage Form Design Considerations: Advances in Pharmaceutical Product Development and Research Series, Vol. I. Academic Press; 2018. p. 399-431. DOI:10.1016/B978-0-12-814423-7.00012-5.

[16] Ye Y, Yu J, Wen D, Kahkoska AR, Gu Z. polymeric microneedles for transdermal protein delivery. Adv Drug Deliv Rev. 2018; 127:106-118. DOI:10.1016/j.addr.2018.01.015

[17] Meredith ME, Salameh TS, Banks WA. Intranasal delivery of proteins and peptides in the treatment of neurodegenerative diseases. AAPS J. 2015; 17(4):780-787. DOI:10.1208/s12248-015-9719-7

[18] Caon T, Jin L, Simoes CM, Norton RS, Nicolazzo JA. Enhancing the buccal mucosal delivery of peptide and protein therapeutics. Pharm Res. 2015; 32(1):1-21. DOI:10.1007/s11095-014-1485-1

[19] Lip Kwok PC, Chan HK. Chapter 2—Pulmonary delivery of peptides and proteins. In: Van Der Walle C, editor. Peptide and Protein Delivery. Boston: Academic Press; 2011. p. 23-46. DOI:10.1016/C2010-0-64887-5

[20] Brown LR. Commercial challenges of protein drug delivery. Expert. Opin. Drug. Deliv. 2005; 2(1):29-42. DOI:10.1517/17425247.2.1.29

[21] Borchardt RT. Optimizing oral absorption of peptides using prodrug strategies. J. Control. Release 1999; 62(1-2):231-238. DOI:10.1016/s0168-3659(99)00042-5

[22] Vilhardt H, Lundin S. In vitro intestinal transport of vasopressin and its analogues. Acta Physiol. 1986; 126(4):601-607. DOI:10.1111/j.1748-1716.1986.tb07861.x

[23] Shaji J, Patole V. Protein and peptide drug delivery: Oral approaches. Indian J. Pharm. Sci. 2008; 70 (3):269-277. DOI:10.4103/0250-474X.42967

[24] Hashimoto M, Takada K, Kiso Y, Muranishi S. Synthesis of palmitoyl derivatives of insulin and their biological activities. Pharm. Res. 1989; 6 (2):171-176. DOI:10.1023/A:1015992828666

[25] Hamman JH, Steenekamp JH. Oral Peptide Drug Delivery: Strategies to Overcome Challenges. Peptide Drug Discovery and Development: Translational Research in Academia and Industry. Wiley; 2011. p. 71-90. DOI:10.1002/9783527636730.ch3

[26] Roberts MJ, Bentley MD, Harris JM. Chemistry for peptide and protein PEGylation. Adv. Drug Deliv. Rev. 2012; 64:116-127. DOI:10.1016/s0169-409x(02)00022-4

[27] Veronese FM. Peptide and protein PEGylation: A review of problems and solutions. Biomaterials 2001; 22(5):405-417. DOI:10.1016/s0142-9612(00)00193-9.

[28] Harris JM, Chess RB. Effect of pegylation on pharmaceuticals. Nat. Rev. Drug Discov. 2003; 2(3):214-221. DOI:10.1038/nrd1033

[29] Gupta H, Sharma A. Recent trends in protein and peptide drug delivery systems. Asian J. Pharm. 2009; 3(2): 69-75. DOI:10.4103/0973-8398.55041

[30] Pasut G, Veronese FM. State of the art in PEGylation: The great versatility achieved after forty years of research. J. Control. Release 2012; 161 (2):461-472. DOI:10.1016/j.jconrel.2011.10.037

[31] Jain A, Jain A, Gulbake A, Shilpi S, Hurkat P, Jain SK. Peptide and protein delivery using new drug delivery systems. Crit. Rev. Ther. Drug Carrier Syst. 2013; 30(4):293-329. DOI:10.1615/critrevtherdrugcarriersyst.2013006955

[32] Hamman JH, Enslin GM, Kotze′ AF. Oral delivery of peptide drugs. BioDrugs 2005;19(3):165-177. DOI:10.2165/00063030-200519030-00003

[33] Ahmad J, Pran Kishore D, Ing HO, Dina El-R, Faridah OS, Rajakumari R.

Design, Synthesis and pharmacological properties of peptidomimetics. Asian J. Chem. 2015; 27(9):3137-3142. DOI:10.14233/ajchem.2015.18962

[34] Pauletti GM, Gangwar S, Siahaan TJ, Aube´ J, Borchardt RT. Improvement of oral peptide bioavailability: Peptidomimetics and prodrug strategies. Adv. Drug Deliv. Rev. 1997; 27(2_3):235-256. DOI:10.1016/s0169-409x(97)00045-8

[35] Ra¨der AF, Reichart F, Weinmu¨ ller M, Kessler H. 2017. Improving oral bioavailability of cyclic peptides by Nmethylation. Bioorg. Med. Chem. 2017; 26(10):2766-2773. DOI:10.1016/j.bmc.2017.08.031.

[36] Silverman R, Holladay M. Lead Discovery and Lead Modifications, the Organic Chemistry of Drug Design and Drug Action., third ed. Elsevier, USA; 2014. p. 19-123. DOI:10.1016/B978-0-12-382030-3.00001-5

[37] Pran Kishore D, Ahmad J, Dina El-R, Tan YH, Elham MN, Mallikarjuna RP. Molecular Docking Studies and Comparative Binding Mode Analysis of FDA Approved HIV Protease Inhibitors. Asian J. Chem. 2014; 26(18):6227-6232. DOI:10.14233/ajchem.2014.17195

[38] Mo'tya'n JA, To´ th F, T˝ozse'r J. Research applications of proteolytic enzymes in molecular biology. Biomolecules 2013; 3(4): 923-942. DOI:10.3390/biom3040923

[39] Park K, Kwon IC, Park K. Oral protein delivery: Current status and future prospect. React. Funct. Polym. 2011; 71(3):280-287. DOI:10.1016/j.reactfunctpolym.2010.10.002

[40] Pivovarova O, Ho¨hn a, Grune T, Pfeiffer AF, Rudovich N. insulin-degrading enzyme: A new therapeutic target for diabetes and Alzheimer's disease? Ann. Med. 2016; 48(8):614-624. DOI:10.1080/07853890.2016.1197416

[41] Renukuntla J, Vadlapudi AD, Patel A, Boddu SH, Mitra AK. Approaches for enhancing oral bioavailability of peptides and proteins. Int. J. Pharm. 2013; 447(1-2):75-93. DOI:10.1016/j.ijpharm.2013.02.030

[42] Williams AC, Barry BW. Penetration enhancers. Adv. Drug Deliv. Rev. 2004; 56 (5):603-618. DOI:10.1016/j.addr.2003.10.025

[43] Choonara BF, Choonara YE, Kumar P, Bijukumar D, du Toit LC, Pillay V. A review of advanced oral drug delivery technologies facilitating the protection and absorption of protein and peptide molecules. Biotechnol. Adv. 2014; 32(7):1269-1282. DOI:10.1016/j.biotechadv.2014.07.006

[44] Sood A, Panchagnula R. Peroral route: An opportunity for protein and peptide drug delivery. Chem. Rev. 2001; 101(11):3275-3304. DOI:10.1021/cr000700m

[45] Lee HJ. Protein drug oral delivery: The recent progress. Arch. Pharm. Res. 2002; 25(5):572-584. DOI:10.1007/BF02976925

[46] Kompella UB, Lee VH. Delivery systems for penetration enhancement of peptide and protein drugs: Design considerations. Adv. Drug Deliv. Rev. 2001; 46(1-3):211-245. DOI:10.1016/s0169-409x(00)00137-x

[47] Balakumar C, Sarah Nedal A, Al-Attraqchi O, Kaushik K, Rakesh KT. Chapter-20: Computer aided prediction of pharmacokinetic (ADMET) properties. In: Tekade, R.K. (Ed.), Dosage Form Design Considerations: Advances in Pharmaceutical Product Development and Research Series, Vol. II. Academic Press; 2018. p. 731-755. DOI:10.1016/B978-0-12-814421-3.00021-X.

[48] Zheng Y, Qiu Y, Lu MYF, Hoffman D, Reiland TL. Permeability and absorption of leuprolide from various intestinal regions in rabbits and rats. Int. J. Pharm. 1999; 185(1):83-92. DOI:10.1016/s0378-5173(99)00146-5

[49] Roldo M, Barbu E, Brown JF, Laight DW, Smart JD, Tsibouklis J. Azo compounds in colon-specific drug delivery. Expert Opin. Drug Deliv. 2007; 4(5):547-560. DOI:10.1517/17425247.4.5.547

[50] Mandava N, Oberoi RK, Minocha M, Mitra AK. Transporter targeted drug delivery. J. Drug Deliv. Sci. Technol. 2010; 20(2):89-99. DOI:10.1016/S1773-2247(10)50012-1

[51] Friedrichsen GM, Nielsen CU, Steffensen B, Begtrup M. Model prodrugs designed for the intestinal peptide transporter. A synthetic approach for coupling of hydroxy-containing compounds to dipeptides. Eur. J. Pharm. Sci. 2001; 14(1):13-19. DOI:10.1016/s0928-0987(01)00137-3

[52] Rubio-Aliaga I, Daniel H. Mammalian peptide transporters as targets for drug delivery. Trends Pharmacol. Sci. 2002; 23(9):434-440. DOI:10.1016/s0165-6147(02)02072-2

[53] Daugherty AL, Mrsny RJ. Transcellular uptake mechanisms of the intestinal epithelial barrier part one. Pharm. Sci. Technol. Today 1999; 2(4):144-151. DOI:10.1016/s1461-5347(99)00142-x

[54] Russell-Jones GJ. The potential use of receptor-mediated endocytosis for oral drug delivery. Adv. Drug Deliv. Rev. 1996; 20(1): 83-97. DOI:10.1016/0169-409X(95)00131-P

[55] Rahamatullah Shaikh TRRS, Garland MJ, Woolfson AD, Donnelly RF. Mucoadhesive drug delivery systems. J. Pharm. Bioallied Sci. 2011; 3(1):89-100. DOI:10.4103/0975-7406.76478

[56] Lehr CM. From sticky stuff to sweet receptors—Achievements, limits, and novel approach to bioadhesion. Eur. J. Drug Metab. Pharmacokinet. 1996; 21(2):139-148. DOI:10.1007/BF03190262

[57] Kreuter J. Peroral administration of nanoparticles. Adv. Drug Deliv. Rev. 1991:7(1):71-86. DOI:10.1016/0169-409X(91)90048-H

[58] Wu ZH, Ping QN, Wei Y, Lai JM. Hypoglycemic efficacy of chitosan-coated insulin liposomes after oral administration in mice. Acta Pharmacol. Sin. 2004; 25:966-972.

[59] Wang LY, Gu YH, Su ZG, Ma GH. Preparation and improvement of release behavior of chitosan microspheres containing insulin. Int. J. Pharm. 2006:311(1-2):187-195. DOI:10.1016/j.ijpharm.2005.12.033

[60] Lowman AM, Morishita M, Kajita M, Nagai T, Peppas NA. Oral delivery of insulin using pH-responsive complexation gels. J. Pharm. Sci. 1999; 88(9):933-937. DOI:10.1021/js980337n

[61] Yun Y, Cho YW, Park K. Nanoparticles for oral delivery: Targeted nanoparticles with peptidic ligands for oral protein delivery. Adv. Drug Deliv. Rev. 2013:65(6):822-832. DOI:10.1016/j.addr.2012.10.007

[62] Sarmento B, Martins S, Ferreira D, Souto EB. Oral insulin delivery by means of solid lipid nanoparticles. Int. J. Nanomedicine 2007; 2:743-749.

[63] Tan ML, Choong PF, Dass CR. Recent developments in liposomes, microparticles and nanoparticles for protein and peptide drug delivery. Peptides 2010; 31(1):184-193. DOI:10.1016/j.peptides.2009.10.002

[64] Su FY, Lin KJ, Sonaje K, Wey SP, Yen TC, Ho YC. Protease inhibition and absorption enhancement by functional nanoparticles for effective oral insulin

delivery. Biomaterials 2012; 33(9): 2801-2811. DOI:10.1016/j.biomaterials.2011.12.038

[65] Faraji AH, Wipf P. Nanoparticles in cellular drug delivery. Bioorg. Med. Chem. 2009; 17(8):2950-2962. DOI:10.1016/j.bmc.2009.02.043

[66] Rawat M, Singh D, Saraf S. Nanocarriers: Promising vehicle for bioactive drugs. Biol. Pharm. Bull. 2006:29:1790-1798. DOI:10.1248/bpb.29.1790

[67] Almeida A J, Souto E. Solid lipid nanoparticles as a drug delivery system for peptides and proteins. Adv. Drug Deliv. Rev. 2007; 59:478-490. DOI:10.1016/j.addr.2007.04.007

[68] Garcia-Fuentes M, Torres D, Alonso MJ. New surface-modified lipid nanoparticles as delivery vehicles for salmon calcitonin. Int. J. Pharm. 2005; 296:122-132. DOI:10.1016/j.ijpharm.2004.12.030

[69] Charman WN, Porter CJ, Mithani S, Dressman JB. Physiochemical and physiological mechanisms for the effects of food on drug absorption: The role of lipids and pH. J. Pharm. Sci. 1997; 86:269-282. DOI:10.1021/js960085v

[70] Charman WN. Lipids, lipophilic drugs, and oral drug delivery-some emerging concepts. J. Pharm. Sci. 2000; 89:967-978. DOI:10.1002/1520-6017(200008)89:8<967::aid-jps1>3.0.co;2-r

[71] Damge C, Reis CP, Maincent P. Nanoparticle strategies for the oral delivery of insulin. Expert Opin. Drug Deliv. 2008; 5:45-68. DOI:10.1517/17425247.5.1.45

[72] Braz L, Rodrigues S, Fonte P, Grenha A, Sarmento B. Mechanisms of Chemical and Enzymatic Chitosan Biodegradability and its Application on Drug Delivery, Biodegradable Polymers: Processing, Degradation and Applications. Nova Publishers, New York, USA; 2011. p. 325-364.

[73] Cano-Cebrian MJ, Zornoza T, Granero L, Polache A. Intestinal absorption enhancement via the paracellular route by fatty acids, chitosans and others: A target for drug delivery. Curr. Drug Deliv. 2005; 2:9-22. DOI:10.2174/1567201052772834

[74] Smith JM, Dornish M, Wood EJ. Involvement of protein kinase C in chitosan glutamate-mediated tight junction disruption. Biomaterials 2005; 26:3269-3276. DOI:10.1016/j.biomaterials.2004.06.020

[75] Fonte P, Nogueira T, Gehm C, Ferreira D, Sarmento B. Chitosan-coated solid lipid nanoparticles enhance the oral absorption of insulin. Drug Deliv. Transl. Res. 2011; 1:299-308. DOI:10.1007/s13346-011-0023-5

[76] Champion JA, Walker A, Mitragotri S. Role of particle size in phagocytosis of polymeric microspheres. Pharm. Res. 2008; 25: 1815-1821. DOI:10.1007/s11095-008-9562-y

[77] Yin Y, Chen D, Qiao M, Wei X, Hu H. Lectin-conjugated PLGA nanoparticles loaded with thymopentin: Ex vivo bioadhesion and in vivo biodistribution. J. Control. Release 2007; 123:27-38. DOI:10.1016/j.jconrel.2007.06.024

[78] Owens DE 3rd. Peppas NA. Opsonization, biodistribution, and pharmacokinetics of polymeric nanoparticles. Int. J. Pharm. 2006; 307:93-102. DOI:10.1016/j.ijpharm.2005.10.010

[79] Lemarchand C, Gref R, Couvreur P. Polysaccharide-decorated nanoparticles. Eur. J. Pharm. Biopharm. 2004; 58:327-341. DOI:10.1016/j.ejpb.2004.02.016

[80] Sarmento B, Mazzaglia D, Bonferoni MC, Neto AP, Monteiro MC, Seabra V. Effect of chitosan coating in overcoming the phagocytosis of insulin loaded solid lipid nanoparticles by mononuclear phagocyte system. Carbohydr. Polym. 2011; 84:919-925. DOI:10.1016/j.carbpol.2010.12.042

[81] Agnihotri SA, Mallikarjuna NN, Aminabhavi TM. Recent advances in chitosan-based micro-and nanoparticles in drug delivery. J. Control. Release 2004; 100(1):5-28. DOI:10.1016/j.jconrel.2004.08.010

[82] Dua K, Bebawy M, Awasthi R, Tekade R, Tekade M, Gupta G. Chitosan and its derivatives in nanocarrier based pulmonary drug delivery systems. Pharm. Nanotechnol. 2017; (4):243-249. DOI:10.2174/221173850566617 0808095258

[83] Dua K, Shukla SD, Tekade RK, Hansbro PM. Whether a novel drug delivery system can overcome the problem of biofilms in respiratory diseases? Drug Deliv. Transl. Res. 2017; 7:179-187. DOI:10.1007/s13346-016-0349-0

[84] Maheshwari RGS, Thakur S, Singhal S, Patel RP, Tekade M, Tekade RK. Chitosan encrusted nonionic surfactant based vesicular formulation for topical administration of ofloxacin. Sci. Adv. Mater. 2015; 7:1163-1176. DOI:10.1166/sam.2015.2245

[85] Amidi M, Mastrobattista E, Jiskoot W, Hennink WE. Chitosan-based delivery systems for protein therapeutics and antigens. Adv. Drug Deliv. Rev. 2010; 62(1):59-82. DOI:10.1016/j.addr.2009.11.009

[86] Kotze AF, Luessen HL, De Boer AG, Verhoef JC, Junginger HE. Chitosan for enhanced intestinal permeability: Prospects for derivatives soluble in neutral and basic environments. Eur. J. Pharm. Sci. 1999; 7(2):145-151. DOI:10.1016/s0928-0987(98)00016-5

[87] Van der Merwe SM, Verhoef JC, Verheijden JHM, Kotze′ AF, Junginger HE. Trimethylated chitosan as a polymeric absorption enhancer for improved peroral delivery of peptide drugs. Eur. J. Pharm. Biopharm. 2004; 58(2):225-235. DOI:10.1016/j.ejpb.2004.03.023

[88] Chin J, Mahmud KF, Kim SE, Park K, Byun Y. The insight of current technologies for oral delivery of proteins and peptides. Drug Discov. Today: Technol. 2012;9(2):e105-e112. DOI:10.1016/j.ddtec.2012.04.005

[89] Morc¸o¨ l T, Nagappan P, Nerenbaum L, Mitchell A, Bell SJD. Calcium phosphate-PEG-insulin-casein (CAPIC) particles as oral delivery systems for insulin. Int. J. Pharm. 2004; 277(1-2):91-97. DOI:10.1016/j.ijpharm.2003.07.015

[90] Umashankar MS, Sachdeva RK, Gulati M. Aquasomes: A promising carrier for peptides and protein delivery. Nanomedicine. 2010; 6(3):419-426. DOI:10.1016/j.nano.2009.11.002

[91] Banerjee S, Sen KK. Aquasomes: a novel nanoparticulate drug carrier. J Drug Deliv Sci Technol. 2018; 43:446-452. DOI:10.1016/j.jddst.2017.11.011

[92] Cherian AK, Rana AC, Jain SK. Self-assembled carbohydrate-stabilized ceramic nanoparticles for the parenteral delivery of insulin. Drug Dev Ind Pharm. 2000; 26(4):459-463. DOI:10.1081/ddc-100101255

[93] Pandey RS, Sahu S, Sudheesh MS, Madan J, Kumar M, Dixit VK. Carbohydrate modified ultrafine ceramic nanoparticles for allergen immunotherapy. Int Immunopharmacol. 2011; 11(8):925-931. DOI:10.1016/j.intimp.2011.02.004

[94] Kossovsky N, Gelman A, Rajguru S, Nguyen R, Sponsler E, Hnatyszyn HJ, et al. Control of molecular polymorphisms

by a structured carbohydrate/ceramic delivery vehicle—Aquasomes. J Control Release. 1996; 39(2):383-388. DOI:10.1016/0168-3659(95)00169-7

[95] Goyal AK, Khatri K, Mishra N, Mehta A, Vaidya B, Tiwari S, et al. Aquasomes—A nanoparticulate approach for the delivery of antigen. Drug Dev Ind Pharm. 2008; 34(12):1297-1305. DOI:10.1080/03639040802071661

[96] Shahabade Gururaj S, Bhosale Ashok V, Mutha Swati S, Bhosale Nilesh R, Khade Prashant H, Bhadane Nishant P, et al. An overview on nanocarrier technology – Aquasomes. J Pharm Res. 2009; 2(7):1174-1177.

[97] Kaushik JK, Bhat R. Why is trehalose an exceptional protein stabilizer? An analysis of the thermal stability of proteins in the presence of the compatible osmolyte trehalose. J Biol Chem. 2003; 278(29):26458-26465. DOI:10.1074/jbc.M300815200

[98] Pandey S, Badola A, Bhatt GK, Kothiyal P. An overview on aquasomes. Int J Pharm Chem Sci. 2013; 2(3):1282-1287.

[99] Rawat M, Singh D, Saraf S, Saraf S. Development and in vitro evaluation of alginate gel–encapsulated, chitosan-coated ceramic nanocores for oral delivery of enzyme. Drug Dev Ind Pharm. 2008; 34(2):181-188. DOI:10.1080/03639040701539479

[100] Ichikawa H, Peppas NA. Novel complexation hydrogels for oral peptide delivery: In vitro evaluation of their cytocompatibility and insulin-transport enhancing effects using Caco-2 cell monolayers. J. Biomed. Mater. Res. A. 2003; 67(2):609-617. DOI:10.1002/jbm.a.10128

[101] Peppas NA, Bures P, Leobandung W, Ichikawa H. Hydrogels in pharmaceutical formulations. Eur. J. Pharm. Biopharm. 2000; 50(1): 27-46. DOI:10.1016/S0939-6411(00)00090-4

[102] Kamei N, Morishita M, Chiba H, Kavimandan NJ, Peppas NA, Takayama K. Complexation hydrogels for intestinal delivery of interferon β and calcitonin. J. Control. Release 2009; 134(2):98-102. DOI:10.1016/j.jconrel.2008.11.014

[103] Koshy ST, Zhang DK, Grolman JM, Stafford AG, Mooney DJ. Injectable nanocomposite cryogels for versatile protein drug delivery. Acta Biomater. 2018; 65:36-43. DOI:10.1016/j.actbio.2017.11.024

[104] Tre'hin R, Merkle HP. Chances and pitfalls of cell penetrating peptides for cellular drug delivery. Eur. J. Pharm. Biopharm. 2004; 58 (2):209-223. DOI:10.1016/j.ejpb.2004.02.018

[105] Morishita M, Peppas NA. Is the oral route possible for peptide and protein drug delivery? Drug Discov. Today 2006; 11(19_20): 905-910. DOI:10.1016/j.drudis.2006.08.005

[106] Judge RA, Forsythe EL, Pusey ML. The effect of protein impurities on lysozyme crystal growth. Biotechnol. Bioeng. 1998; 59 (6):776-785. DOI:10.1002/(sici)1097-0290(19980920)59:6<776::aid-bit14>3.0.co;2-3

[107] Park K, Kwon IC, Park K. Oral protein delivery: Current status and future prospect. React. Funct. Polym. 2011; 71(3):280-287. DOI:10.1016/j.reactfunctpolym.2010.10.002

[108] Layer P, Keller J. Lipase supplementation therapy: Standards, alternatives, and perspectives. Pancreas 2003; 26(1):1-7. DOI:10.1097/00006676-200301000-00001

[109] Arora A, Prausnitz MR, Mitragotri S. Micro-scale devices for

transdermal drug delivery. Int. J. Pharm. 2008; 364(2):227-236. DOI:10.1016/j.ijpharm.2008.08.032

[110] Garland MJ, Caffarel-Salvador E, Migalska K, Woolfson AD, Donnelly RF. Dissolving polymeric microneedle arrays for electrically assisted transdermal drug delivery. J. Control. Release. 2012; 159(1):52-59. DOI:10.1016/j.jconrel.2012.01.003

[111] Wilson, EJ. Three Generations: The past, present, and future of transdermal drug delivery systems. Pharmcon; SC, USA: 2011.

[112] Herwadkar A, Banga AK. Peptide and protein transdermal drug delivery. Drug Discov. Today Technol. 2012; 9(2):e147–e154. DOI:10.1016/j.ddtec.2011.11.007

[113] Lee JW, Gadiraju P, Park JH, Allen MG, Prausnitz MR. Microsecond thermal ablation of skin for transdermal drug delivery. J. Control. Release. 2011; 154(1):58-68. DOI:10.1016/j.jconrel.2011.05.003

[114] Prausnitz MR, Langer R. Transdermal drug delivery. Nat. Biotechnol. 2008; 26(11):1261-1268. DOI:10.1038/nbt.1504

[115] Kalluri H, Banga AK. Transdermal delivery of proteins. AAPS PharmSciTech. 2011; 12(1):431– 441. DOI:10.1208/s12249-011-9601-6

[116] Ghosh B, Iyer D, Nair AB, Sree HN. Prospects of iontophoresis in cardiovascular drug delivery. J. Basic Clin. Pharm. 2013; 4(1):25-30. DOI:10.4103/0976-0105.109407

[117] Denet AR, Vanbever R, Preat V. Skin electroporation for transdermal and topical delivery. Adv. Drug Deliv. Rev. 2004; 56(5):659-674. DOI:10.1016/j.addr.2003.10.027

[118] Pathan IB, Setty CM. Chemical penetration enhancers for transdermal drug delivery systems. Trop. J. Pharm. Res. 2009; 8(2):173-179. DOI:10.4314/tjpr.v8i2.44527

[119] Kim YC, Late S, Banga AK, Ludovice PJ, Prausnitz MR. Biochemical enhancement of transdermal delivery with magainin peptide: Modification of electrostatic interactions by changing pH. Int. J. Pharm. 2008; 362(1-2):20-28. DOI:10.1016/j.ijpharm.2008.05.042

[120] Kim YC, Ludovice PJ, Prausnitz MR. Transdermal delivery enhanced by magainin pore-forming peptide. J. Control. Release. 2007; 122(3):375-383. DOI:10.1016/j.jconrel.2007.05.031

[121] Chen Y, Shen Y, Guo X, et al. Transdermal protein delivery by a coadministered peptide identified via phage display. Nat. Biotechnol. 2006; 24(4):455-460. DOI:10.1038/nbt1193

[122] Cevc G, Blume G. Lipid vesicles penetrate into intact skin owing to the transdermal osmotic gradients and hydration force. Biochim Biophys Acta (BBA)-Biomembr. 1992; 1104:226-232. DOI:10.1016/0005-2736(92)90154-E

[123] Cevc G, Chopra A. Deformable (TransfersomeVR) vesicles for improved drug delivery into and through the skin. In: Dragicevic N, Maibach H, editors. Percutaneous Penetration Enhancers Chemical Methods in Penetration Enhancement. Berlin, Heidelberg: Springer; 2016. p. 39-59. DOI:10.1007/978-3-662-47862-2_3

[124] Guo J, Ping Q, Sun G, et al. Lecithin vesicular carriers for transdermal delivery of cyclosporin a. Int J Pharm. 2000; 194:201-207. DOI:10.1016/s0378-5173(99)00361-0

[125] Cevc G, Gebauer D, Stieber J, et al. Ultraflexible vesicles, transfersomes, have an extremely low pore penetration resistance and transport therapeutic

amounts of insulin across the intact mammalian skin. Biochim Biophys Acta (BBA)-Biomembr. 1998; 1368:201-215. DOI:10.1016/S0005-2736(97)00177-6

[126] Song YK, Kim CK. Topical delivery of low-molecular-weight heparin with surface-charged flexible liposomes. Biomaterials. 2006; 27:271-280. DOI:10.1016/j.biomaterials.2005.05.097

[127] Murdan S. Organogels in drug delivery. Expert Opin Drug Deliv. 2005; 2:489-505. DOI:10.1517/17425247.2.3.489

[128] Russell-Jones G, Himes R. Water-in-oil microemulsions for effective transdermal delivery of proteins. Expert Opin Drug Deliv. 2011; 8:537-546. DOI:10.1517/17425247.2011.559458

[129] Witting M, Obst K, Friess W, et al. Recent advances in topical delivery of proteins and peptides mediated by soft matter nanocarriers. Biotechnol Adv. 2015; 33:1355-1369. DOI:10.1016/j.biotechadv.2015.01.010

[130] Getie M, Wohlrab J, Neubert RH. Dermal delivery of desmopressin acetate using colloidal carrier systems. J Pharm Pharmacol. 2005; 57:423-427. DOI:10.1211/0022357055713

[131] Kreilgaard M. Influence of microemulsions on cutaneous drug delivery. Adv Drug Deliv Rev. 2002; 54(Suppl 1):S77–S98. DOI:10.1016/s0169-409x(02)00116-3

[132] Dreher F, Walde P, Walther P, et al. Interaction of a lecithin microemulsion gel with human stratum corneum and its effect on transdermal transport. J Control Release. 1997; 45:131-140. DOI:10.1016/S0168-3659(96)01559-3

[133] Chaulagain B, Jain A, Tiwari A, Verma A, Jain SK. Passive delivery of protein drugs through transdermal route. Artif Cells Nanomed Biotechnol. 2018; 46(sup1): 472-487. DOI:10.1080/21691401.2018.1430695

[134] Bundgaard H. (C) Means to enhance penetration: (1) Prodrugs as a means to improve the delivery of peptide drugs. Adv Drug Deliv Rev. 1992; 8(1):1-38. DOI:10.1016/0169-409X(92)90014-H

[135] Oliyai R, Stella VJ. Prodrugs of peptides and proteins for improved formulation and delivery. Annu Rev Pharmacol Toxicol. 1993; 33:521-544. DOI:10.1146/annurev.pa.33.040193.002513

[136] van Deurs B, Hansen SH, Olsnes S, et al. Protein uptake and cytoplasmic access in animal cells. In: Audus KL, Raub TJ, editors. Biological Barriers to Protein Delivery. Boston (MA): Springer US; 1993. p. 71-104. DOI:10.1007/978-1-4615-2898-2

[137] Illum L. Nasal drug delivery: New developments and strategies. Drug Discov. Today. 2002; 7(23):1184-1189. DOI:10.1016/s1359-6446(02)02529-1

[138] Maggio ET. Intravail: Highly effective intranasal delivery of peptide and protein drugs. Expert Opin. Drug. Deliv. 2006; 3(4):529-539. DOI:10.1517/17425247.3.4.529

[139] Pillion DJ, Hosmer S, Meezan E. Dodecylmaltoside-mediated nasal and ocular absorption of lyspro-insulin: Independence of surfactant action from multimer dissociation. Pharm. Res. 1998; 15(10):1637-1639. DOI:10.1023/a:1011975721569

[140] Illum L. Nasal drug delivery – Possibilities, problems and solutions. J. Control. Release 2003; 87(1-3):187-198. DOI:10.1016/s0168-3659(02)00363-2.

[141] Illum L. et al. Intranasal delivery of morphine. J. Pharmacol. Exp. Ther. 2002; 301:1-10. DOI:10.1124/jpet.301.1.391

[142] Artursson P. et al. Effect of chitosan on the permeability of

monolayers of intestinal epithelial cells (Caco-2). Pharm. Res. 1994; 11:1358-1361. DOI:10.1023/a:1018967116988

[143] Dodane V. et al. Effect of chitosan on the epithelial permeability and structure. Int. J. Pharm. 1999; 182:21-32. DOI:10.1016/s0378-5173(99)00030-7

[144] Schipper, N.G.M. et al. Chitosan as absorption enhancers for poorly absorbed drugs 2: Mechanism of absorption enhancement. Pharm. Res. 1997; 14:923-929. DOI:10.1023/a:1012160102740

[145] Illum L. Bioadhesive formulations for nasal peptide delivery. In Drug Delivery Issues in Fundamentals, Novel Approaches and Development. (Mathiowitz, E. et al. eds), Marcel Dekker, New York, 1998. p. 507-539

[146] Natsume H. et al. Screening of cationic compounds as an absorption enhancer for nasal drug delivery. Int. J. Pharm. 1999; 5 1-12. DOI:10.1016/s0378-5173(99)00100-3

[147] Ohtake K. et al. Enhancing mechanism of poly-L-arginine in nasal absorption of FITC-dextran. Prooceed. Int. Symp. Control. Rel. Bioact. Mater. 1998; 25:687-688

[148] Wang J. et al. Aminated gelatine as a nasal absorption enhancer for peptide drugs: Evaluation of absorption enhancing effect and nasal mucosa perturbation in rats. J. Pharm. Pharmacol. 2002; 54:181-188. DOI:10.1211/0022357021778367

[149] Merkus FWHM. et al. Cyclodextrins in nasal drug delivery. Adv. Drug Deliv. Rev. 1999; 36:41-57. DOI:10.1016/s0169-409x(98)00054-4

[150] Marttin E. et al. Efficacy, safety and mechanism of cyclodextrins as absorption enhancers in nasal delivery of peptide and protein drugs. J. Drug Target.1998; 6:17-36. DOI:10.3109/10611869808997878

[151] Hilsted J. et al. Intranasal insulin therapy: The clinical realities. Diabetologia 1995; 38:680-684. DOI:10.1007/BF00401839

[152] Shojaei AH. Buccal mucosa as a route for systemic drug delivery: A review. J. Pharm. Pharm. Sci. 1998; 1(1):15-30.

[153] Gandhi P, Patel K. a review article on mucoadhesive buccal drug delivery system. Int. J. Pharm. Res. 2011; 3(5):159-173.

[154] Mujoriya R, Dhamande K, Wankhede U, Angure S. A review on study of buccal drug delivery system. Innovative Syst. Design Eng. 2011; 2(3):1-13.

[155] Agu R, Ugwoke M, Armand M, Kinget R. The lung as a route for systemic delivery of therapeutic proteins and peptides. Respir. Res. 2001; 2(4):198-209. DOI:10.1186/rr58

[156] Niven RW. Delivery of biotherapeutics by inhalation aerosol. Crit. Rev. Ther. Drug Carrier Syst. 1995; 12(2-3):151-231. DOI:10.1615/critrevtherdrugcarriersyst.v12.i2-3.20

[157] Shao Z, Li Y, Mitra AK. Cyclodextrins as mucosal absorption promoters of insulin III: Pulmonary route of delivery. Eur J Pharm Biopharm 1994, 40:283-288. DOI:10.1023/a:1018997101542

[158] Shen Z, Cheny Y, Zhang Q. Lanthanides enhance pulmonary absorption of insulin. Biol Trace Element Res 2000; 75:215-225. DOI:10.1385/BTER:75:1-3:215

[159] Liu FY, Kildsig DO, Mitra AK. Pulmonary biotransformation of insulin in rat and rabbit. Life Sci 1992; 51: 1683-1689. DOI:10.1016/0024-3205(92)90313-e

[160] Shen Z, Zhang Q, Wei S, Nagai T. Proteolytic enzymes as a limitation for

pulmonary absorption of insulin: in vitro and in vivo investigations. Int J Pharm 1999; 192:115-121. DOI:10.1016/s0378-5173(99)00295-1

[161] Fukuda F, Tsuji T, Fujita T, Yamamoto A, Muranishi S. Susceptibility of insulin to proteolysis in rat lung homogenates and its protection from proteolysis by various protease inhibitors. Biol Pharm Bull 1995; 18:891-894. DOI:10.1248/bpb.18.891

[162] Kobayashi S, Kondo S, Juni K. Study of pulmonary delivery of salmon calcitonin in rats: Effects of protease inhibitors and absorption enhancers. Pharm Res 1994; 11:1239-1243. DOI:10.1023/a:1018926007902

[163] Morita T, Yamamoto A, Takakura Y, Hashida M, Sekaki H. Improvement of pulmonary absorption of (ASU1,7)-eel calcitonin by various protease inhibitors in rats. Pharm Res 1994; 11:909-913. DOI:10.1023/a:1018950429341

[164] Yamamoto A, Okumura S, Fukuda Y, Fukui M, Takahashi K, Muranishi S. Improvement of the pulmonary absorption of (ASU1,7)-eel calcitonin by various absorption enhancers and their pulmonary toxicity in rats. J Pharm Sci 1997; 86:1144-1147. DOI:10.1021/js9603764

[165] Edwards DA, Hanes J, Caponetti G, Hrkach J, Ben-Jebria A, Eskew ML, Mintzes J, Deaver D, Lotan N, Langer R. Large porousparticles for pulmonary drug delivery. Science 1997; 276: 1868-1871. DOI:10.1126/science.276.5320.1868

[166] Kawashima Y, Yamamoto H, Takeuchi H, Fujoka S, Hino T. Pulmonary delivery of insulin with nebulized DL-lactide/glycolide copolymer (PLGA) nanosphere to prolong hypoglycemic effect. J Contr Rel 1999; 62:279-287. DOI:10.1016/s0168-3659(99)00048-6

[167] Liu F, Shao Z, Kildsig DO, Mitra AK. Pulmonary delivery of free and liposomal insulin. Pharm Res 1993; 10:228-232. DOI:10.1023/a:1018934810512

[168] Li Y, Mitra AK. Effect of phospholipid chain length, concentration, charge, and vesicle size on pulmonary insulin absorption. Pharm Res 1996; 13:76-79. DOI:10.1023/a:1016029317299

[169] Niven RW, Whitcomb KL, Shaner LD, Ralph LD, Habberfield AD, Wilson JV. Pulmonary absorption of polyethylene glycolated recombinant human granulocyte colony stimulating factor (PEGr-huG-CSF). J Contr Rel 1994; 32:177-189. DOI:10.1016/0168-3659(94)90056-6

[170] Lakshmi P, Deepthi B, Rama N. Rectal drug delivery: A promising route for enhancing drug absorption. Asian J. Res. Pharm. Sci. 2012; 2(4):143-149.

[171] Nishihata T. et al. Enhanced bioavailability of insulin after rectal administration with enamine as adjuvant in depancreatized dogs. J. Pharm. Pharmacol. 37; 1985:22-26. DOI:10.1111/j.2042-7158.1985.tb04925.x

[172] Yoshioka S et al. Enhanced rectal bioavailability of polypeptides using sodium 5-methoxysalicylate as an absorption promoter. J. Pharm. Sci. 71; 1982:593-594. DOI:10.1002/jps.2600710529

[173] Akira Yamamoto, Shozo Muranishi. Rectal drug delivery systems improvement of rectal peptide absorption by absorption enhancers, protease inhibitors and chemical modification. Advanced Drug Delivery Reviews. 1997; 28:275-299. DOI:10.1016/S0169-409X(97)00077-X

[174] Hajime Matsuda, Hidetoshi Arima. Cyclodextrins in transdermal and rectal delivery. Advanced Drug Delivery Reviews. 1999; 36:81-99. DOI:10.1016/s0169-409x(98)00056-8

Chapter 3

Smart Drug-Delivery Systems in the Treatment of Rheumatoid Arthritis: Current, Future Perspectives

Abstract

Rheumatoid arthritis (RA) is a progressive autoimmune inflammatory disorder characterized by cellular infiltration in synovium causing joint destruction and bone erosion. The heterogeneous nature of the disease manifests in different clinical forms, hence treatment of RA still remains obscure. Treatments are limited owing to systemic toxicity by dose-escalation and lack of selectivity. To overcome these limitations, Smart drug delivery systems (SDDS) are under investigation to exploit the arthritic microenvironment either by passive targeting or active targeting to the inflamed joints *via* folate receptor, CD44, angiogenesis, integrins. This review comprehensively deliberates upon understanding the pathophysiology of RA and role of SDDSs, highlighting the emerging trends for RA nanotherapeutics.

Keywords: smart drug delivery systems, active & passive targeting, Stimuli-responsive nanoparticles, polymer-drug conjugates, Arthritic microenvironment

1. Introduction

Rheumatoid arthritis (RA) is an autoimmune-mediated systemic, chronic inflammatory disorder characterized by progressive inflammation of joints, cell infiltration, pannus formation, synovial dysplasia resulting in cartilage destruction and bone erosion [1]. The worldwide prevalence rate of RA in adult population has been predicted between 0.5–1% and 0.92% in India [2]. Generally, prevalent in women when compared to men (3,1) at any age group. According to recent statistics given in 2019 by the Global RA network and WHO, 23 million people are affected by RA, globally [3]. RA etiology is implicated to be linked to metabolic, genetic, environmental factors, and life style of the patient [4]. While it is considered non-lethal, RA is debilitating and severely compromises the quality of life, further reducing life expectancy in patients.

Despite tremendous progress in evolving efficient pharmacological molecules for RA therapy, their efficacious delivery at the diseased joint remains a long-lasting challenge. Over the last two decades, disease-modifying anti-rheumatic drugs (DMARDs: such as methotrexate (MTX), hydroxychloroquine (HCQ), sulfasalazine (SSZ), leflunomide (LFM), have attracted attention for effective attenuation of disease progression. Patient compliance is the primary treatment goal with glucocorticoids(GCs); e.g., prednisolone, dexamethasone, hydrocortisone, triamcinolone acetonide, and NASAID (such as ibuprofen, diclofenac, indomethacin etc) result in reducing pain and curbing disease progression [5]. Unfortunately, the associated toxicity caused by dose-escalation and long-term use with undesirable side-effects are limiting the therapeutic success. Continued medication of NSAIDs causes gastro-intestinal and renal toxicity; glucocorticoids cause hypertension, hyperglycemia, muscle wasting, osteoporosis, etc.; nausea and vomiting are common side-effects of conventional DMARDs, including gastro-intestinal irritations, headaches, insomnia, cytopenia, skin and hair damage, etc.; giving biologicals run the risk of anaphylaxis, infections, malignancy, psoriasis and other autoimmune disorders [6, 7]. Biosimilars/biologicals/Biological response modifiers like infliximab, adalimumab, rituximab etc. that have approval of Food and Drug Administration (FDA), were considered for their selective site-specific action, achieved extensive success in clinics for RA treatment. Prior reports suggest combination therapy with biologics, and synthetic DMARDs were found to be highly effective [8].

To circumvent the off-target drug induced systemic toxicity, direct drug delivery *via* the intra-articular injection to the affected joints was explored. Nevertheless, this mode of administration has several limitations, as it necessitates repeat injections in the joint, risk of infection, and joint disability. Therefore, a concerted effort for development of novel therapies are clearly warranted with a focus on targeting the inflamed joints.

Nanotherapeutics has emerged as an innovative approach enabling efficient delivery of drug for mitigating several diseases. The past decade, has seen an avalanche of publications that have increased our understanding of the pathophysiology of the affected synovial tissue in RA and equivalent progress in nanotechnology and material chemistry, generating tremendous interest in developing Smart drug delivery system (SDDS). Entrapping the anti-inflammatory drugs in SDDS strategically has potential to overcome all the barriers of normal delivery, projecting it as a promising option for site-specific delivery. Currently, RA targeting nanotherapeutics has progressed rapidly because the inflammatory microenvironments of arthritic joints mimic the tumor environment that has typical angiogenic features of neo-vessels coupled with impaired peripheral lymphatic drainage [9, 10]. This review comprehensively deliberates upon the understanding the pathophysiology of RA and role of SDDSs, highlighting the emerging trends for RA nanotherapeutics.

2. RA microenvironment

Chronic inflammation is the hallmark of RA that advances to destructive synovitis [11]. It develops in a genetically susceptible person largely due to environmental factors and related epigenetic mechanisms [12]. It predominantly indicates leukocyte infiltration, dysregulated angiogenesis, proliferation of lining layer, that alters the synovial tissue into an invasive pannus. The microvasculature of synovium is dysregulated, hence, in spite of enhanced flow of blood, the increased metabolic needs outdo the vascular blood supply, thereby creating an intense hypoxic microenvironment. However, rheumatoid factor (RF) and anticitrullinated peptide antibodies(ACPA) are induced and must exist before the onset of this disease. The heterogeneous nature of the disease manifests in different clinical forms, hence treatment of RA still remains obscure. It is well documented that synovial micro-environment has abundance of macrophages, multifaceted crosslink of immune cells secreting granulocyte colony-stimulating factor, pro-inflammatory cytokines, tumor necrosis factor(TNF-α), interleukin (IL-1), IL-6, chemokines, and degrading like MMPs that are particularly responsible for RA pathogenesis [13, 14]. **Figure 1** illustrates the network of cytokines secreted by multitude of cells involved in RA development that can be useful for assessment of disease progression along with biomarkers present on these cells.

2.1 Synovial fibroblasts (SF)

Proliferation and infiltration of SF is the key trigger for disease progression in RA. Under normal conditions fibroblasts are responsible for maintaining tissue homeostasis by modulating the inflammatory response [15]. Transcription factors like activator protein-1 and NF-κB, responsible for proliferation, activation, differentiation of fibroblasts, expression of MMPs, other matrix-degrading enzymes like cysteine proteases and aggrecanases have been observed in the synovium [5]. The genetic analysis of synovium would be useful for biological therapy as synovial tissue has a robust immune-inflammatory gene expression [16].

2.2 B cells

B cells contribute to antibody production *i.e.* RF and anticyclic citrullinated peptide antibody (ACPA), and other effector roles to entail disease progression [17]. RF and/or ACPA promotes severe bone and joint erosions as the citrullinated proteins aggravate RA progression [18]. B cells are pointedly responsible for regulation of inflammatory response by serving as antigen-presenting cells and releasing

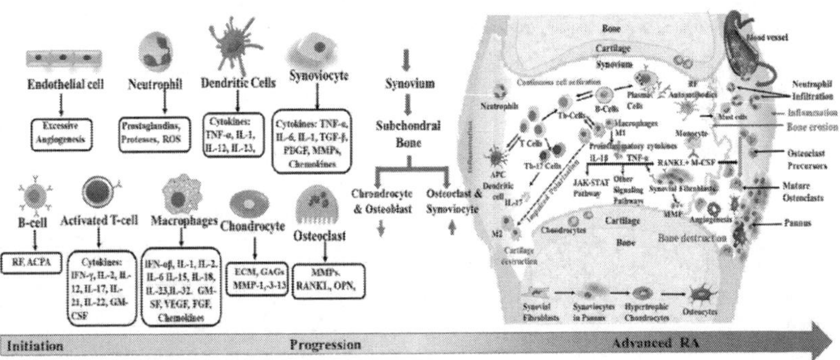

IL interleukin, TNF tumor necrosis factor, MMP matrix metalloproteinase, TGF transforming growth factor, PDGF platelet-derived growth factor, IFN interferon, GM-CSF granulocyte–macrophage colony-stimulating factor, VEGF vascular endothelial growth factor, FGF fibroblast growth factor, RF Rheumatoid Factor, ACPA Anti-Citrullinated Peptide Antibodies

Figure 1.
Schematic illustration indicating the key events and signaling cascades involved in RA pathophysiology. Leukocytes infiltrate synovium and stimulate the inflammatory cascade, characterized by cross-talk of SF and macrophages, monocytes, mast cells, dendritic cells, as well as B and T cells. Endothelial cells facilitate angiogenesis. The advanced stage includes hyperplastic synovium, cartilage damage, bone erosion, and systemic consequence. Bone resorption by osteoclasts practically creates bone erosions. The obliteration of the subchondral bone can ultimately lead to the degeneration of the articular cartilage that is a result of reduced osteoblasts and an increase in the number of osteoclasts and synoviocytes.

pro–/anti-inflammatory cytokines that additionally control T cell differentiation and proliferation, and activation of macrophages [5].

2.3 T cells

Activated T cells comprise ≥50% of RA synovial cells, and majority are memory CD4 T cells. In terms of T cell subsets, the Th1(T helper 1) and Th17(T regulatory) are predominant, but lack Th2 subsets [5]. T cells release cytokines as their effector functions; Th1 release interferon gamma(IFN-γ), that further activate macrophages and increases its phagocytic activity. Likewise, effector cytokines of Th17 cells are IL-17A, IL-17F, IL-21, and IL-22, responsible for cell recruitment, secretion of pro-inflammatory cytokines, initiation of differentiation of B-cell, and activate NK cells [19]. IL-17 may emerge as a beneficial target for RA therapies.

2.4 Macrophages

Macrophages are tightly regulated by microenvironment signals including presence of injured cells, microbial debris, pro/anti-inflammatory cytokine or mechanical forces [19]. Depending on the cues, macrophages tend to polarize into characterized phenotypes like pro-inflammatory or immunomodulatory [20]. Taking advantage of the fundamental homing capability of macrophages to migrate to the injured/inflamed arthritic synovium, macrophages can be exploited as delivery vehicles to target specific macrophage populations to carry payloads.

2.5 Osteoclasts

Enhanced osteoclast activity triggered by disproportionate ratio of Osteoprotegerin (OPG) and receptor activator of nuclear-factor kappa-beta ligand (RANKL) are critical factors for RA progression. When RANKL is overexpressed by activated macrophages, osteoblasts and lymphocytes, it stimulates an imbalance between osteoclast multiplication and anomalous activation triggered by the binding of RANKL to RANK on the mature osteoclasts and on the cell-membranes of precursor cells of osteoclast [21]. In addition, MMP-9 and MMP-14 secreted by the osteoblasts, triggers matrix degradation in cartilage, formation of pannus, and osteoclast migration to surface of the bone. Osteoclasts significantly cause erosion of subchondral bone, articular cartilage, and the synovium.

2.6 Enzymes and other effector molecules

MMPs are the enzymes that irreversibly cause extracellular matrix (ECM) degradation, and slow-destruction of cartilage and bone in diseased joints. MMPs are zinc-dependent endopeptidases that are categorized into five sub-classes: i) gelatinases (MMP-2 and 9), ii) collagenases (MMP-1, –8 and 13), iii) stromelysins (MMP-3, –10 and – 11), iv) matrilysins (MMP-7 and -26) and v) membrane-type MMPs (MMP-14 to –17, –24 and – 25) [22, 23]. MMP-1, 2, 3, and 9 have been directly implicated in RA progression [24]. MMPs, in combination with lipases and esterases, accelerate degradation of ECM, articular cartilage and surface of the subchondral bone [25]. Ever-increasing emerging targets including these enzymes provide more options for anti-arthritic therapy with the help of targeted SDDS for RA.

3. Rationale of SDDS

Enhancement of therapeutic efficiency by 'intelligent/smart' carriers that release drugs in a controlled manner at the site of action to achieve minimal side effects are categorized as "Smart Drug delivery system" (SDDS). Maintaining optimum size and surface properties, the materials can be engineered to create nanoparticles that can maneuver the microenvironment and respond to endogenous stimuli, like increased concentration of some enzymes, redox gradient-enhanced level of glutathione, or variations in interstitial pH [26] and/ or exogenous stimuli that include temperature changes, applying magnetic field or light, and giving high energy radiation.

3.1 pH-responsive

pH, an important parameter linked to pathophysiological conditions, like inflammation can be exploited for enhanced therapeutic efficiency [27]. Reports priori give clarity that pH in normal tissue and blood is maintained around 7.4, but in arthritic microenvironment, extracellular pH values are intrinsically acidic, usually pH 6.8 [28]. The acidic pH can be attributed to the excess infiltration and activation of proinflammatory cells in the synovium, causing increased demand for oxygen and energy. Augmented consumption of glucose *via* glycolysis consequently enhances production of lactic acid, that causes local acidosis [29, 30]. Hence, the nanoparticles should be strategically designed to sensitively distinguish pH changes in inflammatory area where high disease activity and joint destruction correlates with low synovial pH. These pH-responsive nanoparticles encapsulating therapeutic molecules like NSAIDs, DMARDs etc. can be promising for RA treatment. Even at the cellular level, pH-sensitive SDDS can either stimulate drug release into lysosomes, or the late endosomes or may even trigger the escape of nanoparticles from lysosomes into the cytosol [31]. Appropriate size will enable efficient penetration in the inflamed joints, facilitated by angiogenesis during RA progression, that causes endothelial cell discontinuity leading to enhanced vascular permeability [32].

Two strategies are rationally used to design of pH-sensitive SDDS, one using materials with acid-sensitive bonds, that can be cleaved by low pH conditions allowing the release of encapsulated molecules from the nanoparticles; and secondly, using polymers (polyacids or polybases) that have ionizable groups, that undergo pH-dependent transformation and change in solubility [33]. Researchers have engineered a dual-strategy by attributing targeting abilities by surface functionalization and simultaneously using pH responsiveness to enhance therapeutic selectivity in RA.

3.2 Redox-responsive

Intracellular microenvironment can be exploited using redox responsive NPs. Reactive oxygen species (ROS) is generated primarily during oxidative phosphorylation(OXPHOS), but can further be produced by oxidative burst of activated phagocytic cells [34]. Polymers with ROS-sensitive thioketal moiety, or selenium (Se), tellurium (Te), B-based linkers in their monomeric backbone can be utilized as building blocks for the synthesis of stimuli- responsive nanoparticles. Hence, ROS can easily be monitored as an intracellular indicator [35] as chronic inflammation induces continuous production of ROS [36].

ROS concentrations in inflammatory tissues ranges 10- to 100- fold higher than normal tissues [36], thus, promising accuracy and specificity to develop the redox stimuli-responsive DDSs.

3.3 Temperature-responsive

Temperature is another crucial factor essential for release of drug [38], as the normal physiological conditions have lower temperatures compared to the inflamed RA microenvironment [39]. Therefore temperature-responsive functionalized NPs can be used to trigger the release of drug at the inflammatory site. They are designed and fabricated to retain their payloads at physiological temperature (37°C), and quick release it when the temperature is increased around 40–45°C, attributing a more efficient targeted SDDS [40]. Phase-transition behavior of the materials that are thermosensitive are used to design NPs, based on the lower critical solution temperature (LCST) of polymers/lipids whose solubility varies with changes in temperature. All excipients in a mixture are totally miscible in all amounts in LCST. In materials with transitional behavior, increased solubility is observed below LCST; and polymeric constituents are prone to swelling due to the hydrogen bonds being formed between the polymer functional groups with water molecules enabling drug loaded molecules. When temperature is raised above the LCST, a hydrophobic-hydrophilic conversion takes place, that leads to a morphological transformation from a random coil-to-globular form. Because of alterations in temperature, the hydrogen bonds breaks causing the network to collapse, and the polymer becomes insoluble, causing shrinkage in the volume and oozing-out of water molecules from inside. This transition initiates release of the entrapped payload of drugs. The application of thermo-responsive SDDS is based on the concept of exploiting the temperature difference between healthy and diseased tissues [40]. Thermal energy can be given directly, or external utilizing heat sources like NIR that may be indirectly applied in RA, that elicits a thermo-responsive behavior based on the thermo-sensitivity of nanomaterials. Typically, the requisite range of temperature fluctuates from 38–43°C [37]. The temperature-stimuli can originate from within the body, or by localized hypothermia, or hyperthermia, may provoke a response based entirely on the thermo-sensitivity of used nanomaterials. Additional advantages of thermo-sensitive NPs may be attributed to reduction in use of toxic organic solvents during fabrication, the capacity to entrap both lipophilic and hydrophilic molecules, controlled and sustained release properties. A plethora of reports using several polymers have been established for the synthesis of temperature-responsive systems, that include derivatives of poly(N-isopropylacrylamide (PNIPAAm), pluronics (poly(ethylene oxide)- poly(propylene oxide) (PEO-PPO)), poly(N vinyl caprolactam), polysaccharide spinoffs, and derivatives of phosphazene [41–43]. Researchers are making concerted efforts on achieving temperature-responsive NPs stimulated by magnetic action coupled with thermo-responsive effect by light absorption instead of temperature alone.

3.4 Light and magnetic responsive

Light-responsive systems rely on an external stimulus to activate the drug release preferably at the target site using light irradiation. NPs respond to 'on–off drug' release, as it may close/open when stimulated using light radiation. Also termed as photodynamic therapy, SDDS based on magnetic stimuli represents another external way to trigger drug release at the target site under programmable exposure of magnetic field [37]. Iron-oxide NPs have excellent potential for smart drug delivery, as it exhibits a significant response to both light and magnetic stimuli, it can be exploited for triggering a burst release of drug at the inflamed sites of RA termed as the magneto-calorific effect and photothermal effects. Thermal properties of magnetic NPs might be conveniently modulated by modifying their own viscosity in the endo-cellular environment. Photodynamic therapy (PDT) and photothermal therapy (PTT) use photosensitizers as therapeutic molecules. Moreover, near infrared(NIR) light can efficiently infiltrate the inflamed RA joints. $Cu_{7.2}S_4$ nanoparticles triggered with NIR irradiation (808 nm, 1 W cm^{-2}) was suggested to accomplish improved bone mineral density (BMD) and bone structure and volume. It further impedes invasion to synovial tissue, erosion of cartilage and bone *in vivo*.

Huo et al. have prepared optical nanoparticles induced PTT and PDT and documented probable pathways for cell toxicity [44]. During PTT cell necrosis can be induced by NIR laser light irradiation (wavelength:1064 nm), however when given as combination therapies (PTT + PDT), evidence of both necrosis and apoptosis pathways are indicated. Furthermore, PTT-PDT combination given simultaneously, can account for immunogenic cell-death, while fluorophores can be used for optical imaging as a diagnostic tool that can be applied for RA too.

3.5 Enzyme responsive

Specific enzymes like phospholipases, proteases, or glycoside are often overexpressed in different pathological conditions, like inflammation, and can be exploited for enzyme triggered release and accumulation of drugs at the targeted site of interest [37]. Nevertheless, nature of cleavable units, the sensitivity of the delivery system can significantly influence the pharmacokinetics of entrapped payload. Further, it must be ensured that the metabolites or the degraded moieties are non-toxic and biocompatible and are cautiously eliminated from the body. Therefore, in future, enzyme-responsive nanoparticles offer tailor-made therapy according to variations in levels of disease expression. Redox- and enzyme-responsive nanoparticles are coming up as promising therapies in RA treatment.

3.6 Energy upconversion NPs

Nanomaterials with exceptional physico-chemical properties targeting the lesions can be supplemented with precise external stimuli, such as light, microwave, ultrasound, and radiation. Upconversion nanoparticles (UCNPs) synthesized from rare-earth elements that are capable of translating NIR photons that have low-energy to high-energy ultraviolet or visible photons [45]. These extraordinary NIR excitation based optical properties of UCNPs allows penetration to deep tissues with minimum auto-fluorescence background, reinforcing a wide array of diagnostic applications alongwith biomedical imaging system [46, 47]. SDDS can translate the external stimuli and equivalent energy input into beneficial effects or release the payload *via* an energy-upconversion process [48]. Ultrasound-based, photo-dynamic-based, radiation-based and microwave-based, energy-UPNPs have been widely explored in RA treatment as an alternative therapy (**Figure 2**). These developing technologies induce death of synovial fibroblasts and other inflammatory cells by generating hyperthermia, cellular ROS, mechanical and photoelectric effects [49]. Synovial cells can be directly targeted by nanoparticles to decrease bone erosion (**Table 1**) [50].

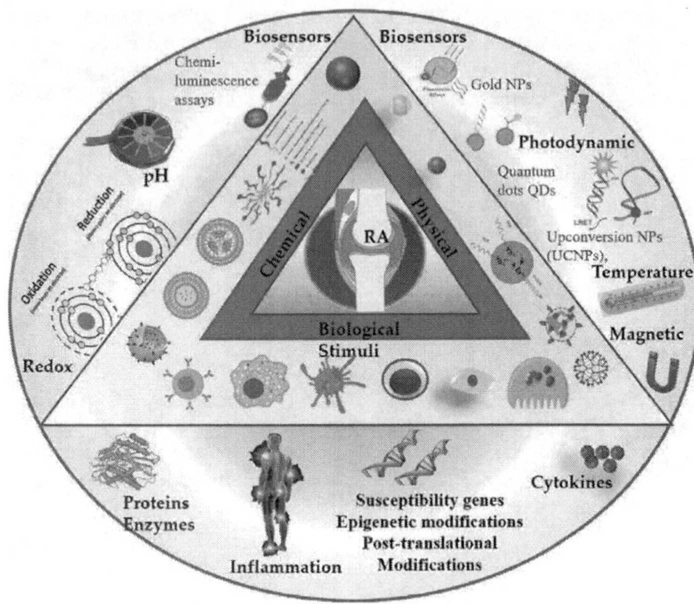

Figure 2.
Schematic representation of stimuli-responsive polymers for nanotherapeutics of rheumatoid arthritis (RA).

Stimuli category	Stimulus	Description of the system	Drug	References
Chemical	pH	PLGA-PK3-lipid-polymer hybrid nanoparticles decorated with stearic acid-octa-arginine and folic acid (Sta-R8-FA-PPLPNs/MTX) [PK3, Folate-PEG-PLGA, egg PC, and Sta-R8]	MTX	[51]
	pH	Polymeric nanoparticles surface modified with Hyaluronic acid (HA)- (HAPNPs) consisting of polyethylenimine, egg phosphatidyl-choline, and PCADK	Dex	[52]
	pH	PEGylated hyaluronic acid(P-HA) mineralized nanoparticles having a hydrophilic shell, 5β-cholanic acid as the hydrophobic core and CaP as the pH-responsive mineral	MTX	[53]
	pH	Lipid nanocarriers formed by PEG-PLGA hydrophilic shell, functionalized with folic acid (FA) ligand for targeting FA-receptor, poly (cyclohexane-1,4-diylacetone dimethylene ketal) (PCADK) & PLGA as the hydrophobic core. PCADK was used as pH-responsive material	MTX	[54]
	pH	Spherical self-assembled micelles of poly (β-amino ester)-graft-poly(ethylene glycol) (PAE-g-PEG) encapsulating MTX into the hydrophobic core.	MTX	[55]
	pH	Acetone-ketal-linked pro-drugs (AKP-dexs) pH-sensitive of dexamethasone nanoparticles	Dex	[56]

Stimuli category	Stimulus	Description of the system	Drug	References
	ROS	Folate conjugated to PEC 100 monostearate as film-forming material, and methotrexate (MTX) and catalase (CAT) co-encapsulated liposomes (FOL-MTX&CAT-L)	MTX	[57]
Physical	NIR	Gold half-shell nanoparticles functionalized with RGD to target the inflammation, encapsulating methotrexate (MTX).	MTX	[58]
	PDT/PTT	Copper (Cu)-based nanomaterials with assistance of L-cystein termed as $Cu_{7.2}S_4$ nanoparticles (NPs)	—	[59]
	Magnetic	Magnetic iron oxide nanoparticles (IONPs)	—	[60]
Multimodal Imaging	Light	Nanoparticles composed of PLGA co-encapsulating Au/Fe/Au- half-shell nanoparticles	MTX	[61]
Biological	Enzyme (MMP)	Lipid nanoparticles with PEG coating, composed of triglycerol monostearate (TGMS) and 1,2-distearoyl-*sn*-glycero-3-phospho-ethanolamine-poly(ethyleneglycol) ($DSPE\text{-}PEG_{2000}$) encapsulating Dexamethasone	Dex	[62]
	Cytokines	Nanoparticle system based on two natural polymers-N-trimethyl chitosan (TMC) and polysialic acid (PSA) encapsulated methotrexate	MTX	[63]
Combinatorial	Temp & pH	MTX loaded Gold nanoparticles and encapsulated in pegylated-poly (DL-lactic-co-glycolic acid) nanospheres	MTX	[64]
	NIR & Magnetic field	MTX-encapsulated poly(lactic-co-glycolic acid) (PLGA) (Au)/iron, (Fe)/gold (Au) half-shell nanoparticles coupled with arginine–glycine–aspartic acid (RGD)	MTX	[61]
	pH & enzyme	Micelles of polyethylene-glycol-phenyl boric acid- triglycerol-monostearate (PEG–PBA–TGMS conjugated PPT) encapsulating Dex	Dex	[65]

Table 1.
List of stimuli-responsive nanoparticles for the treatment of RA.

4. Principle of SDDS

Presently, the conventional treatments exhibit escalation in dose and systemic toxicity upon administration of drug. Most anti-inflammatory therapeutic drugs are equitoxic to both the normal cells and inflamed cells. SDDS has been well recognized in the past few decades owing to its potential for site-specific and targeted delivery [66]. Encapsulation of anti-inflammatory drugs in nanoparticles can enhance the site-specificity, reduce the dose, curtail the systemic toxicity and improve the biodistribution to targeted disease site [67]. To overcome the disadvantage of conventional delivery of drugs, selective delivery whether passive or active can be used for targeting drug to the site of action as SDDS in RA therapy.

4.1 Passive targeting

Passive targeting can be accomplished by targeting the physiological and anatomical changes in inflamed tissues, that occurred due to RA. For passive targeting, NPs do not require any surface modification, either by conjugation or by attaching a surface ligand. Various studies have shown the enhanced permeability and retention (EPR) mechanism for passive accumulation in inflamed tissues [68]. In the inflammatory RA milieu, there is evidence of angiogenesis but no evidence of displaying an abnormal lymphatic drainage [69]. The long-circulating delivery vehicles have been evidenced to specifically accumulate within the pannus of the inflamed synovium [70]. The hyperplasia in pannus exhibits a leaky vasculature due to high vascular permeability comparable to solid tumors. Consequently, taking advantage of leaky vasculature may for passive targeting is a promising option [71]. EPR allows NPs in size range from 20 to 200 nm to selectively accumulate in pannus and display on the surface of inflamed tissue. In addition to the EPR effect, hypoxic and acidic environment of inflamed joint also favors passive targeting [70]. Arthritic inflamed joint has poor oxygen delivery and increased metabolic rate due to meager perfusion into the diseased synovial joint. Therefore, the two conditions can easily be used as method of passive drug targeting in less oxygen and acidic microenvironment of RA affected inflamed tissue. NPs administrated in blood stream with hydrophobic surface are easily recognized by reticuloendothelial system (RES) such as spleen and liver, and engulfed by macrophages, consequently quickly eliminated from systemic circulation.

4.2 Active targeting

Targeted delivery involves active targeting to specific cells in the microenvironment of arthritic joints. Overexpressed receptors on particular immune cells can be targeted with its complimentary ligand that is decorated on nanoparticle surface. Several receptors are expressed by different cells, we shall be discussing a few including CD44, folate and beta-3 integrins. Targeting angiogenic vascular endothelial cells are also under investigation, with E-selectin as a promising target molecule [72]. Receptor mediated endocytosis is responsible for efficient uptake of the ligand decorated carrier molecule (ligand-receptor interaction) (**Figure 3**).

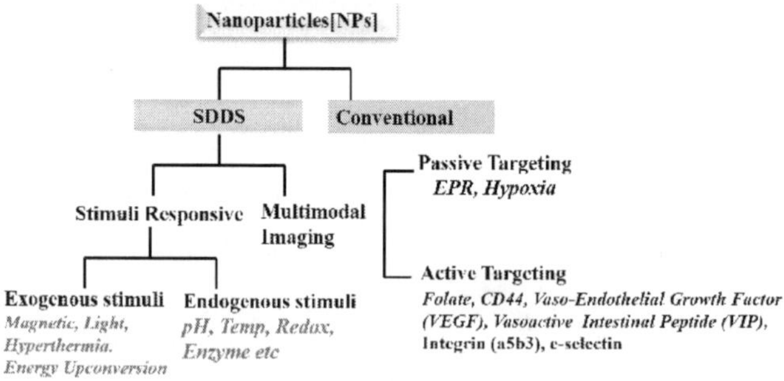

Figure 3.
Outline of the targeting strategies for nanoparticulate drug delivery systems used in RA.

4.2.1 Folic acid (FA) based active targeting

Activated macrophages overexpress folate receptor β(FR-β) in the arthritic joints [73]. Owing to post-translational modifications, the folate expressed on neutrophils are incapable of binding to FR-β [74]. Alternatively, a functional FR-β has been identified on the activated macrophages having nanomolar affinity for folate. Hence, the FR-β receptor emerges as a useful target in various diseases including RA, osteoarthritis [75], systemic lupus erythematosus [76], atherosclerosis [77] and Crohn's disease [78]. Macrophages are key players of RA pathogenesis, as they secrete pro-inflammatory cytokines, metalloproteinases, ROS and prostaglandins. Folate is an attractive option for ease of surface modification, hydrophilicity, and stability in different solvents. Methotrexate (MTX) encapsulated folate-conjugated glycol chitosan (MFGCN) have been targeted to inflamed joint in adjuvant-induced arthritic rat model [79]. Likewise, surface of MTX-loaded liposomes was decorated with folate and were evaluated both *in vitro* and *in vivo* (DBA/1 J mice strain) [80, 81], and targeted against the FR-β on activated macrophages. Clinical efficacy of MTX in the DBA/1 J arthritic mice indicated significant expression of CD73. Since, low doses were required, this nanoformulation was economical and cost-effective. MTX loaded dendrimer nanoparticles with folic acid (FA) surface functionalization were reported to reduce progression of disease [82]. Further, authors suggested a ~ 7.5-fold increase in the maximum-tolerated dose of the MTX, when given as the formulation compared to the free MTX.

4.2.2 Hyaluronic acid (HA) based active targeting

CD44 is a glycoprotein, overexpressed on the surface of activated macrophages, present in the inflamed joints of RA. CD44 can be exploited as a prospective target in RA treatment. HA, a biocompatible natural polymer has ben explored as a ligand that effectively binds to CD44 receptor. HA coated hydroxyapatite NPs (HA-NPs) encapsulating methotrexate (MTX) and teriflunomide (TEF) - (HYA-HAMT-NP) were reported for RA treatment [83]. Results suggested that HYA-HAMT-NP could emerge as an effective delivery vehicle to circumvent hepatotoxicity caused by drugs in RA.

4.2.3 Anti-angiogenesis

Hypoxia in a critical factor in inflamed synovium that triggers neo-vascularization from existing vessels termed as angiogenesis [84]. The neo-vascularization preserves the chronic inflammatory state by engaging cells to the inflammatory site, provides nutrition and oxygen to the multiplying cells. Additionally, the enlarged surface of endothelium triggers secretion of adhesion molecules, cytokines and stimulates neutrophil infiltration as well as synovial membrane into the cartilage, causing cartilage destruction and bone erosion [85]. Promising therapies based on angiogenesis are emerging for RA therapy, where VEGF and integrins are the therapeutic targets.

4.2.3.1 Vascular endothelial growth factor (VEGF)

Vascular endothelial growth factor (VEGF) is an endothelial-cell-specific angiogenic factor principally secreted by SFs in the pannus. In angiogenesis, VEGF triggers multiplication and migration of endothelial cells. Further, it enhanced blood vascular permeability, stimulates maturation and maintenance of the neo-vessels [86]. TNF-α and IL-1, the pro-inflammatory cytokines induce the SFs and other cells to secrete VEGF, and VEGF is overexpressed at the inflamed joint owing to angiogenesis [87]. Therefore, VEGF and VEGF receptor inhibition can be an attractive strategy for RA treatment as it may effectively decrease inflammation by inhibiting angiogenesis.

4.2.3.2 Vasoactive intestinal peptide (VIP)

Vasoactive intestinal peptide (VIP) is a neuropeptide of the central and peripheral nervous system that has vasodilatory, anti-proliferative, anti-inflammatory, cell protective agent and broncho-dilatory role. The activity of VIP binds to high affinity VIP receptors, that are overexpressed on T-lymphocytes and several inflammatory cells. VIP inhibits the secretion of pro-inflammatory cytokines to act as anti-inflammatory molecule. It also promotes the secretion of anti-inflammatory molecules by stimulated innate cells [88]. Proliferating synoviocytes and activated macrophages overexpress VIP receptors in inflamed RA. Therefore, VIP receptor specific ligands can be conjugates to nanoparticles to specifically target the diseased site. Therefore, VIP can be exploited as a therapeutic agent for active targeting to RA joint.

4.2.3.3 Integrins

Integrins are the biogenic markers of endothelium undergoing angiogenesis and play a vital effector role in it. Integrin alpha-V-beta 3 ($\alpha v\beta 3$ integrin), also referred to as vitronectin receptor are overexpressed on osteoclasts and activated macrophages of the inflamed synovium. Integrin receptor promotes angiogenesis, helps in osteoclast-mediated bone resorption, and induces pathological neo-vascularization [89]. Inhibition of $\alpha v\beta 3$ integrin activity stimulates endothelial cell apoptosis, thereby inhibiting angiogenesis [90]. Hence, $\alpha v\beta 3$ is considered a reliable maker for targeted delivery to RA patients.

4.2.3.4 E-selectin

E- Selectin is a glycoprotein that is associated with leukocyte rolling and adhesion and is expressed on vascular endothelium of the inflamed synovium, and promotes angiogenesis [91]. The inflammatory cytokines maintain its upregulated expression in the inflamed tissue. Therefore, expression of e-selectin can be a useful molecular target for RA therapy. Therefore, e-selectin serves as yet another attractive strategy for active targeting of the chosen delivery of drug to the diseased RA joint [92].

5. Nanotherapeutics

The assembly of stimuli-sensitive nanoparticles necessities the usage of biocompatible constituents, that can undergo supra-molecular changes in conformation, a hydrolytic cleavage, and precise protonation, etc. Polymers have maximum suitability and has been widely explored class of materials that have incredible potential. Polymers may be of natural or synthetic origin. The flexibility of the polymer sources and its ability for synthesis of various combinations of polymers has facilitated manipulation of the polymer sensitivity to specific stimuli within a narrow range [93]. Nanoparticles could be synthesized by lipid, metals and polymers. NPs decoy pro-inflammatory molecules like cytokines and ROS and sometimes osteoclast differentiation factors. Moreover, surface modification of NPs with target moiety is a extensive application in site specific drug delivery by enhancing the bioavailability of drug and reducing non-target side effects [94].

5.1 Polymer-drug conjugate (PDC)

PDC based DDS has been proposed by Ringsdrof in 1975 [95], in which a low molecular weight drug, targeting moiety and solubilizer are attached to polymeric backbone covalently *via* bioresponsive linkers. PDC improves drug bioavailability, reduces drug toxicity, and are less toxic in nature, can easily be fabricated in regulated sizes that escape through renal filtration, exhibit increased retention time in blood circulation [96]. PDCs under investigation include N-(2-hydroxypropyl) methacrylamide, poly(vinylpyrrolidone) (PVP), hyaluronic acid (HA) and poly (ethylene glycol) (PEG) [11, 97]. N-(2-hydroxypropyl) methacrylamide (HPMA) shows improved biodegradability, biocompatibility and increased efficacy in treating RA [11, 97]. HPMA-Dex conjugates were administered intravenously into CIA induced RA model, that resulted in accumulation at the inflamed joints [98]. PEG has been used for its hydrophilicity and biocompatible properties. PEG-DEX have been developed *via* acid-labile hydrazine bond and given to arthritic rats leading to decrease in joint inflammation [99]. Recently, FDA approved two PEGylated proteins for the treatment of RA: Pegloticase (Krystexxa®) and certolizumab pegol (CIMZIA®). Although, PEG attributes stealth properties to the NPs, there are some concerns regarding PEG conjugates that include low biodegradability and the possibility to elicit an anti-PEG IgM antibody [100].

5.2 Nanoparticles

Nanoparticles are solid colloidal particles with unique physico-chemical properties such as ultra-small size, surface charge, large surface area to mass ratio Unlike polymer-drug conjugates, NPs allow encapsulation/absorption/entrapment of drug without modification. The high reactivity, diffusivity, solubility, toxicity, immunogenicity and drug release characteristics can be manipulated to make efficient delivery system. Polymeric, liposomes, micelles and metallic nanoparticles are the most commonly used nanoparticles [101].

5.2.1 Biopolymeric nanoparticles

The biodegradable backbone in biopolymeric NPs protects the drug from *in vitro* and *in vivo* degradation. Alginate, Gelatin, Pectin, Chitosan, are natural biopolymers that are highly investigated as they are biocompatible and biodegradable. Chitosan is polycationic in nature, that allows surface modification with ease and is a natural mucoadhesive. Kumar et al. reported Chitosan nanoparticles encapsulating Dexamethasone (DEX) and Methotrexate (MTX) for their *in vitro* efficacy in RAW264.7 cells and *in vivo* efficacy in arthritic rat model. Results convincingly indicated reduced toxicity and high efficacy in arthritic model [28]. The main drawback of chitosan is insoluble in alkaline and neutral medium due to absence of free amino group, but due to protonation of free amino group in acidic medium, there is enhanced solubility.

Glycol chitosan has enhanced water solubility and functional groups for further chemical modifications making it better suited as a potent drug carrier [102]. Glycol-chitosan nanoparticles(GCNPs) are biocompatible, pH responsive and biodegradable. Methotrexate (MTX) encapsulated folate-conjugated glycol chitosan (MFGCN) have been reported to target the overexpressed folate receptors β (FR-β) on activated macrophages in the inflamed joint in adjuvant-induced arthritic rat model. **Figure 4** gives a pictorial description of MFGCN that reduced the arthritic index, improved the antioxidant response and decreases pro-inflammatory cytokines and suggesting its potential in targeting activated macrophages of synovium [79].

5.2.2 Gold nanoparticles(GNPs)

GNPs can be surface functionalized through covalent bonding, by cationic polymers or physical or ionic absorption [103], functional groups like e.g. thiol, amine, and carboxyl groups that are reactive [104]. GNPs were strategically planted

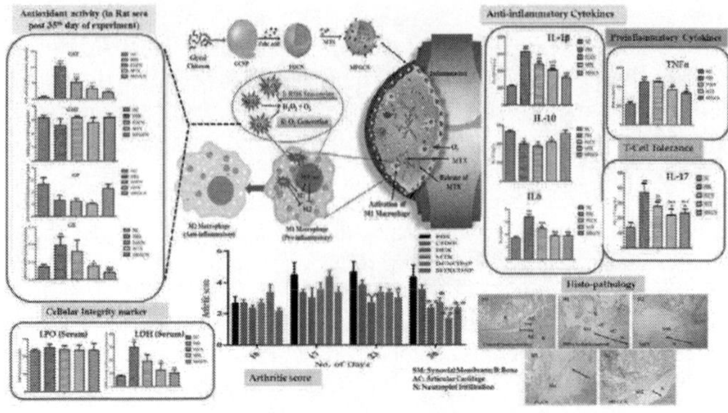

Figure 4.
*Pictorial representation of utilization of folate functionalized methotrexate loaded glycol chitosan nanoparticles (MFGCN) in treating CIA rats targeting inflammation and ROS in rat serum post 21 days of treatment (n = 6). [A] MFGCN development and active targeting of M1 macrophages in the inflammatory synovium. [B] LPO and LDH activity [C] panel showing antioxidant potential (activity quantification of GST, GSH, GP and GR) [D] quantification of TNF-α, IL-4, IL-1β, IL-10 and IL-17 [E] Representative H&E staining images of study groups comparing healthy and arthritic control groups with the treatment groups (n = 6). Data was analyzed by one-way ANOVA *$p < 0.05$, **$p < 0.01$, ***$p < 0.001$.*

in macrophages to target thioredoxin reductase to evaluate its antiangiogenic impact by binding to the vascular endothelial growth factor (VEGF) [105]. Lee et al. suggested MTX encapsulated RGD-attached gold half-shell NP system for RA treatment [106]. On irradiation with near-infrared (NIR), these GNPs delivered MTX to the inflamed joints, maximizing its efficacy with minimal side effects. GNPs were modified physically with Tocilizumab(TCZ) and chemically altered with an end-group thiolated hyaluronate(HA). This complex of HA-GNP-TCZ indicated a synergistic effect for its dual-functional effect on VEGF and IL-6R (receptors for IL-6) in RA treatment [107]. GNPs may block the RANKL induced osteoclast formation which leads to cartilage and bone destruction [108].

5.2.3 Liposomes

Liposomes are bilayered lipids with an aqueous core. Both hydrophobic as well as hydrophilic drugs can be encapsulated within phospholipids and the water phase cavity, making them SDDS [109]. Particle size determines the extent of accumulation at the synovium, with maximum accumulation of liposomes reported with size <100 nm diameter [110]. Therapeutic efficacy is limited due to rapid clearance from circulation *via* the RES in the liver/spleen. Surface modification by PEG enhances its hydrophilicity, makes them sterically stabilized, circumvent rapid clearance, and enhance the retention time in blood circulation [110]. Corvo et al. reported enhanced circulation and accumulation of PEG-coated SOD entrapped liposomes (mean diameter ~ 0.11 μm) at the arthritic joints [111]. Considering the dynamic microenvironment of the diseased synovium, liposomal surface can be modified with ligands, antibodies/antibody fragments or for site-specific delivery of encapsulated cargo. Recently, dexamethasone encapsulated PEG-liposome treated arthritic rats indicated accumulation of liposomes, down regulation of pro-inflammatory cytokines along with reduced inflammation of the arthritic joints [112]. Liposome tagged with a peptide sequence (CKPFDRALC-called ART-2 ligand) encapsulating DEX significantly inhibited RA progression [113].

5.2.4 Micelles

Micelles can be synthesized in small size with narrow size distribution from amphiphilic molecules that self-assemble into NPs in aqueous solution with a distinct hydrophobic cavity and an exterior hydrophilic surface. This makes them apt for intravenous injection and targeted delivery into the inflamed synovium as a consequence of extravasation through leaky vasculature and subsequent inflammatory cell-mediated sequestration (ELVIS) [114]. Wang et al. reported self-assembled micelles with an amphiphilic copolymer PEG-poly-e-caprolactone (PEG-PCL), which displayed ELVIS in inflamed joints [115], but the non-biodegradable backbone of synthetic polymers caused non-specific accumulation in liver. Bader et al. [116] developed micelles from polysialic acid (PSA)-the hydrophilic polymer and synthesized micelles by altering it with N-decylamine (DA) and PCL, that formed the hydrophobic fragment. Prolonged circulation was observed with these micelles that accumulated passively at the inflamed tissue. PSA-DA micelles exhibited *in-vitro* cytotoxicity towards a synovial fibroblast cell line, the PSA-PCL micelles displayed negligible *in-vivo* cytotoxicity [117]. Further modifications were reported to improve the blood kinetic profile of the micelles. Core-cross-linked micelles were developed based on copolymer PEG-b-poly [N-(2-hydroxypropyl) methacrylamide-lactate] for targeted delivery of glucocorticoids to the RA affected joints. Here, dexamethasone was modified by methacrylated linkers *via* ester bonds, and covalently encapsulated within the polymeric structure, leading to tailorable release of dexamethasone [118]. Targeted delivery of aqueous-synthesized MTX-PEI@HA NPs to mitigate inflammatory arthritis was reported [114]. Li et al. formulated pH-sensitive micelles by conjugating hydrophobic prednisolone to PEG-derivative that confers acid-sensitive sites for attachment by forming hydrazone bonds [119]. Dual-drug loading of nimesulide and MTX in RGD-modified micelles to target αvβ3-integrin validated efficient site-specific delivery, decreased angiogenesis with minimal dose of nimesulide and MTX [120].

6. Conclusion

Multifactorial pathogenesis is the hallmark in RA causing bone fragility and functional erosion linked disability in extreme conditions. Although, conventional therapeutic formulations alone or in combination may relieve the symptoms, these are associated with complex adverse reactions. Dose-escalation, immunogenicity, systemic toxicity, and non-specific biodistribution in tissues warrant SDDS development. Stimuli-responsive NPs target specific inflammatory intermediaries, thereby suppressing the pathophysiological cascade, that may alleviate RA symptoms and delay joint destruction. Therefore, both the approaches may be exploited for achieving dose reduction coupled with drug accumulation at the targeted inflamed joint.

Acknowledgements

LB is thankful to UGC, and VS is thankful to ICMR, Govt of India for Senior Research Fellowship. VK is thankful to Individual Fellowship from European Union's Research and Innovation program, Marie Skłodowska-Curie grant agreement No. 890507.

Authors contributions

Writing—original draft preparation, AKV, LB, VS and VK; visualization, AKV; conceptualization, writing—review and editing, supervision and project administration, AKV. All authors have read and agreed to the published version of the manuscript.

Funding

This research received no external funding.

Conflicts of interest

The authors declare no conflict of interest.

References

[1] Aletaha D, Smolen JS. Diagnosis and management of rheumatoid arthritis: a review. Jama. 2018 2;320(13):1360-72.

[2] Burmester GR, Bijlsma JW, Cutolo M, McInnes IB. Managing rheumatic and musculoskeletal diseases—past, present and future. Nature Reviews Rheumatology. 2017;13(7):443.

[3] Global RA Network. About Arthritis and RA. https://globalranetwork.org/project/disease-info/

[4] Mahdi H, Fisher BA, Källberg H, Plant D, Malmström V, Rönnelid J, Charles P, Ding B, Alfredsson L, Padyukov L, Symmons DP. Specific interaction between genotype, smoking and autoimmunity to citrullinated α-enolase in the etiology of rheumatoid arthritis. Nature genetics. 2009;41(12): 1319-24.

[5] Koga T, Kawakami A, Tsokos GC. Current insights and future prospects for the pathogenesis and treatment for rheumatoid arthritis. Clinical Immunology. 2021;225:108680.

[6] Lühder F, Reichardt HM. Novel drug delivery systems tailored for improved administration of glucocorticoids. International journal of molecular sciences. 2017;18(9):1836.

[7] Horton HM, Bernett MJ, Peipp M, Pong E, Karki S, Chu SY, Richards JO, Chen H, Repp R, Desjarlais JR, Zhukovsky EA. Fc-engineered anti-CD40 antibody enhances multiple effector functions and exhibits potent in vitro and in vivo antitumor activity against hematologic malignancies. Blood, The Journal of the American Society of Hematology. 2010;116(16): 3004-12.

[8] Gabay C, Riek M, Scherer A, Finckh A. Effectiveness of biologic DMARDs in monotherapy versus in combination with synthetic DMARDs in rheumatoid arthritis: data from the Swiss Clinical Quality Management Registry. Rheumatology. 2015;54(9): 1664-72.

[9] Shi J, Ying H, Du J, Shen B. Serum sclerostin levels in patients with ankylosing spondylitis and rheumatoid arthritis: a systematic review and meta-analysis. Biomed Res Int;2017:9295313.

[10] Müller-Ladner U, Ospelt C, Gay S, Distler O, Pap T. Cells of the synovium in rheumatoid arthritis. Synovial fibroblasts. Arthritis research & therapy. 2007;9(6):1-0.

[11] Gorantla S, Singhvi G, Rapalli VK, Waghule T, Dubey SK, Saha RN. Targeted drug-delivery systems in the treatment of rheumatoid arthritis: recent advancement and clinical status. Therapeutic Delivery. 2020;11(4):269-84.

[12] Neumann E, Hasseli R, Ohl S, Lange U, Frommer KW, Müller-Ladner U. Adipokines and Autoimmunity in Inflammatory Arthritis. Cells. 2021 Feb;10(2):216.

[13] Bui VL, Brahn E. Cytokine targeting in rheumatoid arthritis. Clinical Immunology (Orlando, Fla.). 2018 3;206:3-8.

[14] O'Shea JJ, Schwartz DM, Villarino AV, Gadina M, McInnes IB, Laurence A. The JAK-STAT pathway: impact on human disease and therapeutic intervention. Annual review of medicine. 2015;66:311-28.

[15] Orr C, Vieira-Sousa E, Boyle DL, Buch MH, Buckley CD, Cañete JD, Catrina AI, Choy EH, Emery P, Fearon U, Filer A. Synovial tissue research: a state-of-the-art review. Nature Reviews Rheumatology. 2017;13(8):463.

[16] Lliso-Ribera G, Humby F, Lewis M, Nerviani A, Mauro D, Rivellese F, Kelly S, Hands R, Bene F, Ramamoorthi N, Hackney JA. Synovial tissue signatures enhance clinical classification and prognostic/treatment response algorithms in early inflammatory arthritis and predict requirement for subsequent biological therapy: results from the pathobiology of early arthritis cohort (PEAC). Annals of the rheumatic diseases. 2019;78(12): 1642-52.

[17] Davis III JM, Crowson CS, Knutson KL, Achenbach SJ, Strausbauch MA, Therneau TM, Matteson EL, Gabriel SE, Wettstein PJ. Longitudinal relationships between rheumatoid factor and cytokine expression by immunostimulated peripheral blood lymphocytes from patients with rheumatoid arthritis: New insights into B-cell activation. Clinical Immunology. 2020;211:108342.

[18] Scherer HU, Huizinga TW, Krönke G, Schett G, Toes RE. The B cell response to citrullinated antigens in the development of rheumatoid arthritis. Nature Reviews Rheumatology. 2018; 14(3):157.

[19] Arango Duque G, Descoteaux A. Macrophage cytokines: involvement in immunity and infectious diseases. Frontiers in immunology. 2014;5:491

[20] Xu X, Gao W, Cheng S, Yin D, Li F, Wu Y, Sun D, Zhou S, Wang D, Zhang Y, Jiang R. Anti-inflammatory and immunomodulatory mechanisms of atorvastatin in a murine model of traumatic brain injury. Journal of neuroinflammation. 2017;14(1):1-5.

[21] Kotake S, Yago T, Kawamoto M, Nanke Y. Human receptor activator of NF-κB ligand (RANKL) induces osteoclastogenesis of primates in vitro. In Vitro Cellular & Developmental Biology-Animal. 2012;48(9):593-8.

[22] Itoh Y. Membrane-type matrix metalloproteinases: Their functions and regulations. Matrix Biology. 2015;44: 207-23.

[23] Conigliaro P, Triggianese P, De Martino E, Fonti GL, Chimenti MS, Sunzini F, Viola A, Canofari C, Perricone R. Challenges in the treatment of rheumatoid arthritis. Autoimmunity reviews. 2019;18(7):706-13.

[24] Konttinen YT, Ainola M, Valleala H, Ma J, Ida H, Mandelin J, Kinne RW, Santavirta S, Sorsa T, López-Otín C, Takagi M. Analysis of 16 different matrix metalloproteinases (MMP-1 to MMP-20) in the synovial membrane: different profiles in trauma and rheumatoid arthritis. Annals of the rheumatic diseases. 1999;58(11):691-7.

[25] Srivastava S, Singh D, Patel S, Parihar AK, Singh MR. Novel carters and targeted approaches: Way out for rheumatoid arthritis quandrum. Journal of Drug Delivery Science and Technology. 2017 Aug 1;40:125-35.

[26] Liu D, Yang F, Xiong F, Gu N. The smart drug delivery system and its clinical potential. Theranostics. 2016;6(9):1306.

[27] Wu L, Shen S. What potential do magnetic iron oxide nanoparticles have for the treatment of rheumatoid arthritis? Nanomedicine. 2019;14(8): 927-30.

[28] Kumar V, Leekha A, Tyagi A, Kaul A, Mishra AK, Verma AK. Preparation and evaluation of biopolymeric nanoparticles as drug delivery system in effective treatment of rheumatoid arthritis. Pharmaceutical research. 2017;34(3):654-67.

[29] Rajamäki K, Nordström T, Nurmi K, Åkerman KE, Kovanen PT, Öörni K, Eklund KK. Extracellular acidosis is a novel danger signal alerting innate

immunity via the NLRP3 inflammasome. Journal of Biological Chemistry. 2013;288(19):13410-9.

[30] Roiniotis J, Dinh H, Masendycz P, Turner A, Elsegood CL, Scholz GM, Hamilton JA. Hypoxia prolongs monocyte/macrophage survival and enhanced glycolysis is associated with their maturation under aerobic conditions. The Journal of Immunology. 2009;182(12):7974-81.

[31] Karimi M, Ghasemi A, Zangabad PS, Rahighi R, Basri SM, Mirshekari H, Amiri M, Pishabad ZS, Aslani A, Bozorgomid M, Ghosh D. Smart micro/nanoparticles in stimulus-responsive drug/gene delivery systems. Chemical Society Reviews. 2016;45(5):1457-501.

[32] Wang L, Zhu B, Huang J, Xiang X, Tang Y, Ma L, Yan F, Cheng C, Qiu L. Ultrasound-targeted microbubble destruction augmented synergistic therapy of rheumatoid arthritis via targeted liposomes. Journal of Materials Chemistry B. 2020;8(24):5245-56.

[33] Yang L, Shao Y, Han HK. Improved pH-dependent drug release and oral exposure of telmisartan, a poorly soluble drug through the formation of drug-aminoclay complex. International journal of pharmaceutics. 2014;471 (1-2):258-63.

[34] Fonseca LJ, Nunes-Souza V, Goulart MO, Rabelo LA. Oxidative stress in rheumatoid arthritis: What the future might hold regarding novel biomarkers and add-on therapies. Oxidative medicine and cellular longevity. 2019;2019.

[35] Mortezaee K, Najafi M, Samadian H, Barabadi H, Azarnezhad A, Ahmadi A. Redox interactions and genotoxicity of metal-based nanoparticles: A comprehensive review. Chemico-biological interactions. 2019;312:108814.

[36] Kuang M, Zheng G. Nanostructured bifunctional redox electrocatalysts. Small. 2016;12(41):5656-75.

[37] De La Rica R, Aili D, Stevens MM. Enzyme-responsive nanoparticles for drug release and diagnostics. Advanced drug delivery reviews. 2012;64(11): 967-78.

[38] Goyal AK, Rath G, Faujdar C, Malik B. Application and perspective of pH-responsive nano drug delivery systems. In Applications of Targeted Nano Drugs and Delivery Systems. 2019;15-33.

[39] Karimi M, Sahandi Zangabad P, Ghasemi A, Amiri M, Bahrami M, Malekzad H, Ghahramanzadeh Asl H, Mahdieh Z, Bozorgomid M, Ghasemi A, Rahmani Taji Boyuk MR. Temperature-responsive smart nanocarriers for delivery of therapeutic agents: applications and recent advances. ACS applied materials & interfaces. 2016;8 (33):21107-33.

[40] Singh A, Amiji MM, editors. Stimuli-responsive Drug Delivery Systems. Royal Society of Chemistry; 2018.

[41] Behrens MA, Lopez M, Kjøniksen AL, Zhu K, Nyström B, Pedersen JS. The effect of cationic and anionic blocks on temperature-induced micelle formation. Journal of Applied Crystallography. 2014;1;47(1):22-8.

[42] Chen YC, Xie R, Chu LY. Stimuli-responsive gating membranes responding to temperature, pH, salt concentration and anion species. Journal of membrane science. 2013;442:206-15.

[43] Zhang X, Hou Y, Xiao X, Chen X, Hu M, Geng X, Wang Z, Zhao J. Recent development of the transition metal complexes showing strong absorption of visible light and long-lived triplet excited state: From molecular structure

design to photophysical properties and applications. Coordination Chemistry Reviews. 2020;417:213371.

[44] Huo, Y; Yang, X; Liu, R; Zhao,D; Guo, C; Zhu, A; Wen, M; Liu, Z, Qu, G; Meng, H; "Pathological Mechanism of Photodynamic Therapy and Photothermal Therapy Based on Nanoparticles"International Journal of Nanomedicine. 2020:15 6827-6838

[45] Chen G, Qiu H, Prasad PN, Chen X. Upconversion nanoparticles: design, nanochemistry, and applications in theranostics. Chemical reviews. 2014;114(10):5161-214.

[46] Xu J, Xu L, Wang C, Yang R, Zhuang Q, Han X, Dong Z, Zhu W, Peng R, Liu Z. Near-infrared-triggered photodynamic therapy with multitasking upconversion nanoparticles in combination with checkpoint blockade for immunotherapy of colorectal cancer. ACS nano. 2017;11(5):4463-74.

[47] Kwon OS, Song HS, Conde J, Kim HI, Artzi N, Kim JH. Dual-color emissive upconversion nanocapsules for differential cancer bioimaging in vivo. ACS nano. 2016;10(1):1512-21.

[48] Xiang H, Chen Y. Energy-converting nanomedicine. Small. 2019;15(13):1805339.

[49] Chen X, Zhu X, Ma L, Lin A, Gong Y, Yuan G, Liu J. A core–shell structure QRu-PLGA-RES-DS NP nanocomposite with photothermal response-induced M2-macrophage polarization for rheumatoid arthritis therapy. Nanoscale. 2019;11(39):18209-23.

[50] Tang Q, Cui J, Tian Z, Sun J, Wang Z, Chang S, Zhu S. Oxygen and indocyanine green loaded phase-transition nanoparticle-mediated photo-sonodynamic cytotoxic effects on rheumatoid arthritis fibroblast-like synoviocytes. International journal of nanomedicine. 2017;12:381.

[51] Zhao J, Zhang X, Sun X, Zhao M, Yu C, Lee RJ, Sun F, Zhou Y, Li Y, Teng L. Dual-functional lipid polymeric hybrid pH-responsive nanoparticles decorated with cell penetrating peptide and folate for therapy against rheumatoid arthritis. European Journal of Pharmaceutics and Biopharmaceutics. 2018;130:39-47.

[52] Yu C, Li X, Hou Y, Meng X, Wang D, Liu J, Sun F, Li Y. Hyaluronic acid coated acid-sensitive nanoparticles for targeted therapy of adjuvant-induced arthritis in rats. Molecules. 2019;24(1):146.

[53] Alam MM, Han HS, Sung S, Kang JH, Sa KH, Al Faruque H, Hong J, Nam EJ, San Kim I, Park JH, Kang YM. Endogenous inspired biomineral-installed hyaluronan nanoparticles as pH-responsive carrier of methotrexate for rheumatoid arthritis. Journal of Controlled Release. 2017;252:62-72.

[54] Zhao J, Zhao M, Yu C, Zhang X, Liu J, Cheng X, Lee RJ, Sun F, Teng L, Li Y. Multifunctional folate receptor-targeting and pH-responsive nanocarriers loaded with methotrexate for treatment of rheumatoid arthritis. International journal of nanomedicine. 2017;12:6735.

[55] Moon SJ, You DG, Li Y, Um W, Jung JM, Kim CH, Oh BH, Park JH, Lee DS. pH-Sensitive Polymeric Micelles as the Methotrexate Carrier for Targeting Rheumatoid Arthritis. Macromolecular Research. 2020;28(2): 99-102.

[56] Xu Y, Mu J, Xu Z, Zhong H, Chen Z, Ni Q, Liang XJ, Guo S. Modular acid-activatable acetone-based ketal-linked nanomedicine by dexamethasone prodrugs for enhanced anti-rheumatoid arthritis with low side effects. Nano letters. 2020;20(4):2558-68.

[57] Chen M, Daddy JC KA, Su Z, Guissi NE, Xiao Y, Zong L, Ping Q. Folate receptor-targeting and reactive oxygen species-responsive liposomal formulation of methotrexate for treatment of rheumatoid arthritis. Pharmaceutics. 2019;11(11):582.

[58] Lee SM, Kim HJ, Ha YJ, Park YN, Lee SK, Park YB, Yoo KH. Targeted chemo-photothermal treatments of rheumatoid arthritis using gold half-shell multifunctional nanoparticles. ACS nano. 2013, 22;7(1):50-7.

[59] Lu Y, Li L, Lin Z, Wang L, Lin L, Li M, Zhang Y, Yin Q, Li Q, Xia H. A new treatment modality for rheumatoid arthritis: combined photothermal and photodynamic therapy using Cu7. 2S4 nanoparticles. Advanced healthcare materials. 2018;7 (14):1800013.

[60] Wu, K; Su, D; Liu J, Saha R and Wang, J.P. Magnetic nanoparticles in nanomedicine: a review of recent advances; 2019 *Nanotechnology* **30** 502003.

[61] Kim HJ, Lee SM, Park KH, Mun CH, Park YB, Yoo KH. Drug-loaded gold/iron/gold plasmonic nanoparticles for magnetic targeted chemo-photothermal treatment of rheumatoid arthritis. Biomaterials. 2015;61:95-102.

[62] He L, Fan D, Liang W, Wang Q, Fang J. Matrix Metalloproteinase-Responsive PEGylated Lipid Nanoparticles for Controlled Drug Delivery in the Treatment of Rheumatoid Arthritis. ACS Applied Bio Materials. 2020;3(5):3276-84.

[63] Wardwell PR, Forstner MB, Bader RA. Investigation of the cytokine response to NF-κB decoy oligonucleotide-coated polysaccharide based nanoparticles in rheumatoid arthritis:*in vitro* models. Arthritis research & therapy. 2015(1):1-1.

[64] Lima SA, Reis S. Temperature-responsive polymeric nanospheres containing methotrexate and gold nanoparticles: a multi-drug system for theranostic in rheumatoid arthritis. Colloids and Surfaces B: Biointerfaces. 2015;133:378-87.

[65] He L, Qin X, Fan D, Feng C, Wang Q, & Fang J. Dual-Stimuli Responsive Polymeric Micelles for the Effective Treatment of Rheumatoid Arthritis. ACS Appl Mater Interfaces 2021;13(18):21076-21086.

[66] Yang M, Feng X, Ding J, Chang F, Chen X. Nanotherapeutics relieve rheumatoid arthritis. Journal of Controlled Release. 2017;252:108-24.

[67] Prasad LK, O'Mary H, Cui Z. Nanomedicine delivers promising treatments for rheumatoid arthritis. Nanomedicine. 2015;10(13):2063-74.

[68] Maeda H. The enhanced permeability and retention (EPR) effect in tumor vasculature: the key role of tumor-selective macromolecular drug targeting. Adv. Enzyme Regul. 2001;41:189-207

[69] Walsh DA. Angiogenesis and arthritis. Rheumatology (Oxford, England).999;38(2):103-12.

[70] Girdhar V, Patil S, Banerjee S, Singhvi G. Nanocarriers for drug delivery: mini review. Current Nanomedicine (Formerly: Recent Patents on Nanomedicine). 2018;8(2):88-99.

[71] Xu H, Edwards J, Banerji S, Prevo R, Jackson DG, Athanasou NA. Distribution of lymphatic vessels in normal and arthritic human synovial tissues. Annals of the rheumatic diseases. 2003;62(12):1227-9.

[72] Gao C, Huang Q, Liu C, Kwong CH, Yue L, Wan JB, Lee SM, Wang R.

Treatment of atherosclerosis by macrophage-biomimetic nanoparticles via targeted pharmacotherapy and sequestration of proinflammatory cytokines. Nature communications. 2020;11(1):1-4.

[73] Nakashima-Matsushita N, Homma T, Yu S, Matsuda T, Sunahara N, Nakamura T, Tsukano M, Ratnam M, Matsuyama T. Selective expression of folate receptor β and its possible role in methotrexate transport in synovial macrophages from patients with rheumatoid arthritis. Arthritis & Rheumatism: Official Journal of the American College of Rheumatology. 1999;42(8):1609-16.

[74] Hao H, Qi H, Ratnam M. Modulation of the folate receptor type β gene by coordinate actions of retinoic acid receptors at activator Sp1/ets and repressor AP-1 sites. Blood. 2003;101(11):4551-60.

[75] Tsuneyoshi Y, Tanaka M, Nagai T, Sunahara N, Matsuda T, Sonoda T, Ijiri K, Komiya S, Matsuyama T. Functional folate receptor beta-expressing macrophages in osteoarthritis synovium and their M1/M2 expression profiles. Scandinavian journal of rheumatology. 2012;41(2):132-40.

[76] Varghese B, Haase N, Low PS. Depletion of folate-receptor-positive macrophages leads to alleviation of symptoms and prolonged survival in two murine models of systemic lupus erythematosus. Molecular pharmaceutics. 2007;4(5):679-85.

[77] Ayala-López W, Xia W, Varghese B, Low PS. Imaging of atherosclerosis in apoliprotein e knockout mice: targeting of a folate-conjugated radiopharmaceutical to activated macrophages. Journal of Nuclear Medicine. 2010;51(5):768-74.

[78] Low PS, Antony AC. Folate receptor-targeted drugs for cancer and inflammatory diseases. Advanced drug delivery reviews. 2004;56(8).

[79] Kumar V, Leekha A, Kaul A, Mishra AK, Verma AK. Role of folate-conjugated glycol-chitosan nanoparticles in modulating the activated macrophages to ameliorate inflammatory arthritis: *in vitro* and *in vivo* activities. Drug delivery and translational research. 2020;10(4):1057-75.

[80] Nogueira E, Lager F, Le Roux D, Nogueira P, Freitas J, Charvet C, Renault G, Loureiro A, Almeida CR, Ohradanova-Repic A, Machacek C. Enhancing methotrexate tolerance with folate tagged liposomes in arthritic mice. Journal of biomedical nanotechnology. 2015;11(12): 2243-52.

[81] Thomas TP, Goonewardena SN, Majoros IJ, Kotlyar A, Cao Z, Leroueil PR, Baker Jr JR. Folate-targeted nanoparticles show efficacy in the treatment of inflammatory arthritis. Arthritis & Rheumatism. 2011;63(9):2671-80.

[82] Pandey P.K. ; Maheshwari, R; Raval, N; Raval P; Kalia, G. K.; Tekade, R.K.; Nanogold-core multifunctional dendrimer for pulsatile chemo-, photothermal- and photodynamic-therapy of rheumatoid arthritis; 2019; 544, 15, 61-77.

[83] Pandey S, Rai N, Mahtab A, Mittal D, Ahmad FJ, Sandal N, Neupane YR, Verma AK, Talegaonkar S. Hyaluronate-functionalized hydroxyapatite nanoparticles laden with methotrexate and teriflunomide for the treatment of rheumatoid arthritis. International Journal of Biological Macromolecules. 2021;28;171:502-13.

[84] Szekanecz Z, Koch AE. Mechanisms of disease: angiogenesis in inflammatory diseases. Nature clinical practice Rheumatology. 2007; 3(11):635-43.

[85] Marrelli A, Cipriani P, Liakouli V, Carubbi F, Perricone C, Perricone R, Giacomelli R. Angiogenesis in rheumatoid arthritis: a disease specific process or a common response to chronic inflammation? Autoimmunity reviews. 2011;10(10):595-8.

[86] Shibuya M. Vascular endothelial growth factor-dependent and-independent regulation of angiogenesis. BMB reports. 2008;41(4):278-86.

[87] Szekanecz Z, Koch AE. VEGF as an activity marker in rheumatoid arthritis. International Journal of Clinical Rheumatology. 2010;5(3):287.

[88] Ganea D, Hooper KM, Kong W. The neuropeptide vasoactive intestinal peptide: direct effects on immune cells and involvement in inflammatory and autoimmune diseases. Acta Physiologica. 2015;213(2):442-52.

[89] Teitelbaum SL. Bone resorption by osteoclasts. Science. 2000;289(5484): 1504-8.

[90] Wilder RL. Integrin alpha V beta 3 as a target for treatment of rheumatoid arthritis and related rheumatic diseases. Annals of the rheumatic diseases. 2002;61(suppl 2):ii,96-9.

[91] Jamar F, Chapman PT, Harrison AA, Binns RM, Haskard DO, Peters AM. Inflammatory arthritis: imaging of endothelial cell activation with an indium-111-labeled F (ab') 2 fragment of anti-E-selectin monoclonal antibody. Radiology. 1995;194(3):843-50.

[92] Jubeli E, Moine L, Vergnaud-Gauduchon J, Barratt G. E-selectin as a target for drug delivery and molecular imaging. Journal of controlled release. 2012;158(2):194-206.

[93] James HP, John R, Alex A, Anoop K. Smart polymers for the controlled delivery of drugs–a concise overview. Acta Pharmaceutica Sinica B. 2014;4(2): 120-7.

[94] Ulbrich W, Lamprecht A. Targeted drug-delivery approaches by nanoparticulate carriers in the therapy of inflammatory diseases. Journal of The Royal Society Interface. 2010;7(suppl_1):S55-66.

[95] Bader RA. The development of targeted drug delivery systems for rheumatoid arthritis treatment. Rheumatoid Arthritis–Treatment. Rijeka and Shanghai: InTech. 2012;18:111-32.

[96] Syed A, Devi VK. Potential of targeted drug delivery systems in treatment of rheumatoid arthritis. Journal of Drug Delivery Science and Technology. 2019;1;53:101217.

[97] Wang Q, Sun X. Recent advances in nanomedicines for the treatment of rheumatoid arthritis. Biomaterials science. 2017;5(8):1407-20.

[98] Wang D, Miller SC, Liu XM, Anderson B, Wang XS, Goldring SR. Novel dexamethasone-HPMA copolymer conjugate and its potential application in treatment of rheumatoid arthritis. Arthritis research & therapy. 2007;9(1):1-9.

[99] Liu XM, Quan LD, Tian J, Laquer FC, Ciborowski P,Wang D. Syntheses of click PEG–dexamethasone conjugates for the treatment of rheumatoid arthritis. Biomacromolecules. 2010;11(10): 2621-2628.

[100] Li Q, Cao J, Li Z, Chu X. Cubic liquid crystalline gels based on glycerol monooleate for intra-articular injection. AAPS PharmSciTech. 2018;19(2):858-65.

[101] Junkai Zhao, Xuan Chen, Kwun-Hei Ho, Chao Cai, Cheuk-Wing Li, Mo Yang, Changqing Yi. Nanotechnology for diagnosis and therapy of rheumatoid arthritis: Evolution towards theranostic approaches. Chinese Chemical Letters, 2021;32(1): 66-86.

[102] Yang H, Tang C, Yin C. Estrone-modified pH-sensitive glycol chitosan nanoparticles for drug delivery in breast cancer. Acta biomaterialia. 2018;73: 400-11.

[103] Vigderman L, Zubarev ER. Therapeutic platforms based on gold nanoparticles and their covalent conjugates with drug molecules. Advanced drug delivery reviews. 2013;65(5):663-76.

[104] Jeong EH, Jung G, Am Hong C, Lee H. Gold nanoparticle (AuNP)-based drug delivery and molecular imaging for biomedical applications. Archives of pharmacal research. 2014;37(1):53-9.

[105] James LR, Xu ZQ, Sluyter R, Hawksworth EL, Kelso C, Lai B, Paterson DJ, de Jonge MD, Dixon NE, Beck JL, Ralph SF. An investigation into the interactions of gold nanoparticles and anti-arthritic drugs with macrophages, and their reactivity towards thioredoxin reductase. Journal of inorganic biochemistry. 2015 1;142:28-38.

[106] Lee SM, Kim HJ, Ha YJ, Park YN, Lee SK, Park YB, Yoo KH. Targeted chemo-photothermal treatments of rheumatoid arthritis using gold half-shell multifunctional nanoparticles. ACS nano. 2013; 22;7(1):50-7.

[107] Lee H, Lee MY, Bhang SH, Kim BS, Kim YS, Ju JH, Kim KS, Hahn SK. Hyaluronate-gold nanoparticle/tocilizumab complex for the treatment of rheumatoid arthritis. ACS Nano. 2014;8(5):4790-8.

[108] Pirmardvand CS, Varshosaz J, & Taymouri S. Recent approaches for targeted drug delivery in rheumatoid arthritis diagnosis and treatment. Artificial cells, nanomedicine, and biotechnology. 2018;46(sup2):502-514.

[109] Wang WX, Feng SS, Zheng CH. A comparison between conventional liposome and drug-cyclodextrin complex in liposome system. International journal of pharmaceutics. 2016;513(1-2):387-92.

[110] Mastrotto F, Brazzale C, Bellato F, De Martin S, Grange G, Mahmoudzadeh M, Magarkar A, Bunker A, Salmaso S, Caliceti P. In vitro and in vivo behavior of liposomes decorated with PEGs with different chemical features. Molecular pharmaceutics. 2019;17(2):472-87.

[111] Corvo ML, Boerman OC, Oyen WJG, et al. Intravenous administration of superoxide dismutase entrapped in long circulating liposomes II. In vivo fate in a rat model of adjuvant arthritis. BBA Membranes. 1999;1419:325-334

[112] Wang Q, He L, Fan D, Liang W, Fang J. Improving the anti-inflammatory efficacy of dexamethasone in the treatment of rheumatoid arthritis with polymerized stealth liposomes as a delivery vehicle. Journal of Materials Chemistry B. 2020;8(9):1841-51.

[113] Meka RR, Venkatesha SH, Acharya B, Moudgil KD. Peptide-targeted liposomal delivery of dexamethasone for arthritis therapy. Nanomedicine. 2019;14(11):1455-69.

[114] Zhong, S.; Liu, P.; Ding, J.; Zhou, W. Hyaluronic Acid-Coated MTX-PEI Nanoparticles for Targeted Rheumatoid Arthritis Therapy. Crystals. 2021;11:321.

[115] Wang Q, Jiang J, Chen W, Jiang H, Zhang Z, Sun X. Targeted delivery of low-dose dexamethasone using PCL–PEG micelles for effective treatment of rheumatoid arthritis. Journal of Controlled Release. 2016;230:64-72.

[116] Bader RA, Silvers AL, Zhang N. Polysialic acid-based micelles for encapsulation of hydrophobic drugs. Biomacromolecules. 2011;12(2):314-20.

[117] Wilson DR, Zhang N, Silvers AL, Forstner MB, Bader RA. Synthesis and evaluation of cyclosporine A-loaded polysialic acid–polycaprolactone micelles for rheumatoid arthritis. European Journal of Pharmaceutical Sciences. 2014;51:146-56.

[118] Crielaard BJ, Rijcken CJ, Quan L, Van Der Wal S, Altintas I, Van Der Pot M, Kruijtzer JA, Liskamp RM, Schiffelers RM, Van Nostrum CF, Hennink WE. Glucocorticoid-loaded core-cross-linked polymeric micelles with tailorable release kinetics for targeted therapy of rheumatoid arthritis. Angewandte Chemie. 2012;124(29):7366-70.

[119] Li C, Li H, Wang Q, Zhou M, Li M, Gong T, Zhang Z, Sun X. pH-sensitive polymeric micelles for targeted delivery to inflamed joints. Journal of Controlled Release. 2017;246:133-41

[120] Wang Y, Liu Z, Li T, Chen L, Lyu J, Li C, Lin Y, Hao N, Zhou M, Zhong Z. Enhanced therapeutic effect of RGD-modified polymeric micelles loaded with low-dose methotrexate and nimesulide on rheumatoid arthritis. Theranostics. 2019;9(3):708.

Chapter 4

Phosphoplipid Based Nano Drug Delivery Systems of Phytoconstituents

Abstract

The development of phytochemistry and phyto-pharmacology has enabled elucidation of composition and biological activities of several medicinal plant constituents. However phytoconstituents are poorly absorbed due to their low aqueous solubility, large molecular size and poor membrane permeability when taken orally. Nanotechnology based drug delivery systems can be used to improve the dissolution rate, permeability and stability of these phytoconstituents. The current chapter aims to present the extraction of phytoconstituents, their identifications, and development/utilization of phospholipid based nano drug delivery systems (PBNDDS). The content of the chapter also provides characteristic features, *in-vitro, in-vivo* evaluations and stability performance of PBNDDS. The results from the UHPLC and GC-MS showed different phytoconstituents in the extracted samples with quantitative value. Dynamic light scattering (DLS) data showed PBNDDS of different phytoconstituents in the range of 50–250 nm with PDI value of 0.02–0.5, which was also confirmed by the electron microscopic data. Phytoconstituents loading or entrapment for PBNDDS was in the range of 60–95%. PBNDDS exhibited better *in-vitro* and *in-vivo* performance with improved Physico-chemical stability.

Keywords: phospholipid, liposome, phytosome, epigallocatechin gallate (EGCG), phytol, *Aphanamixis polystachia*, thymoquinone

1. Introduction

Phospholipid based nano drug delivery systems (PBNDDS) are becoming more promising due to its biocompatibility, amphiphilic characteristics, Physico-chemical stability and can be prepared for different diseases with sustain release and targeted delivery of different drugs [1]. PBNDDS can protect the drug from biodegradation, transformation and reduce cell toxicity by altering the bio-distribution. PBNDDS are easy to scale-up, sterilize in product development and cost effective. PBNDDS performance depends on size, morphology of particles and possesses some unique properties like surface area to mass ratio which is larger than other colloidal systems. Controlled release and targeted drug delivery depend on the rate and mechanism of drug release from the carrier based drug delivery systems like PBNDDS, which can vary depending on the formulation, processing and routes of administration [1–6].

Phospholipids are heterolipids which can be extracted from both animal and plant origin, have been shown to generate lipid matrices of low crystallinity.

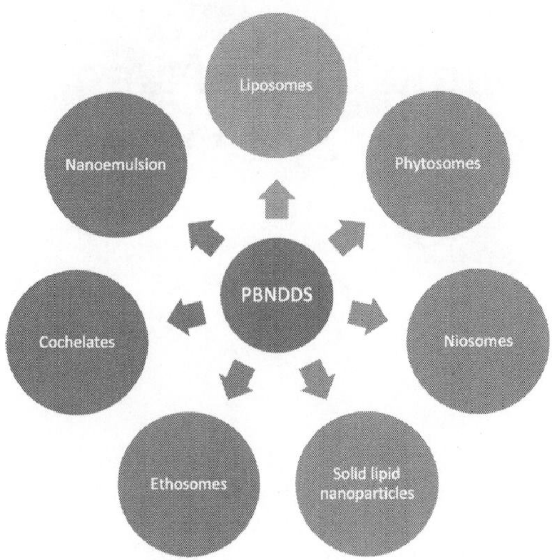

Figure 1.
Phospholipid based nano drug delivery systems (PBNDDS) [1–3].

Different types of phospholipid based nano drug delivery systems (**Figure 1**) are used for both synthetic and natural source of drugs [7, 8].

Natural source of medicines have been used from ancient time [9]. Phytoconstituents present in plants having different pharmacological properties are useful substitutes to synthetic drugs. There are over 100 active ingredients derived from natural plants for use as drugs and medicines. Chronic inflammatory (stroke, chronic respiratory diseases and heart disorders), and central nervous system (CNS) diseases are major cause of global mortality. Different synthetic drugs used to treat these diseases results in severe adverse effects. Research is going on for the development of new drugs from natural medicinal plants [10].

Phytoconstituents showed strong anti-inflammatory activities due to their strong free radical scavenging action [11] and have shown beneficial effects on cancers, diabetes, cardiovascular diseases, stroke and obesity etc. Phytoconstituents also exhibit activity against neurodegenerative diseases (Alzheimer's disease, and Parkinson's disease) through different pathways [12–21].

2. Natural plant extract and phytoconstituents

In this chapter four different plant extracts and its phytoconstituents (Black seed oil containing thymoquinone, Jute leaf extract containing phytol, *Aphanamixis polystachia* leaf extract, green tea extract containing EGCG) are discussed (**Figure 2**), which were formulated as phospholipid based nano drug delivery systems (PBNDDS).

Thymoquinone a natural component of Black seed oil, which can be obtained from the seeds of *Nigella sativa*, found to have different pharmacological activity for the treatment of various diseases [22–26]. However, despite the various pharmacological properties of thymoquinone, its administration *in-vivo* remains crucial due to its poor water solubility and stability issues. Therefore an advanced drug

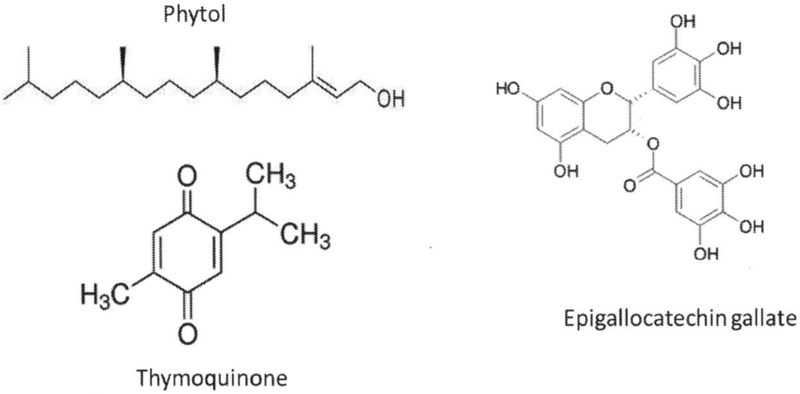

Figure 2.
Chemical structure of phytol, thymoquinone and epigallocatechin gallate.

delivery system is required to improve the therapeutic outcome of thymoquinone by enhancing the solubility and stability in water [27].

Jute leaf obtained from *Corchorus olitorius L.* [28, 29] has been used as traditional medicine. Jute leaf extract contains different phytoconstituents which are medicinally active and exhibits pharmacological effects against different diseases [30–33]. Phytol is one of the main phytoconstituents found in jute leaf extract demonstrates pharmacological activity against different diseases and in different *in-vitro* cell line studies [29, 34]. Phytol due to its multiple ring structure shows poor water solubility and absorption through the intestinal wall.

Aphanamixis polystachya a natural plant which contains phytoconstituents found to have different medicinal activities [35–38]. Leaf extract of *A. polystachya* plant showed CNS activities [39], therefore in this chapter *A. polystachya* leaf extracts and its phospholipid based nano drug delivery system (PBNDDS) activity against animal model of dementia is discussed.

Epigallocatechin-3-gallate (EGCG) is a main potent constituent of green tea extract (*Camellia sinensis*), which is one of the major catechins [40]. EGCG exhibit pharmacological activity against different diseases [41, 42] and also showed activity against carcinogenic effects in different animal models with different cancers [43–46]. EGCG has high water solubility however it exhibits low permeability across the gastrointestinal tract (GIT) leading to poor bioavailability [47, 48].

3. Issues with natural phytoconstituents

Phytoconstituents showed a range of pharmacological activity and less side effects compared to synthetic drugs; however phytoconstituents exhibit low water solubility, poor permeability through gastrointestinal tract and impede fast systemic clearance [49]. Physical and chemical stability of phytochemicals is another issue [50–54]. Treatment of CNS and cancer diseases require targeted drug delivery for better therapeutic outcome. Nano drug delivery systems may be a promising platform for the improvement of aforementioned issues of natural plant extracts and their phytoconstituents. Therefore phospholipid based nano drug delivery systems of natural phytoconstituents could be the potential delivery system with better performance and stability [55].

4. Nanoparticle based drug delivery of phytoconstituents

Novel nano drug delivery systems can improve the solubility, permeability, physicochemical stability and reduce toxicity of drugs [52]. Previous studies showed that the phospholipid based nano drug delivery systems can improve the oral delivery of thymoquinone [56, 57], and effective against breast cancer cell line. Mesoporous silica and chitosan nanoparticles are developed for delivery of thymoquinone to the brain [58]. In other study self nanoemulsifying and alginate beads delivery system were developed to improve the bioavailability, stability and targeted delivery of black seed oil [59].

Nanoparticulate based drug delivery system of phytol was used for Alzheimer's disease [60]. Previous research also showed strong cytotoxic, anti-phytopathogenic and hepatoprotective effect of phytol loaded nano drug delivery systems [61, 62]. Phospholipid based nano formulation of EGCG are developed to enhance the release characteristics, bioavailability, and stability [63–66]. Previous study data suggest that nanoparticulate based delivery of EGCG showed better cytotoxic and *in-vivo* performance compared to pure EGCG [67–69].

5. Phospholipid based nano drug delivery systems (PBNDDS) of plant extracts and phytoconstituents

Two types of phospholipid based nano drug delivery systems (PBNDDS) have been discussed in this chapter for four different natural extracts and its phytoconstituents, which are liposomes and phytosomes.

Liposome is a phospholipid based lipid bilayer vesicles where both hydrophilic and lipophilic drugs can be entrapped. Liposomal drug delivery system has become a budding technology for delivering drugs to improve the bioavailability, efficacy, safety and stability of both synthetic and natural source of medicines [70, 71]. Liposomal drug delivery system can be used to deliver drugs for neurodegenerative diseases through blood brain barrier (BBB) [72–74].

Phytosomes are structures prepared using natural plant extract with phospholipid matrix. Phytosomal delivery system can improve the absorption and bioavailability of phytoconstituents. In phytosome drug form complex with phospholipid like matrix formation while in liposomes, drug is entrapped in the core or lipid bilayer of phospholipids. Phytoconstituents of plant extracts showed better biological activity when delivered through phytosomes [75–79].

This chapter is mainly focused on the development, preparation and solid state characterization of liposomal drug delivery systems of black seed oil, *A. polystachya* leaf extracts and *Corchorus olitorius* leaf extracts and their main phytoconstituents. Phytosomal delivery system development of green tea extract and EGCG is also discussed with different solid state characterizations. Finally stability, *in-vitro* and *in-vivo* studies were discussed for phospholipids based nano preparations of all extracts and their phytoconstituents.

Phospholipid can be extracted from both plant and animal source of origin. Phospholipid used in these studies was extracted from egg yolk, which is known as lecithin or egg lecithin. Results (UHPLC data) showed the presence of phosphatidylcholine (PC) peak (the main phospholipid component for liposome) and suggest that per gram of egg lecithin contain 100–200 mg of PC, where filtrate of egg phospholipid contain the most of the PC content compared to solid residue (**Table 1**) [80]. Phosphatidylcholine (PC) content was also quantified for peanut using UHPLC analysis and results demonstrate that less amount of PC is present in per gram of peanut (**Table 1**).

Sample no/name	Mass (mg/g)	%
Egg sample 1 (filtrate)	212.80 ± 3.22	21.38
Egg sample 2 (solid residue)	9.71 ± 1.19	0.97
Peanut	5.56 ± 0.27	0.56

Table 1.
Amount of PC present in egg yolk. Sample 1 represents extracted PC as filtrate and sample 2 represents PC as solid residue. Data are mean ± SD (N = 3).

6. Plant extraction, identification and quantification by UHPLC and GC-MS

All four plants described in this chapter was extracted using maceration method (**Figure 3**). Plant extraction, its phytoconstituents identification and quantification were performed using UHPLC and GC-MS analytical methods [80–83]. Results from UHPLC data showed that the concentration of thymoquinone was 2.28 ± 0.68 mg/g of black seed oil [80].

Table 2 shows main phytoconstituents determined for *Aphanamixis polystachya* leaf extracts using GC-MS including Octadec-9-enoic acid, hexadecanoic acid, 2-Pentanone, 2-hydrazino-2-imidazoline and beta-elemene etc. [81]. Previous researches in this area suggest that these phytoconstituents exhibit strong antioxidant, anticancer and anti-inflammatory property [84–88], which found to have impact in neurodegenerative disorders including stroke [89–92]. However few of these phytoconstituents have poor solubility in water.

Major phytoconstituents present in the methanolic extract of *Corchorus olitorius* leaf are mentioned in **Table 3**, which are oleic acid, hexadecanoic acid, and

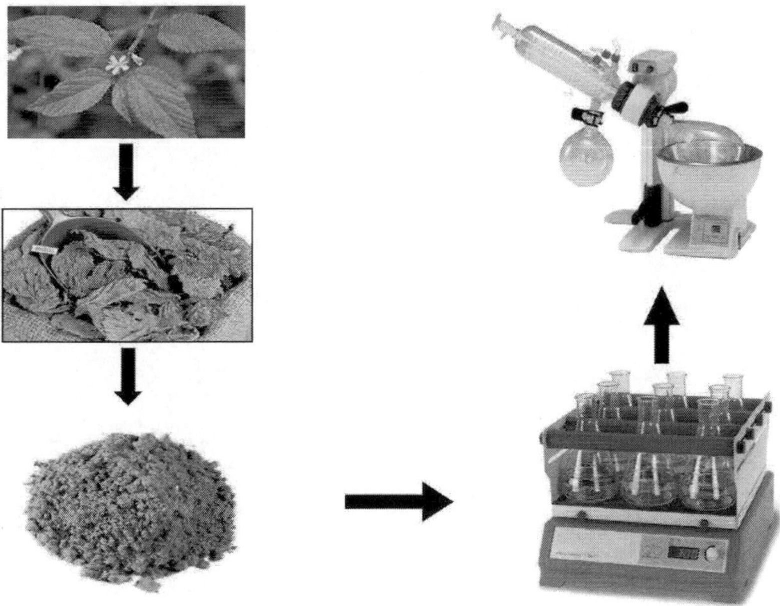

Figure 3.
Plant extraction process using maceration method.

No.	Name	RT	Area %	N area %
1	4-hexen-2-one	4.68	1.72	6
2	Acetic acid, butyl ester	5.06	2.36	8.24
3	3-acetoxydodecane	5.68	1.83	6.39
4	2-pentanone	5.88	14.62	51.08
5	4,4-dimethyl-1-hydroxy-2-cyclo	8.94	2.55	8.92
6	Acetic acid, hexyl ester	10.78	4.73	16.53
7	1,2-cyclohexanediol	13.76	4.12	14.39
8	Acetic acid	15.4	4.05	14.14
9	2-hydrazino-2-imidazoline	17.6	3.41	11.91
10	Beta-elemene	22.4	0.4	1.39
11	5-hydroxypipecolic acid	29	1.88	6.56
12	2-hexadecen-1-ol, 3,7,11,15-TE	33.36	0.63	2.19
13	Octadecanal	33.48	0.67	2.36
14	9-hexadecenoic acid	35.88	5.66	19.77
15	Hexadecanoic acid	36.32	8.83	30.84
16	4-hydroxytetradec-2-ynal	38.96	1.69	5.89
17	Octadec-9-enoic acid	39.72	28.63	100
18	1.beta.-allylperhydro-2.alpha.	44.32	1.32	4.6
19	Cyclopentadecanone	44.86	4.02	14.02
20	1-tetradecene	45.82	3.18	11.09
21	Tridec-4-en-2-ynal	50.06	3.71	12.96

Table 2.
List of major components present in the ethanolic leaf extract of Aphanamixis polystachya (adapted from [81]).

No.	Name	RT	Area %	N area %
1	2,3-dihydro-3,5-dihydroxy-6-me	15.1	4.58	8.08
2	D-neoisomenthol	15.9	1.21	2.14
3	Neophytadiene	33.36	1.15	2.02
4	Tetradecanoic acid	35.3	3.25	5.72
5	14-pentadecenoic acid	35.9	4.31	7.6
6	Hexadecanoic acid	36.36	16.16	28.48
7	Hexadecanoic acid	37.28	1.54	2.72
8	Caryophyllene diepoxide	38.7	1.76	3.1
9	2-hexadecen-1-ol	38.96	6.48	11.41
10	Oleic acid	39.76	56.75	100
11	9-tricosene	41.84	2.81	4.94

Table 3.
List of major components present in the methanolic leaf extract of Corchorus olitorius (adapted from [82]).

2-hexadecan-1-ol (phytol) etc [82]. Chromatographic results also suggest that 500 μg EGCG was present in one milliliter of green tea leaf, which was extracted using water as solvent at different temperatures [83]. Results also suggest that

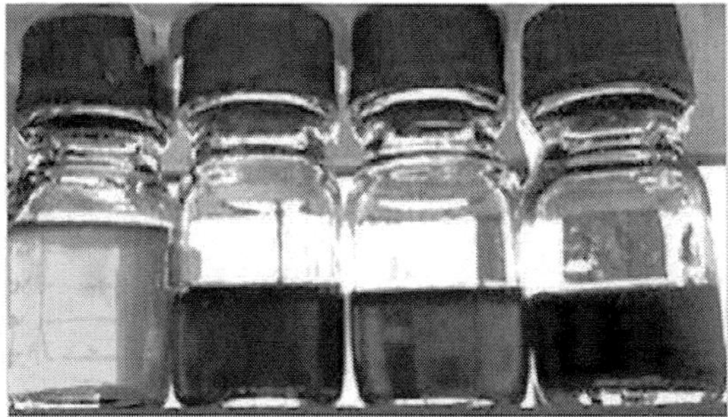

Figure 4.
Green tea leaf extracted at different temperature using water as solvent.

extraction process performed at high temperature (80°C) exhibited high content of EGCG, which was also observed by other research study (**Figure 4**) [83].

7. Preparation of PBNDDS of plant extracts and its phytoconstituents

Phospholipid based nano drug delivery systems using liposomes & phytosomes were prepared for plant extracts and phytoconstituents. Phospholipid based nano drug delivery systems (PBNDDS) batches of plant extracts and its phytoconstituents showed average particle size of 50–250 nm, PDI value of 0.02–0.5 and entrapment efficiency up to 90% (**Figures 5** and **6**). It was observed that the average size, polydispersity and entrapment efficiency of PBNDDS were markedly affected by the process and formulation factors used in different studies.

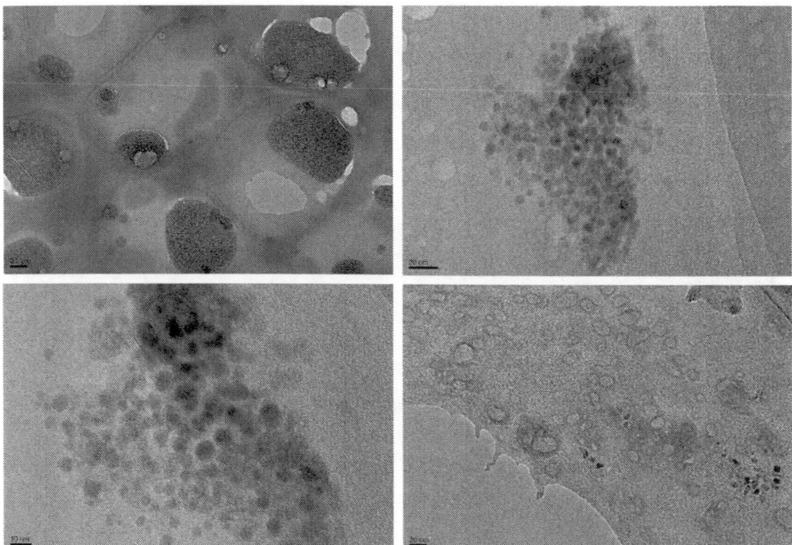

Figure 5.
TEM images for PBNDDS of phytoconstituents.

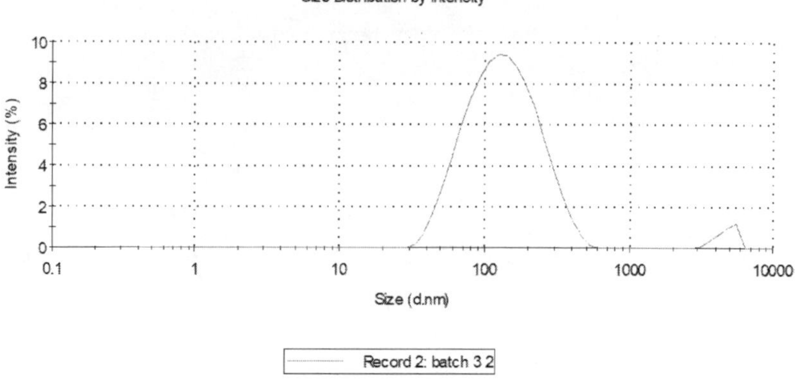

Figure 6.
DLS data of PBNDDS of phytoconstituents.

Entrapment efficiency of black seed oil loaded liposomes was increased markedly while cryoprotectant (sugar) and cholesterol were used in the preparation of liposomes. It was also observed that entrapment efficiency of liposomes was high for larger sized liposomes compared to small average size of liposomes.

8. Effect of process parameters and formulation attributes on development of PBNDDS of plant extracts and its phytoconstituents

Process parameters perspective injection rate, stirring speed, stirring time and processing temperature (solvent-antisolvent mixing) found to have marked impact on the average particle size, polydispersity and entrapment efficiency of PBNDDS [80–83, 93, 94]. It was observed that high injection rate and processing temperature found to have major impact leading to low average size of phospholipid based nano drug delivery systems (PBNDDS). Low stirring speed (<1000 rpm) and stirring time exhibit low average size of PBNDDS. Interactions between process parameter also have marked impact on average size of PBNDDS, where batches prepared using high injection rate and slow stirring speed demonstrate low average size (**Figure 7a** and **b**).

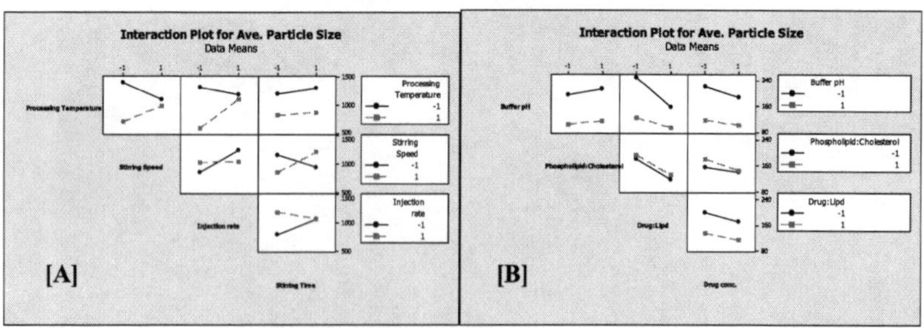

Figure 7.
Two way interaction plots of [A] process parameters and [B] formulation attributes for average particle size of PBNDDS.

Processing temperature found to be the most important process parameters which have significant impact on entrapment efficiency or loading of phytoconstituents on PBNDDS [83]. PBNDDS prepared using high temperature and injection rate leading to low entrapment efficiency. This phenomenon also probably related to low average size of PBNDDS developed at these conditions, while PBNDDS with high average particle size having high entrapment or loading efficiency. Polydispersity of PBNDDS was markedly affected by processing temperature and stirring speed and suggesting that batches processed at low temperature and high stirring speed found to be lessly polydispersed [81, 82].

Formulation attributes - ratio of drug: phospholipid and phospholipid: cholesterol, solvent system and its properties (phytoconstituents solubility, pH of the solvent), drug concentration found to have major impact on average particle size, polydispersity and entrapment efficiency of PBNDDS of phytoconstituents [80–83].

It is very imperative to find out the optimum level and amount of each of these process parameters and formulation attributes to achieve low average size with high entrapment or loading of phytoconstituents for PBNDDS. It was evident that not only the impact of individual parameters but its interactions also exhibited marked impact on the average size and loading of phytoconstituents for PBNDDS (**Figure** 7) [81–83].

9. Stability study of PBNDDS of phytoconstituents

Stability study data suggest that PBNDDS of phytoconstituents prepared using egg phospholipid were stable at 25°C and 65% RH for three months compared to accelerated conditions (10°C/45% RH and 40°C/75% RH) [80]. However previous research study suggested that PBNDDS developed using DPPC was more stable at 10°C/45% RH compared to other storage conditions [95]. This phenomenon probably related to egg phospholipid composition which is different from DPPC. DPPC is only one type of phosphatidylcholine, while egg phospholipid (lecithin) contains multiple types of phosphatidylcholine and phospholipids. PBNDDS blank and phytoconstituents loaded PBNDDS were studied using gastric media (pH 1.2) to evaluate the physical stability of PBNDDS. It was observed that PBNDDS batches of phytoconstituents were stable in gastric medium after 4 hours (maximum transit time in the stomach) and also suggests that no physical changes (precipitation or degradation) were observed for PBNDDS prepared using egg phospholipid even after 24 hrs [81].

10. *In-vitro* and *in-vivo* study of PBNDDS of phytoconstituents

Sustain release of phytoconstituents was observed when delivered through PBNDDS, which can be utilized for better therapeutic outcome against certain diseases. PBNDDS of phytoconstituents demonstrate better performance during *in-vitro* cancer cell line study performed on different cell lines. *In-vitro* cell line study data suggest that PBNDDS of phytoconstituents showed better activity in terms of % cell viability against AML and leukemia cell line compared to pure

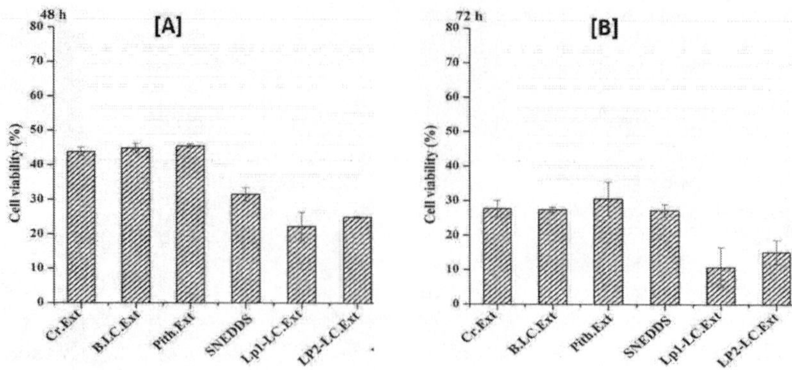

Figure 8.
In-vitro cell line study of plant extracts and PBNDDS of different plant extracts after [A] 48 h and [B] 72 h.

phytoconstituents only. It was also observed that PBNDDS of phytoconstituents showed better activity against specific AML and leukemia cell lines compared to all cell lines used in the study. This is possibly due to more permeability of PBNDDS occurred through those specific cell lines, which suggest that PBNDDS may be selective for specific cancer cell lines which may be related to the phospholipid composition, type and drug delivered through PBNDDS [82]. PBNDDS of different phytoconstituents also exhibited better activity against breast cancer cell line (MCF7) study compared to phytoconstituents in isolation (**Figure 8**).

Significant improvement was observed for *in-vivo* analgesic activity for the PBNDDS of black seed oil containing thymoquinone compared to black seed oil only and control groups. This phenomenon probably related to the improve bioavailability of thymoquinone when delivered through PBNDDS. Previous research study also showed analgesic and anti-inflammatory activity for black seed oil containing thymoquinone [80, 96].

Strong anti-inflammatory activity was observed for different plant extracts and its phytoconstituents against carrageenan induced paw edema (**Table 4**). It was also observed that plant extract and phytoconstituents delivered through PBNDDS exhibit better anti-inflammatory activity, which is possibly due to enhancement of dissolution, bioavailability and stability of phytoconstituents when delivered through PBNDDS [81–83].

Neurobehavioral study of PBNDDS of phytoconstituents was performed using open field, arm maze and water maze studies (**Figure 9**). Marked improvement in locomotor activity, ambulatory performance and memory function of dementia induced mice model was observed for PBNDDS of phytoconstituents compare to disease and plant extract groups [81]. This phenomenon probably related to strong anti-inflammatory along with antioxidant activities observed for the plant extract in different research studies. CNS inflammation is one of the pathway for developing neurodegenerative disorders, therefore by reducing inflammation significantly through PBNDDS of plant phytoconstituents in dementia induced mice model might be an option to treat neurodegenerative disease. Natural phytoconstituents may contain some ingredients which also can be effective against neurodegenerative disease through another mechanism of action which need to be confirmed in future study.

Time	Positive control	*Corchorus olitorius* leaf extract		Extract PBNDDS		Standard	
	Paw volume (ml)	Paw volume (ml)	(%) Reduction	Paw volume (ml)	(%) Reduction	Paw volume (ml)	(%) Reduction
5 h (1 day)	1.95 ± 0.15	1.31 ± 0.24	30.98	1.31 ± 0.35	33.5	0.75 ± 0.08	59.32
2 days	1.74 ± 0.32	1.20 ± 0.30	29.6	0.88 ± 0.34	50	0.20 ± 0.04	88.04
4 days	1.08 ± 0.20	0.45 ± 0.22	55.57	0.30 ± 0.27	79.06	0.14 ± 0.05	89.1
Time	**Positive control**	**Green tea leaf extract**		**Extract PBNDDS**		**Standard**	
	Paw volume (ml)	**Paw volume (ml)**	**(%) Reduction**	**Paw volume (ml)**	**(%) Reduction**	**Paw volume (ml)**	**(%) Reduction**
5 h (1 day)	1.92 ± 0.14	1.40 ± 0.12	25.8	1.80 ± 0.11	7.5	0.78 ± 0.08	59.02
2 days	1.70 ± 0.30	1.05 ± 0.10	37.52	1.35 ± 0.12	21.93	0.34 ± 0.09	80.67
4 days	1.05 ± 0.20	0.48 ± 0.13	52.53	0.51 ± 0.15	67.64	0.12 ± 0.05	88.78
Time	**Positive control**	***A. polystachya* leaf extract**		**Extract PBNDDS**		**Standard**	
	Paw volume (ml)	**Paw volume (ml)**	**(%) Reduction**	**Paw volume (ml)**	**(%) Reduction**	**Paw volume (ml)**	**(%) Reduction**
5 h (1 day)	1.90 ± 0.15	1.12 ± 0.18	39.8	0.62 ± 0.17	68.54	0.76 ± 0.08	61.02
2 days	1.71 ± 0.32	0.90 ± 0.07	46.56	0.34 ± 0.13	80.68	0.37 ± 0.09	79.05
4 days	1.06 ± 0.20	0.63 ± 0.06	40.21	0.08 ± 0.05	92.73	0.12 ± 0.05	88.79

Table 4.
Anti-inflammatory studies of plant extracts, and its PBNDDS (adapted from [81–83]).

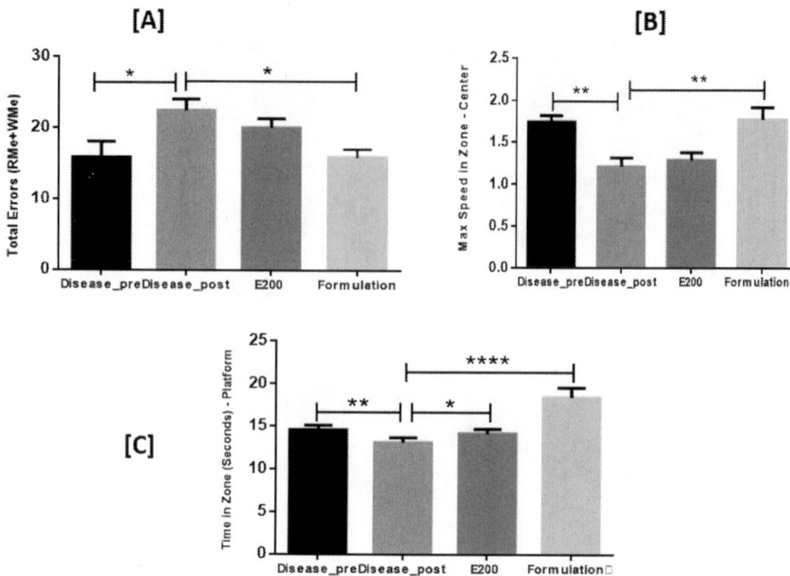

Figure 9.
*[A] Number of total errors for different mouse groups in arm maze study [B] maximum speed into central zone for different mouse groups in open field study [C] time spent on platform for different mice groups in water maze study (where **** means p ≤ 0.0001, **means p ≤ 0.01 and * mean p ≤ 0.05) [four different groups—1. Pre disease group 2. Post disease group 3. E 200 - extract group and 4. Formulation—PBNDDS of extracts] (adapted from [81]).*

11. Conclusion

Plant extract found to have a range of major phytoconstituents which were identified and quantified by UHPLC and GC-MS. Major phytoconstituents emonstrate marked pharmacological activities which were evident by different *in-vitro* and *in-vivo* studies. Phytoconstituents delivered through PBNDDS exhibit better performance compared to phytoconstituents in isolation. It was observed that process parameters and formulation attributes showed significant impact on average size, polydispersity and entrapment or loading of phytoconstituents for PBNDDS. Processing temperature, injection rate, solvent system properties (pH, solubility level), phospholipd concentration related to drug and cholesterol are major factors affecting the quality output of PBNDDS. PBNDDS prepared using egg phospholipid was physico-chemically stable even at ambient conditions (25°C, 60% RH). This phenomenon might be a great advantage for developing PBNDDS of different phytoconstituents for improving the bioavialabilty, stability and targeted drug delivery. PBNDDS also exhibit better selective activity against cancer cell lines which is an indication for treating different types of cancer by developing PBNDDS using different formulation attributes. PBNDDS also showed better analgesic, anti-inflammatory and neurobehavioral activities compared to phytoconstituents only. Therefore PBNDDS can be a promising platform for delivering phytoconstituents with better therapeutic outcome. PBNDDS having average size of <150 nm with ≥85% entrapment or loading might exhibit desirable performance to treat chronic inflammatory disease, cancer, and CNS diseases.

Acknowledgements

This work was funded by National plan of Science, Technology and Innovation (MAARIFAH), King Abdul Aziz city for Science and Technology, Kingdom of Saudi Arabia, Award Number (13NAN929-02).

Conflict of interest

The authors declare no conflict of interest.

References

[1] Singh RP, Gangadharappa HV, Mruthunjaya K. Phospholipids: Unique carriers for drug delivery systems. Journal of Drug Delivery Science and Technology. 2017;**39**:166-179. DOI: 10.1016/j.jddst.2017.03.027

[2] Attama A, A, Momoh MA, Builders PF. Chapter 5: Lipid nanoparticulate drug delivery systems: A revolution in dosage form design and development. In: Sezer AD, editor. Recent Advances in Novel Drug Carrier Systems. InTech; 2012. pp. 107-140. DOI: 10.5772/50486

[3] Rahman HS, Othman HH, Hammadi NI, Yeap SK, Amin KM, Abdul Samad N, et al. Novel drug delivery systems for loading of natural plant extracts and their biomedical applications. International Journal of Nanomedicine. 2020;**15**:2439-2483. DOI: 10.2147/IJN.S227805

[4] Lipid Based Drug Formulation. Northern Lipids Inc; 2008. Available from: http://www.northernlipids.com/ourfacilities.htm [Accessed: April 17, 2012]

[5] Muller RH, Radtke M, Wissing SA. Solid lipid nanoparticles (SLN) and nanostructured lipid carriers (NLC) in cosmetic and dermatological preparations. Advanced Drug Delivery Reviews. 2002;**54**(Suppl. 1):S131-S155

[6] Muller RH. Medicament Vehicle for the Controlled Administration of an Active Agent, Produced from Lipid Matrix-Medicament Conjugates. 2000; WO0067800

[7] Stuchlík M, Žák S. Lipid-based vehicle for oral drug delivery. Biomedical Papers. 2001;**145**(2):17-26

[8] Attama AA, Müller-Goymann CC. Investigation of surface-modified solid lipid nanocontainers formulated with a heterolipid-templated homolipid. International Journal of Pharmaceutics. 2007;**334**(1):179-189

[9] Atmakuri LR. Current trends in herbal medicines. Journal of Pharmacy Research. 2010;**3**:109-113

[10] Bjarnason I, Hayllar J, MacPherson AJ, Russell AS. Side effects of nonsteroidal anti-inflammatory drugs on the small and large intestine in humans. Gastro-enterology. 1993;**104**:1832-1847. DOI: 10.1016/0016-5085(93)90667-2

[11] Zhang YJ, Gan RY, Li S, et al. Antioxidant phytochemicals for the prevention and treatment of chronic diseases. Molecules. 2015;**20**(12):21138-21156. DOI: 10.3390/molecules201219753

[12] Atanasov AG et al. Discovery and resupply of pharmacologically active plant-derived natural products: A review. Biotechnology Advances. 2015;**33**:1582-1614. DOI: 10.1016/j.biotechadv.2015.08.001

[13] Yan JJ et al. Protection against beta-amyloid peptide toxicity in vivo with long-term administration of ferulic acid. British Journal of Pharmacology. 2001;**133**:89-96. DOI: 10.1038/sj.bjp.0704047

[14] de la Puerta R, Forder RA, Hoult JR. Inhibition of leukocyte eicosanoid generation and radical scavenging activity by gnaphalin, a lipophilic flavonol isolated from Helichrysum picardii. Planta Medica. 1999;**65**:507-511. DOI: 10.1055/s-1999-14005

[15] Harborne JB, Baxter H, Webster FX. Phytochemical dictionary: A handbook of bioactive compounds from plants. Journal of Chemical Ecology. 1994;**20**:815-818

[16] Howes MJR, Perry NS, Houghton PJ. Plants with traditional uses and activities, relevant to the management of Alzheimer's disease and other

cognitive disorders. Phytotherapy Research. 2003;**17**:1-18

[17] Perry EK et al. Neocortical cholinergic activities differentiate Lewy body dementia from classical Alzheimer's disease. Neuroreport. 1994;**5**:747-749

[18] Loizzo MR, Tundis R, Menichini F, Menichini F. Natural products and their derivatives as cholinesterase inhibitors in the treatment of neurodegenerative disorders: an update. Current Medicinal Chemistry. 2008;**15**:1209-1228

[19] Ahmad S et al. Chemical composition, antioxidant and anticholinesterase potentials of essential oil of D. Don collected from Rumex hastatus the North West of Pakistan. BMC Complementary & Alternative Medicine. 2016;**16**:29

[20] Rajakrishnan V, Viswanathan P, Rajasekharan K, Menon VP. Neuro-protective role of curcumin from *Curcuma longa* on ethanol-induced brain damage. Phytotherapy Research. 1999; **13**:571-574

[21] Perry N, Court G, Bidet N, Court J, Perry E. European herbs with cholinergic activities: Potential in dementia therapy. International Journal of Geriatric Psychiatry. 1996;**11**:1063-1069

[22] Abdelwahed W, Degobert G, Stainmesse S, Fessi H. Freeze-drying of nanoparticles: Formulation, process and storage considerations. Advanced Drug Delivery Reviews. 2006;**58**(15):1688-1713

[23] Ahmad A, Husain A, Mujeeb M, Khan SA, Najmi AK, Siddique NA, et al. A review on therapeutic potential of Nigella sativa: A miracle herb. Asian Pacific Journal of Tropical Biomedicine. 2013;**3**(5):337-352

[24] Al-Awadi F, Fatania H, Shamte U. The effect of a plant mixture extract on liver gluconeogenesis in streptozotocin-induced diabetic rats. Diabetes Research. 1991;**18**(4):163-168

[25] Al-Ghamdi MS. Anti-inflammatory, analgesic and anti-pyretic activity of Nigella sativa. Journal of Ethno-pharmacology. 2001;**76**(1):45-48

[26] Alijabre SHM, Alakloby OM, Randhawa MA. Dermatological effect of nagellasative. Journal of Dermatology and Dermatologic Surgery. 2015;**19**(2):92-98

[27] Salmani JMM, Asghar S, Lv H, Zhou J. Aqueous solubility and degradation kinetics of the phyto-chemical anticancer thymoquinone; probing the effects of solvents, pH and light. Molecules. 2014;**19**(5):5925-5939

[28] Hand R. Supplementary notes to the flora of Cyprus III. Willdenowia. 2003;**33**:305-325

[29] Işeri OD, Yurtcu E, Sahin FI, Haberal M. *Corchorus olitorius* (jute) extract induced cytotoxicity and genotoxicity on human multiple myeloma cells (ARH-77). Pharmaceutical Biology. 2013;**51**(6):766-770

[30] Das AK, Bag S, Sahu R, Dua TK, Sinha MK, Gangopadhyay M, et al. Protective effect of *Corchorus olitorius* leaves on sodium arsenite-induced toxicity in experimental rats. Food and Chemical Toxicology. 2010;**48**(1):326-335

[31] Al Batran R, Al-Bayaty F, Abdulla MA, Al-Obaidi MM, Hajrezaei M, Hassandarvish P, et al. Gastroprotective effects of *Corchorus olitorius* leaf extract against ethanol-induced gastric mucosal hemorrhagic lesions in rats. Journal of Gastro-enterology and Hepatology. 2013;**28**(8): 1321-1329

[32] Patil DK, Jain AP. In-vivo antidiabetic activity of methanolic extract of *Corchorus olitorius* for the management of type 2 diabetes. Journal of Pharmacognosy and Phytochemistry. 2019;**8**(3):3213-3218

[33] Airaodion AI, Akinmolayan JD, Ogbuagu EO, Airaodion EO, Ogbuagu U,

Awosanya OO. Effect of methanolic extract of corchorus olitorius leaves on hypoglycemic and hypolipidaemic activities in albino rats. Asian Plant Research Journal. 2019;**2**(4):1-13

[34] Soykut G, Becer E, Calis I, Yucecan S, Vatansever H. Apoptotic effects of *Corchorus olitorius* L. leaf extracts in colon adenocarcinoma cell lines. Progress in Food & Nutrition Science. 2018;**20**:689-698

[35] Snigdha HSH, Ali R, Das DK, Wadud MA. Biological evaluation of ethanolic extract of Aphanamixis polystachya (Wall.) Parker leaf. International Journal of Recent Advances in Multidisciplinary Research. 2016;**3**: 13-21

[36] Mishra AP et al. Aphanamixis polystachya (wall.) Parker, phytochemistry, pharmacological properties and medicinal uses: An overview. World Journal of Pharmaceutical Sciences. 2014;**3**: 2242-2252

[37] Apu AS et al. Phytochemical analysis and bioactivities of Aphanamixis polystachya (Wall.) R. Parker leaves from Bangladesh. Journal of Biological Sciences. 2013;**13**:393-399

[38] Krishnaraju AV, Rao CV, Rao TV, Reddy K, Trimurtulu G. In vitro and in vivo antioxidant activity of Aphanamixis polystachya bark. American Journal of Infectious Diseases. 2009;**5**:60-67

[39] Hossain MM, Biva IJ, Jahangir R, Vhuiyan MMI. Central nervous system depressant and analgesic activity of Aphanamixis polystachya (Wall.) parker leaf extract in mice. African Journal of Pharmacy and Pharmacology. 2009;**3**: 282-286

[40] Singh BN, Shankar S, Srivastava RK. Green tea catechin, epigallocatechin-3-gallate (EGCG): Mechanisms, perspectives and clinical applications. Biochemical Pharmacology. 2011;**82**:1807-1821. DOI: 10.1016/j.bcp.2011.07.093

[41] Prasanth MI, Sivamaruthi BS, Chaiyasut C, Tencomnao T. A review of the role of green tea (*Camellia sinensis*) in antiphotoaging, stress resistance, neuroprotection, and autophagy. Nutrients. 2019;**11**:474. DOI: 10.3390/nu11020474

[42] Crespy V, Williamson G. A review of the health effects of green tea catechins in in vivo animal models. The Journal of Nutrition. 2004;**134**:3431S-3440S. DOI: 10.1093/jn/134.12.3431s

[43] Conney AH, Lu YP, Lou YR, Xie JG, Huang MT. Inhibitory effect of green and black tea on tumor growth. Experimental Biology and Medicine. 1999;**220**:229-233. DOI: 10.3181/00379727-220-44371

[44] Mantena SK, Meeran SM, Elmets CA, Katiyar SK. Orally administered green tea polyphenols prevent ultraviolet radiation-induced skin cancer in mice through activation of cytotoxic T cells and inhibition of angiogenesis in tumors. The Journal of Nutrition. 2005;**135**:2871-2877. DOI: 10.1093/jn/135.12.2871

[45] Yokozawa T, Nakagawa T, Kitani K. Antioxidative activity of green tea polyphenol in cholesterol-fed rats. Journal of Agricultural and Food Chemistry. 2002;**50**:3549-3552. DOI: 10.1021/jf020029h

[46] Murase T, Nagasawa A, Suzuki J, Hase T, Tokimitsu I. Beneficial effects of tea catechins on dietinduced obesity: Stimulation of lipid catabolism in the liver. International Journal of Obesity and Related Metabolic Disorders. 2002; **26**:1459-1464

[47] Patel AR, Seijen-ten-Hoorn J, Velikov KP. Colloidal complexes from associated water soluble cellulose

derivative (methylcellulose) and green tea polyphenol (*Epigallocatechin gallate*). Journal of Colloid and Interface Science. 2011;**364**(2):317-323

[48] Cai ZY, Li XM, Liang JP, Xiang LP, Wang KR, Shi YL, et al. Bioavailability of tea catechins and its improvement. Molecules. 2018;**23**:2346. DOI: 10.3390/molecules23092346

[49] Amin T, Bhat SV. A review on phytosome technology as a novel approach to improve the bioavailability of nutraceuticals. International Journal of Advanced Research in Science and Technology. 2012;**1**:1-5

[50] Musthaba SM, Baboota S, Ahmed S, Ahuja A, Ali J. Status of novel drug delivery technology for phyto-therapeutics. Expert Opinion in Drug Delivery. 2009;**6**:625-637

[51] Bonifacio BV et al. Nanotechnology-based drug delivery systems and herbal medicines: A review. International Journal of Nanomedicine. 2014;**9**:1

[52] Saraf AS. Applications of novel drug delivery system for herbal formulations. Fitoterapia. 2010;**81**:680-689

[53] Li S et al. Catanionic lipid nanosystems improve pharmacokinetics and anti-lung cancer activity of curcumin. Nanomedicine. 2016;**12**:1567-1579

[54] Bansal SS, Goel M, Aqil F, Vadhanam MV, Gupta RC. Advanced drug delivery systems of curcumin for cancer chemoprevention. Cancer Prevention Research. 2011;**4**:1158-1171

[55] Fonseca-Santos B, MPD G, Chorilli M. Nanotechnology-based drug delivery systems for the treatment of Alzheimer's disease. International Journal of Nanomedicine. 2015;**10**:4981-5003

[56] Odeh F, Ismail SI, Abu-Dahab R, Mahmoud IS, Al BA. Thymoquinone in liposomes: A study of loading efficiency and biological activity towards breast cancer. Drug Delivery. 2012;**19**(8):371-377. DOI: 10.3109/10717544.2012.727500

[57] Ravindran J, Nair HB, Sung B, Prasad S, Tekmal RR, Aggarwal BB. Thymoquinone poly (lactide-co-glycolide) nanoparticles exhibit enhanced anti-proliferative, anti-inflammatory, and chemosensitization potential. Biochemical Pharmacology. 2010;**79**(11):1640-1647. DOI: 10.1016/j.bcp.2010.01.023

[58] Fahmy HM, Fathy MM, Abd-elbadia RA, Elshemey WM. Targeting of Thymoquinone-loaded mesoporous silica nanoparticles to different brain areas: In vivo study. Life Sciences. 2019;**222**:94-102

[59] Azad AK, Al-Mahmood SMA, Chatterjee B, Wan Sulaiman WMA, Elsayed TM, Doolaanea AA. Encapsulation of black seed oil in alginate beads as a pH-sensitive carrier for intestine-targeted drug delivery: In vitro, in vivo and ex vivo study. Pharmaceutics. 2020;**12**(3):219

[60] Sathya S, Shanmuganathan B, Saranya S, Vaidevi S, Ruckmani K, Devi KP. Phytol-loaded PLGA nanoparticle as a modulator of Alzheimer's toxic Aβ peptide aggregation and fibrillation associated with impaired neuronal cell function. Artificial Cells Nanomedicine and Biotechnology. 2018;**46**(8):1719-1730

[61] Ismail EH, Saqer AMA, Assirey E, Naqvi A, Okasha RM. Successful green synthesis of gold nanoparticles using a *Corchorus olitorius* extract and their antiproliferative effect in cancer cells. International Journal of Molecular Sciences. 2018;**19**(9)

[62] Azeez L, Lateef A, Wahab AA, Rufai MA, Salau AK, Ajayi EIO, et al. Phytomodulatory effects of silver nanoparticles on Corchorus olitorius: Its

antiphytopathogenic and hepato-protective potentials. Plant Physiology and Biochemistry. 2019;**136**:109-117

[63] Zhang J, Nie S, Wang S. Nanoencapsulation enhances epigallocatechin-3-gallate stability and its antiatherogenic bioactivities in macrophages. Journal of Agricultural and Food Chemistry. 2013;**61**:9200-9209. DOI: 10.1021/jf4023004

[64] Dube A, Nicolazzo JA, Larson I. Chitosan nanoparticles enhance the intestinal absorption of the green tea catechins (+)-catechin and (−)-epigallocatechin gallate. European Journal of Pharmaceutical Sciences. 2010;**41**:219-225. DOI: 10.1016/j.ejps.2010.06.010

[65] Hu B, Ting Y, Yang X, Tang W, Zeng X, Huang Q. Nanochemoprevention by encapsulation of (−)-epigallocatechin-3-gallate with bioactive peptides/chitosan nanoparticles for enhancement of its bioavailability. Chemical Communications. 2012;**48**:2421-2423. DOI: 10.1039/c2cc17295j

[66] Smith A, Giunta B, Bickford PC, Fountain M, Tan J, Shytle RD. Nanolipidic particles improve the bioavailability and α-secretase inducing ability of epigallocatechin-3-gallate (EGCG) for the treatment of Alzheimer's disease. International Journal of Pharmaceutics. 2010;**389**:207-212. DOI: 10.1016/j.ijpharm.2010.01.012

[67] Song Q, Li D, Zhou Y, Yang J, Yang W, Zhou G, et al. Enhanced uptake and transport of (+)-catechin and (−)-epigallocatechin gallate in niosomal formulation by human intestinal Caco-2 cells. International Journal of Nanomedicine. 2014;**9**:2157-2165. DOI: 10.2147/ijn.s59331

[68] Yeh MK, Chen CC, Hsieh DS, Huang KJ, Chan YL, Hong PD, et al. Improving anticancer efficacy of (−)-epigallocatechin-3-gallate gold nanoparticles in murine B16F10 melanoma cells. Drug Design, Development and Therapy. 2014;**8**:459-474. DOI: 10.2147/dddt.s58414

[69] Lambert JD, Sang S, Hong J, Kwon SJ, Lee MJ, Ho CT, et al. Peracetylation as a means of enhancing in vitro bioactivity and bioavailability of epigallocatechin-3-gallate. Drug Metabolism and Disposition. 2006;**34**:2111-2116. DOI: 10.1124/dmd.106.011460

[70] Schnyder A, Huwyler J. Drug transport to brain with targeted liposomes. NeuroRx. 2005;**2**(1):99-107. DOI: 10.1602/neurorx.2.1.99

[71] Li C, Zhang Y, Su T, Feng L, Long Y, Chen Z. Silica coated flexible liposomes as a nanohybrid delivery system for enhanced oral bioavailability of curcumin. International Journal of Nanomedicine. 2012;7:5995-6002. DOI: 10.2147/IJN.S38043

[72] Kesarwani K, Gupta R. Bioavailability enhancers of herbal origin: An overview. Asian Pacific Journal of Tropical Biomedicine. 2013;**3**:253-266

[73] Akbarzadeh A et al. Liposome: classification, preparation, and applications. Nanoscale Research Letters. 2013;**8**:102

[74] Sułkowski W, Pentak D, Nowak K, Sułkowska A. The influence of temperature, cholesterol content and pH on liposome stability. Journal of Molecular Structure. 2005;**744**:737-747

[75] Manach C, Scalbert A, Morand C, Rémésy C, Jiménez L. Polyphenols: Food sources and bioavailability. The American Journal of Clinical Nutrition. 2004;**79**:727-747. DOI: 10.1093/ajcn/79.5.727

[76] Scalbert A, Williamson G. Dietary intake and bioavailability of polyphenols. The Journal of Nutrition. 2000;**130**:2073S-2085S. DOI: 10.1093/jn/130.8.2073s

[77] Kidd P, Head K. A review of the bioavailability and clinical efficacy of milk thistle phytosome: A silybin-phosphatidylcholine complex (Siliphos). Alternative Medicine Review. 2005;**10**:193-203

[78] Semalty A, Semalty M, Rawat MSM, Franceschi F. Supramolecular phospholipids–polyphenolics interactions: The PHYTOSOME® strategy to improve the bioavailability of phytochemicals. Fitoterapia. 2010;**81**:306-314. DOI: 10.1016/j.fitote.2009.11.001

[79] Pietta PG, Simonetti P, Gardana C, Brusamolino A, Morazzoni P, Bombardelli E. Relationshipbetween rate and extent of catechin absorption and plasma antioxidant status. Biochemistry and Molecular Biology International. 1998;**46**:895-903. DOI: 10.1080/15216549800204442

[80] Rushmi ZT, Akter N, Mow RJ, Afroz M, Kazi M, de Matas M, et al. The impact of formulation attributes and process parameters on black seed oil loaded liposomes and their performance in animal models of analgesia. Saudi Pharm Journal. 2017;**25**(3):404-412. DOI: 10.1016/j.jsps.2016.09.011

[81] Shariare MH, Rahman M, Lubna SR, et al. Liposomal drug delivery of Aphanamixis polystachya leaf extracts and its neurobehavioral activity in mice model. Scientific Reports. 2020;**10**:6938. DOI: 10.1038/s41598-020-63894-9

[82] Shariare MH, Noor HB, Khan JH, Uddin J, Ahamad SR, Altamimi MA, et al. Liposomal drug delivery of Corchorus olitorius leaf extract containing phytol using design of experiment (DoE): In-vitro anticancer and in-vivo anti-inflammatory studies. Colloids and Surfaces B: Biointerfaces. 2021;**199**: 111543

[83] Shariare MH, Afnan K, Iqbal F, Altamimi MA, Ahamad SR, Aldughaim MS, et al. Development and optimization of epigallocatechin-3-gallate (egcg) nano phytosome using design of experiment (DoE) and their in vivo anti-inflammatory studies. Molecules. 2020;**25**(22):5453. DOI: 10.3390/molecules25225453

[84] Jiang Z, Jacob JA, Loganathachetti DS, Nainangu P, Chen B. β-Elemene: Mechanistic studies on cancer cell interaction and its chemosensitization effect. Frontiers in Pharmacology. 2017;**8**:105

[85] Liu J et al. β-Elemene-induced autophagy protects human gastric cancer cells from undergoing apoptosis. BMC Cancer. 2011;**11**:183

[86] Zhang Y et al. The role of E3 ubiquitin ligase Cbl proteins in β-elemene reversing multi-drug resistance of human gastric adenocarcinoma cells. International Journal of Molecular Sciences. 2013;**14**:10075-10089

[87] Zhong Y et al. β-Elemene reduces the progression of atherosclerosis in rabbits. Chinese Journal of Natural Medicines. 2015;**13**:415-420

[88] Meng X et al. Beneficial effect of β-elemene alone and in combination with hyperbaric oxygen in traumatic brain injury by inflammatory pathway. Translational Neuroscience. 2018;**9**:33-37

[89] Kinney JW et al. Inflammation as a central mechanism in Alzheimer's disease. Alzheimer's Dementia. 2018;**4**:575-590

[90] Hertz L, Chen Y, Waagepetersen HS. Effects of ketone bodies in Alzheimer's disease in relation to neural hypo-metabolism, β-amyloid toxicity, and astrocyte function. Journal of Neurochemistry. 2015;**134**:7-20

[91] Chen H et al. Hydroxycarboxylic acid receptor 2 mediates dimethyl fumarate's protective effect in EAE. Journal of Clinical Investigation. 2014;**124**:2188-2192

[92] Rahman M et al. The β-hydroxybutyrate receptor HCA 2 activates a neuroprotective subset of macrophages. Nature Communications. 2014;**5**:1-11

[93] Song J, Shi F, Zhang Z, Zhu F, Xue J, Tan X, et al. Formulation and evaluation of celastrol-loaded liposomes. Molecules. 2011;**16**:7880-7892. DOI: 10.3390/molecules16097880

[94] Laouini A, Charcosset C, Holdich RG, Vladisavljevic GT. Preparation of liposomes: A novel application of microengineered membranes-investigation of the process parameters and application to the encapsulation of vitamin E. RSC Advances. 2013;**3**(15):4985-4994

[95] Khan D, Rezler E, Lauer J, Fields G. Effects of drug hydrophobicity on liposomal stability. Chemical Biology & Drug Design. 2008;**71**:3-7. DOI: 10.1111/j.1747-0285.2007.00610.x

[96] Hajhashemi V, Ghannadi A, Jafarabadi H. Black cumin seed essential oil, as a potent analgesic and anti-inflammatory drug. Phytotherapy Research: PTR. 2004;**18**:195-199

Chapter 5

Aliphatic Polyester Nanoparticles for Drug Delivery Systems

Abstract

Drug delivery systems using aliphatic polyester nanoparticles are usually prepared via an emulsion process. These nanoparticles can control drug release and improve pharmacokinetics. Aliphatic polyesters are linear polymers containing ester linkages, showing sensitivity to hydrolytic degradation. The byproducts then promote autocatalytic degradation. These byproducts could enter the Krebs cycle and be eliminated from the body, resulting in the high biocompatibility of these nanoparticles. The properties of these polyesters are linked to the drug release rate due to biodegradation, i.e., polymer crystallinity, glass transition temperature, polymer hydrophobicity, and molecular weight (MW), all of which relatively influence hydrolysis. Mathematical equations have been used to study the factors and mechanisms that affect drug dissolution compared to experimental release data. The equations used as models for predicting the kinetics of drug release include the *zero-order*, *first-order*, *Higuchi*, *Hixson-Crowell*, and *Korsmeyer-Peppas* equations. Aliphatic polyester-based controlled drug delivery has surrounded much of the current activity in the estimation parameters of nanoparticles and stimulated additional research. Polymeric nanoparticles have potential in a wide range of applications, such as in biotechnology, vaccine systems, and the pharmaceutical industry. The main goal of this chapter is to discuss aliphatic polyester nanoparticles as drug carrier systems.

Keywords: aliphatic polyester, nanoparticles, emulsion, drug release kinetics, drug delivery systems

1. Introduction

Our inspiration for the examples contained within this chapter comes from our direct experience. Chumnanvej et al. retrospectively investigated the clinical outcomes of patients treated after ruptured cerebral arteriovenous malformation (AVM) admitted to Ramathibodi Hospital, Thailand. The results showed that approximately 50% and 7% of cases had symptoms of intracranial hemorrhage and hemorrhage associated with aneurysms, respectively [1]. A subarachnoid hemorrhage (SAH) is a hemorrhage that occurs in the subarachnoid space and leads to rupture. After cerebral surgery, these patients carry the risk of developing vasospasms within 4–14 days after surgery, with the peak occurring at 7 days [2]. Vasospasms can result from a reduction in the rapid release of blood escape from the cerebrum. Nicardipine hydrochloride (NCH) is a calcium channel blocker that is used to treat this vascular condition; nevertheless, the half-life of NCH is approximately 8 h and provides an insufficient dose to treat vasospasms.

From a biomedical engineering point of view, polymers can be employed, particularly in neurosurgery, as surgical sutures, vascular grafts, stents, implants, tissue substitutes, or drug delivery systems. Additionally, these polymers could be biopolymers. Polymers must have the required physical properties and also be biocompatible for their intended purpose. Biopolymers are biocompatible polymeric materials that could be appropriate for treating certain neurosurgical complications. Biopolymers can respond to both the physiological and biological environments, and the kind of response is the main characteristic that determines whether the biopolymer should be used to construct biomedical devices or be applied in advanced neurosurgical applications. To our knowledge, there are three classifications of biopolymer medical-associated applications: (i) synthetic polymers, (ii) tissue engineering, and (iii) controlled-release agents. For cerebrovascular surgery applications, biopolymers have been applied to create new types of responsive delivery systems. This kind of polymer is needed to treat certain complications during cerebrovascular surgery, such as cerebrovascular spasms. When polymers are fabricated as controlled-release agents, they must have the appropriate mechanical characteristics that are suitable for use as drug delivery agents to treat vasospasms [3–5].

Due to the short biological half-life of NCH, we were able to modify the NCH pharmacokinetics via carboxymethyl cellulose/poly(D,L-lactide-co-glycolide) (NCH-CMC/PLGA) nanoparticles using a contemporary emulsion process [6]. PLGA is an aliphatic polyester with hydrophobic properties that is highly biocompatible and biodegradable. The insolubility of PLGA was improved by the addition of CMC to increase the hydrophilicity of these nanoparticles to enhance the therapeutic index. These nanoparticles gave rise to a new drug delivery system that was capable of solving some of the major bottlenecks of the NCH-PLGA microparticles prepared by the double emulsion process in our previous research [7]. The NCH-CMC/PLGA nanoparticles were flexibly designed to protect the developed delivery system against the drug degradation observed in the absence of a delivery system and improve the insufficient drug release during the first 6 days of microparticle treatment. These nanoparticles had a rate of drug release and a daily dose that was sufficient to treat vasoconstriction during the 4–14 days that this condition could occur. The results demonstrated that the designed aliphatic polyester nanoparticles had wide application prospects in drug delivery systems. These polymeric nanoparticles could release drugs on demand and are easily customized depending on the desired application. Potentially, these same nanoparticles could be extended to many fields and fulfill the different purposes of delivery systems; for example, in the food, pharmaceutical, cosmetics, biotechnology, and sustainable agriculture industries. Consequently, this chapter focuses mainly on describing the core characteristics of aliphatic polyester nanoparticles fabricated using an emulsion process.

2. Aliphatic polyesters

Currently, biodegradable polymers are utilized as a component of drug delivery systems. There are a large number of literature reports that have studied aliphatic polyesters, and their high biocompatibility and biodegradability potential has been demonstrated. Most of these polyesters have been approved for use as drug delivery devices by the Food and Drug Administration (FDA) [8]. Among these studies, aliphatic polyesters have been used to circumvent several major challenges that occur during drug delivery applications. In the 1960s, these polymers were initially used with drug delivery systems to control drug release [9]. They can improve pharmacokinetics by maintaining the concentration of the drug at a therapeutic level and minimizing side effects.

Aliphatic polyesters are linear polymers with repeating units formed through ester linkages (R_1–COO–R_2). They are classified into two types according to the structure of their repeating units, poly(alkylene dicarboxylate)s and poly(hydroxy acid)s, as summarized in **Figure 1**. Poly(alkylene dicarboxylate)s consists of two types of repeating units between succinic acid (HOOC–$(CH_2)_2$–COOH) and alkanediol (HO–R–OH) and are prepared by esterification [10, 11]. Examples include poly(eth ylene succinate) (PES), poly(butylene succinate) (PBS), and poly(butylene succinate-co-butylene adipate) (PBSA). Additionally, poly(hydroxy acid)s are aliphatic polyesters that have hydroxy acid (HO–R–COOH) repeating units that consist of carboxylic acid (–COOH) and hydroxyl (–OH) groups. These polymers can be further classified according to the bonding position of the hydroxyl group (α, β, or ω) in the polymer chain. As a result, these hydroxy acids containing hydroxyl groups can be classified as poly(α-hydroxy acid)s, poly (β-hydroxyalkanoate)s, and poly(ω-hydroxyalkanoate)s.

Poly(α-hydroxy acid)s have a hydroxyl group attached to the α-carbon (or first carbon) atom bonded to the carboxylic acid. Poly(lactide) (PLA) and poly(glycolide) (PGA) are members of the poly(α-hydroxy acid) family with repeating lactic acid and glycolic acid units, respectively. PLA has three stereoisomers: poly(L-lactide) (PLLA), poly(D-lactide) (PDLA), and poly(D,L-lactide) (PDLLA). Furthermore, poly(D,L-lactide-co-glycolide) (PLGA), another member of this family, is formed from a block copolymer containing both PDLLA and PGA [10, 12, 13]. Poly(β-hydroxyalkanoate) has a hydroxyl group bonded to the β-carbon of the carboxylic acid, which is the carbon atom next to the α-carbon.

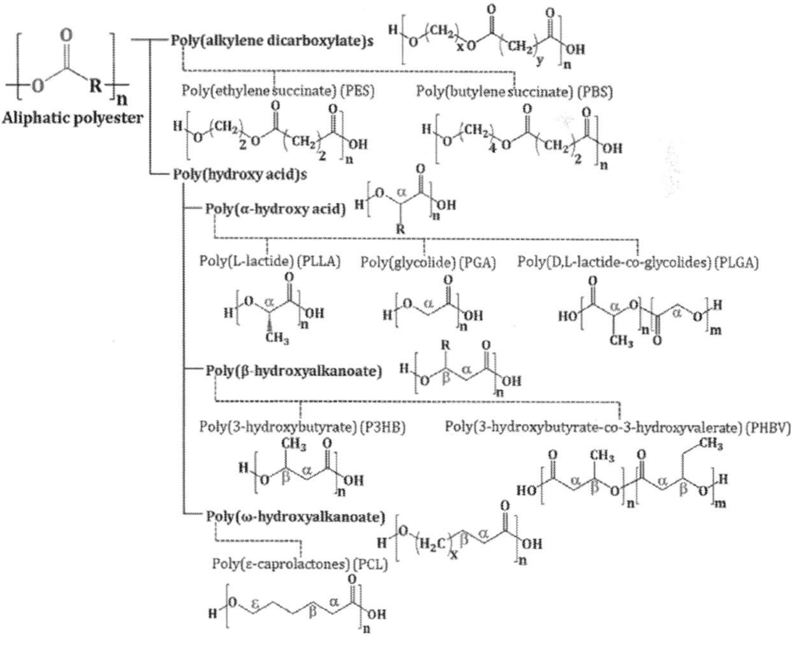

Figure 1.
Classification and examples of aliphatic polyesters [10].

This family includes poly(hydroxyalkanoate), i.e., poly(3-hydroxybutyrate) (P3HB), poly(3-hydroxyvalerate) (P3HV) and poly(3-hydroxybutyrate-co-3-hydroxyvalerate) (PHBV), etc. Additionally, hydroxyl groups attached to a carbon that is three or more carbon atoms away from the carbonyl are poly(ω-hydroxyalkanoate)s, such as poly(ε-caprolactones) (PCL) [10, 13]. The ester linkages of these polymers can be degraded under physiological conditions, and their degradation products are nontoxic to human connective tissue.

2.1 Biodegradation and biocompatibility of aliphatic polyesters

The ester linkages of aliphatic polyesters are sensitive to hydrolytic attacks in aqueous media. The water molecules break down the long polymer chains into small molecules with increased water solubility. Alternatively, aliphatic polyesters degraded via enzymatic hydrolysis have been reported. Esterase and lipase are important hydrolytic enzymes that can cleave the internal ester bonds of these polyesters. In addition to both of these enzymes, proteases can degrade the members of the poly(α-hydroxy acid) family as a result of the α-ester linkages in their backbone [14]. These degradation products (i.e., PLA, PGA, and PLGA) can enter the Krebs cycle and be eliminated from the body as carbon dioxide (CO_2) and water, resulting in the high biocompatibility of aliphatic polyesters [12]. **Figure 2** shows the biodegradation mechanism in which these polyesters are converted into carbon dioxide and water.

The hydrolysis of polyesters happens in three stages. During the first stage, water is absorbed onto the exterior surface and matrix swelling and polymer chain transfer occur. This absorption results from the hydrophobic properties of aliphatic polyesters and leads to surface erosion. In the next stage, an amorphous region becomes swollen followed by stress relaxation of the polymer chain [6]. Next, the matrix can absorb additional water molecules via a diffusion mechanism that leads to the hydrolysis of the polymeric chains in the matrix, creating matrix porosity. After the final stage, the hydrolysis products are acid derivatives (R–COOH), which are catalyzed by acids that trigger polyester hydrolysis. The parent derivatives can cause dissociation of the carboxyl end groups into their conjugate carboxylate anions ($R{-}COO^-$) also forming the acidic proton (H^+) byproducts. The acid produced catalyzes the hydrolytic reaction, generating additional acid. Continuous mass loss occurs via the formation of these fresh acids, resulting in the autocatalytic degradation of the polyester. Moreover, the addition of acidic compounds (i.e., drugs or additives) and environmental pH can modify the rate of polymer degradation for catalytic hydrolysis [15, 16].

An example of the above process is that of PLGA degradation. Synthesized PLGA has two different structures, as it can be acid-terminated or ester-terminated. Acid-terminated PLGA and ester-terminated PLGA have end-group structures of carboxylic acids (PLGA–COOH) and esters ($PLGA{-}COOCH_3$), respectively. End group functionalization causes differences in PLGA biodegradation.

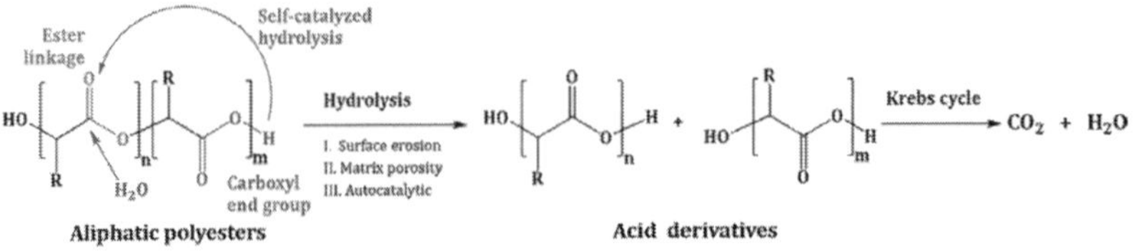

Figure 2.
Hydrolytic degradation of aliphatic polyesters.

Acid-terminated PLGA is degraded rapidly in comparison with the more hydrophobic ester-terminated PLGA. Carboxylic end-capped PLGA can be used as an acid to initiate autocatalytic degradation; thus, these acids have been applied to catalyze acid hydrolysis and promote autocatalytic degradation. Therefore, acid-terminated PLGA hydrolyzes the ester linkages more easily than ester-terminated PLGA as a result of the carboxylic end groups that are capable of producing acidic byproducts, as shown in **Figure 3** [17].

Furthermore, the rate of degradation of PLGA is dependent on the PDLLA:PGA ratio as determined by the weight percentages of PDLLA and PGA, such as 50:50, 65:35, 75:25, and 95:5. The decelerated degradation of PLGA occurs at a high amount of PDLLA, whereas a higher amount of PGA indicates rapid degradation. PDLLA, with methyl groups in its structure, has reduced chain mobility (chain configuration), leading to more hydrophobicity than PGA, which is devoid of these methyl groups (**Figure 1**). PGA is a highly hydrophilic polymer that can absorb more water molecules [6, 13]. Thus, PGA hydrolysis is more complimentary than PDLLA hydrolysis. As a rule, the drug release of PLGA is affected by the biodegradation of PDLLA and PGA. A 50:50 ratio of PDLLA:PGA has been shown to prompt degradation and produce higher rates of drug release [18, 19].

2.2 The properties of aliphatic polyesters properties in delivery systems

Following an earlier example, these differences in chemical structure illustrate how the changes in the physicochemical properties of the polymers are linked to the drug release rate via aliphatic polyester biodegradation. The biodegradation characteristics are controlled by polymer crystallinity, glass transition temperature (T_g), polymer hydrophobicity, and molecular weight (MW), all of which influence hydrolysis.

2.2.1 Polymer crystallinity

The crystalline regions of polymers consist of regular and orderly arranged polymeric chains that result in nanoparticles with high drug-loading abilities. Highly crystalline polymers present difficult mass transfer of both water and drug molecules. Water molecules are strongly absorbed and restricted within the

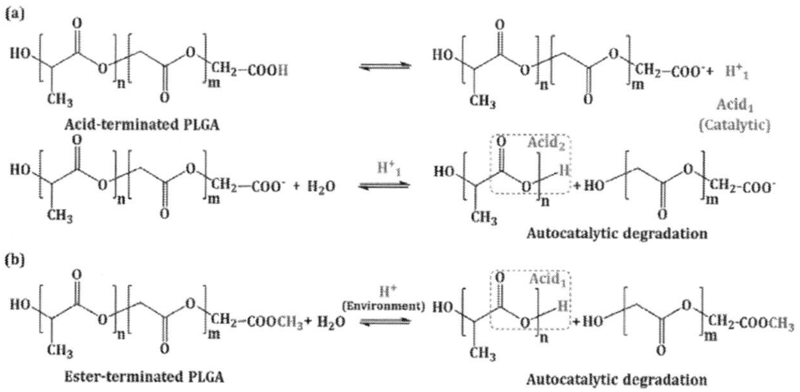

Figure 3.
Proposed hydrolysis reactions of acid-terminated PLGA (a) and ester-terminated PLGA (b) by autocatalytic degradation.

orderly polymeric chains of the crystalline regions, leading to a lower swelling rate. Crystalline polymer regions are resistant to hydrolysis compared to amorphous regions [16, 20]. As a result, the crystalline regions display delayed degradation. The byproducts of later hydrolysis still contain a very large number of high MW compounds in the polymer in the matrix, resulting in a high degree of chain entanglement. Polymer chain entanglement has an important effect on the drug release rate. High amounts of entanglement cause the drug release rate to be slower than that of highly disordered amorphous polymer materials.

2.2.2 T_g

The T_g value may impact the kinetics of drug release from delivery systems. For instance, PLGA micro/nanoparticles were prepared via the emulsion solvent evaporation method [6, 7, 21–23]. The residual solvent was removed via evaporation to harden the nanoparticles. Solvent evaporation promotes the transition to the glassy state from the rubbery state, as observed by hardening. As a result, the removal of solvents is comparable to the glass transition caused by reducing the temperature below T_g. Additionally, drug loading in micro/nanoparticles can decrease T_g through plasticizing effects. Increased drug loading leads to drug dispersion throughout the polymeric matrix, which increases the distance between polymeric chains. This causes the free volume to increase and reduces the T_g of the polymer [23]. The formation of glassy PLGA affects delivery systems by, for example, lowering the elastic modulus and transfer rates of water and the drug molecules and slowing the degradation and drug release rates. In comparison, the formation of the rubbery state facilitates higher mass transfer rates, and a higher elastic modulus leads to faster degradation and drug release rates.

2.2.3 Polymer hydrophobicity

The hydrophobicity of aliphatic polyesters is key to their hydrolytic degradation. When aliphatic polyesters are more hydrophobic, they are less water-sensitive and less susceptible to ester linkage hydrolysis than more hydrophilic polyesters. This causes a decrease in nanoparticle swelling, which results from the low water uptake. These polymers have high hydrolytic resistance and a slower degradation rate. Additionally, a large number of entanglements causes a slower release rate.

2.2.4 Polymer MW

The MW of a polymer is the molecular mass of its polymeric chains and affects the delivery system properties. High MW polymers have a large amount of chain entanglement and low chain mobility. Compared with low MW polymers, high MW polymers show the benefits of lower mass transfer rates, a lower swelling rate, a lower elastic modulus, and reduced solubility. Low MW polymers have a reduced number of polymeric chain entanglements, leading to greater molecular mobility. Water molecules can be comfortably absorbed in the polymeric matrix of these low MW polymers, resulting in faster hydrolytic degradation and a faster drug release rate.

3. Polymeric nanoparticle drug delivery systems

Nanoparticles in drug delivery systems normally have sizes ranging from 1 to 1000 nm. In essence, nanoparticles with sizes in this range have a high surface area to volume ratio and their behavior in the body could cause increases in the absorption potential and cytotoxicity as the expanded surface is proportional to cytotoxicity [24]; thus, these nanoparticles could potentially lead to an increase in cytotoxicity. Nevertheless, nanoparticles prepared from aliphatic polyesters could possibly lead to a reduction in cytotoxicity, as they are highly biocompatible and biodegradable. Aliphatic polyester nanoparticles play key roles in improving the pharmacokinetics, drug bioavailability, specific delivery at the site of action, and stability in the bloodstream. Their high surface area can adsorb drug molecules and encapsulate a large number of drugs in their matrix, effectively carrying drugs, proteins, DNA, and organs. Therefore, the development of aliphatic polyester nanoparticles is one of the most successful ideas for drug delivery innovation.

3.1 Polymeric nanoparticles

Polymeric nanoparticle delivery systems refer to both nanospheres and nanocapsules. Their classification is based on the positional characteristics of the drugs and polymers, as shown schematically in **Figure 4a** and **b.** Nanospheres contain drug molecules within a uniformly dispersed polymeric matrix, while nanocapsules entrap the drug molecules inside their core, a cavity surrounded by a polymeric membrane that acts as a shell [25].

Regarding the molecular orientation surface, we propose a possible schematic of the polyester chain on the nanoparticle surface as shown in **Figure 4**. In the case of PLGA nanospheres, the polymeric chains ignore water molecules, which is consistent with computational simulation results that demonstrated that PLGA is strictly hydrophobic [26]. At both the surface and interface, the carbon backbones clump together rather than being distributed in the aqueous solution. This causes the hydrophobic molecules to have minimal contact with hydrophilic molecules. On the other hand, the oxygen atoms of the hydroxyl groups (–OH), carboxylic acids (–COOH), and ester groups (–COO–) interact with the water molecules residing near the water-PLGA interface, and the hydrogen atoms in the polymer chain resemble the oxygen atoms. Hydrophobic drugs display the tendency to accumulate

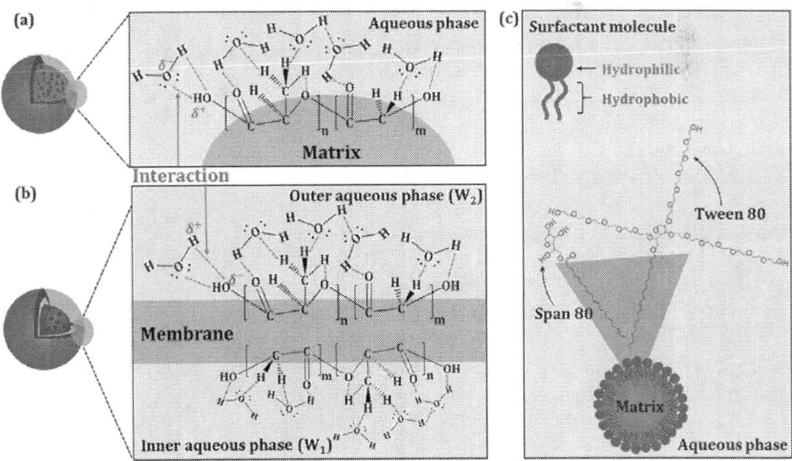

Figure 4.
Schematic representation of the structures and molecular orientations of PLGA nanospheres (a), PLGA nanocapsules (b), and the packing of emulsifiers (Span 80 and Tween 80) at the interface of the dispersed polymer droplets (c).

on the surface, with a few drug molecules migrating to the core, leading to the uniform distribution of drug molecules within the polymeric matrix, especially in the vicinity of the nanosphere surface (**Figure 4a**). The nanocapsules have contact with both the inner and outer aqueous solutions. Thus, the molecular orientation of aliphatic polyesters on the inner and outer membrane surfaces corresponded to nanospheres. Nevertheless, the hydrophilic drugs tend to be entrapped inside the core of a cavity surrounded by the polymeric membrane due to the insolubility between the drug and the polymer (**Figure 4b**).

3.2 Polymeric nanoparticle preparation

The preparation of nanospheres and nanocapsules follows an uncomplicated basic principle, the emulsification solvent evaporation method. The guiding principles are that the drug and polymer dissolve in each other during nanosphere preparation. As a result, the drug molecules are uniformly distributed in the polymeric matrix. Examples of hydrophobic drugs with hydrophobic polymers were previously discussed in the section on nanosphere molecular orientation. However, nanocapsules are prepared from drugs and polymers that are essentially insoluble in each other. This property promotes the formation of core-shell structures to load drugs.

The preparation of both types of nanoparticles depends upon drug solubility and polymer solubility. Therefore, drug solubility is a strict limitation in the use of aliphatic polyesters, as drug solubility affects the type of nanoparticles that can be prepared because polyesters are hydrophobic polymers. This indicates that the use of water-soluble drugs could produce nanocapsules, but insoluble drugs yield nanospheres. In addition to drug solubility, nanoparticles of aliphatic polyesters can be easily prepared. This section describes the preparation of nanoparticles via emulsification methods for these polyester-controlled drug delivery systems.

3.2.1 Single emulsion method

Oil-in-water emulsification (O/W emulsion) can be used to prepare nanospheres that are ideal for entrapping hydrophobic drugs (i.e., steroids) [19] or water-soluble drugs entrapped on nanosphere surfaces [27]. Examples include amoxicillin-loaded PCL micro/nanospheres modified surface by chitosan for antibacterial applications. The amino groups ($-NH_3^+$) of chitosan interact with PCL via carboxylate anions ($-COO^-$) on the micro/nanosphere surface. Amoxicillin is encapsulated by the electrostatic interactions between the negative charges of the drug and the residual positive charge on the surface of chitosan, as observed by the zeta potential values of −20.03 mV and +53.93 mV, respectively. This study varied the ratios of PCL:chitosan to be 1:1, 1:3, and 1:5, and the results showed that increasing the ratio improved the encapsulation efficiency (~73–83%) and controlled drug release (~5.76–6.56 mg) over 7 days compared to amoxicillin-loaded PCL micro/nanospheres, which showed rapid drug release within 12 h due to the low encapsulation efficiency (~5.4%). Additionally, the amoxicillin-loaded PCL micro/nanosphere modification inhibited microbial growth, but the chitosan-free micro/nanospheres were less effective [27].

3.2.2 Double emulsion method

Water-in-oil-in-water ($W_1/O/W_2$) double emulsions could be used to prepare nanocapsules for the loading of water-soluble molecules, such as hydrophilic drugs, proteins, peptides, and vaccines [19]. This system is an extraordinarily complex dispersion system of liquid membranes. In addition, the contemporary $W_1/O/W_2$ double emulsion method led to the preparation of PLGA nanocapsules. This emulsion method can enhance the solubility of poorly soluble drugs in the medium. As mentioned previously in the introduction, we prepared NCH-CMC/PLGA nanocapsules via a contemporary emulsion process. The composition of phase W_1 included NCH and CMC. Notably, NCH dissolves in citric acid solution, but CMC is insoluble in acidic solutions, as citric acid is a crosslinking agent of CMC. This method fabricated two systems, citric acid crosslinking droplets and CMC droplets. To generate the crosslinking droplets, solid NCH was first dissolved in citric acid mixed poly(vinyl alcohol) (PVA) solution (W_1). This solution was then added to an organic solution of PLGA with stirring (O). Similarly, the CMC solution (W_1) was added to PLGA solution with stirring, forming CMC droplets. Both droplets were added together and ultrasonicated to form crosslinked droplets (W_1/O single emulsion). This single emulsion was again added and ultrasonicated, forming the $W_1/O/W_2$ double emulsion. This unique synthesis enhanced the drug loading of the nanoparticles for controlled drug release for up to 16 days. As a result, NCH-CMC/PLGA nanoparticles containing calcium channel blockers were created. This method paved the way to generate a treatment for the prevention of vasospasm complications after surgery for ruptured intracranial aneurysms. There are several applications for calcium channel blocker prolonged-release implants. This application involves the binding of calcium channel blockers in composite polymer formulations for slow release at a rate that is effective to treat cerebral vasospasm in animal models. This drug delivery system is objectively locally positioned at the surgical site after the intracranial aneurysm is secured. These nanoparticles are located around the inflamed vessels and can avoid being washed away. The strategy for controlled release is based on polymer degradation at a rate that is effective for the treatment of cerebral vasospasms for 4–14 days. However, a clinical scenario needs to be investigated in the future [6].

3.3 Polymeric nanoparticle stabilization

Stabilizing the produced nanoparticles is a key factor in the delivery systems because the nanoparticles need to protect the encapsulated drugs from degradation. Agglomeration and flocculation are the destruction methods of nanoparticles and can produce macroscopic lumps that lead to the diffusion of drug molecules and their degradation in the residence environment. To stabilize these nanoparticles, an emulsion stabilizer is required, and this can be efficiently accomplished with amphiphilic molecules. These molecules contain two components, a hydrophilic part, and a lipophilic side. Typical examples of amphiphilic molecules include Span 80 and Tween 80 as nonionic emulsifiers. Additionally, anionic emulsifiers, cationic emulsifiers, and zwitterionic emulsifiers provide structural diversity.

The most commonly used rule for emulsifier selection is the hydrophilic-lipophilic balance (HLB) scale (HLB scale ranges from 0 to 20). This scale indicates the relative fraction of hydrophilic to lipophilic parts within the emulsifier molecule. High HLB values (8.0–18.0) are more suitable for use in O/W emulsions because they have a higher degree of hydrophilicity. In this case, O/W emulsions with a large amount of water are required to allow the formation of polymer dispersion droplets. As a result, these emulsifiers can widely expand the applications of the hydrophilic molecule for nanoparticle isolation, which then leads to interrupted agglomeration. Emulsifiers that have HLB values between 3.5 and 6.0 are most commonly used in W/O emulsions because they are more lipophilic [28, 29]. **Figure 4c** illustrates the expansion of the hydrophilic molecules of Span 80 (HLB = 4.3) and Tween 80 (HLB = 15.0) [7] at the interface of dispersed polymer droplets.

Furthermore, polymers have been used as emulsion stabilizers during emulsifier preparation methods, i.e., PVA, chitosan, and alginate [22, 30]. High MW polymers (>10 kDa) show driving forces that are equivalent to or greater than van der Waals-London (VDWL) forces. These VDWL forces are the primary source of attraction between nanoparticle surfaces and cause them to clump together. Through the addition of polymers, the polymeric chains can stabilize the nanoparticles via electrostatic, steric, and depletion forces. Electrostatic stabilization can be applied to charged polymers based on the simple principle that similar electric charges repel each other. Nanoparticle surfaces with zeta potential values greater than +30 mV or less than −30 mV are normally considered stable, as presented in **Figure 5a**. Steric stabilization is achieved on the surfaces of nanoparticles via adsorbed or chemically attached nonionic/ionic polymers. These uncharged polymers have a steric barrier due to a long chain that prevents the nanoparticles from sticking together (**Figure 5b**). Moreover, the addition of a high concentration of polymer for stabilization could lead to a high amount of free polymer in the dispersion medium. These free polymers establish repulsive forces between the nanoparticles to prevent nanoparticle aggregation and act as depletion stabilizers (**Figure 5c**) [31].

For example, PVA is an uncharged polymer that is commonly used as an emulsion stabilizer for the preparation of PLGA nanoparticles. The hydroxyl groups on the PVA chains are adsorbed at the interface with the PLGA chains via the hydroxyl, carboxylic acid, and ester groups. The interface between PLGA and PVA is an area with strong interactions, resulting in high nanoparticle stabilization [32, 33]. This interaction corresponds to the molecular orientation of PLGA nanospheres and PLGA nanocapsules (**Figure 4**). **Figure 5d** proposes a schematic representation of the molecular orientation of PVA at the surface of PLGA nanoparticles.

The use of polymers as stabilizers affects the characteristics of the nanoparticles to a greater extent than the use of other emulsifiers; as a result, these nanoparticles have a high MW. As a result, the use of low MW polymers or polymers at a low concentration results in reduced stability, lower drug loading, a rapid release rate, and a smaller size compared with high MW polymers or polymers present in high concentrations [6]. In addition, the charged polymers affect aliphatic polyester

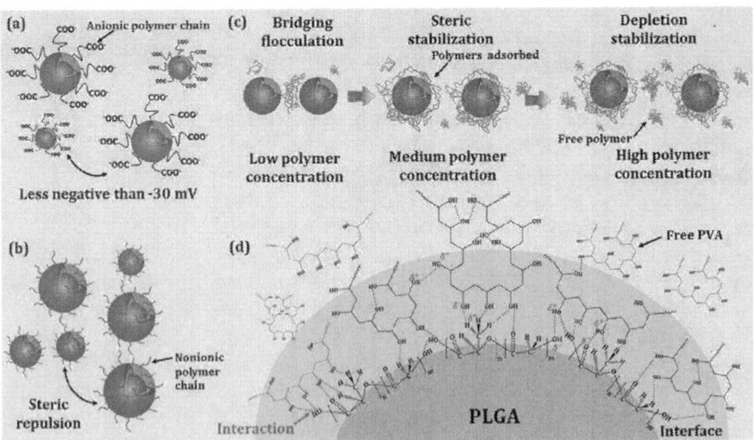

Figure 5.
Schematic representation of the molecular interactions of electrostatic stabilization (a), steric stabilization (b), depletion stabilization (c), and PVA at the surface of PLGA nanoparticles (d), based on information from a review article [31–33].

nanoparticles. Alginate is an anionic polymer and contains carboxylate anions ($-COO^-$) on its polymer chains. These anions repel the anions of the aliphatic polyesters, resulting in a larger size and permitting an increase in the retention of cationic drugs. However, cationic polymers (i.e., chitosan with a $-NH_3^+$ groups) interact with the carboxylate anions of the stabilizing polymers, leading to reduced particle size and increased retention of anionic drugs [30].

3.4 Mathematical models of drug release

Mathematical knowledge could assist in clarifying the drug release mechanism from polymer-based nanoparticles for controlled delivery. The exact mass transport and the relationship between drug release as a function of time can be described through various mathematical models. These models are able to predict analytics via data obtained from the drug release experiments to explain drug release kinetics. The coefficient of determination (R^2) and adjusted coefficient of determination (adj.-R^2) are investigated by statistical analysis to determine the relationship that the equation explains. The highest values of R^2 and adj.-R^2 from curve fitting involving describing the optimal relations (maximum accuracy) as a function of release time can be predicted with these Equations [6, 21]. This chapter will discuss some of the most commonly used equations to predict the kinetics of release from polymeric nanoparticles, including the *zero-order*, *first-order*, *Higuchi*, *Hixson-Crowell*, and *Korsmeyer-Peppas* equations, as summarized in **Table 1**.

When predicting drug release rates, the *zero-order model* represents controlled drug release that occurs at a constant rate depending on only the time and is independent of the amount of polymer. In the *first-order model*, the amount of drug released tends to depend on the polymer concentration, which affects the swelling and porosity of the nanoparticles. The *Hixson-Crowell model* describes the rate of drug release according to the cube root of its volume, in which matrix dissolution occurs. As a result, the diameter and surface area of the nanoparticles decreases proportionally over time according to the cube root of the weight at that particular time [34]. The *Higuchi model* predicts the release rate via diffusion control based on Fick's first law, which is square root time-dependent ($t^{1/2}$) [35].

Generally, the release mechanism can be predicted by the *Korsmeyer-Peppas model*. This model determines the exponential relationship between the rate of drug release and time. It is based on polymeric matrices with different geometries, following the released exponential (n). The exponential n-value indicates three types

Model	Equation	Graphical representation
Zero-order	$Q_t = K_0 t$	Cumulative release vs time
First-order	$\log M_t = \log M_0 + \frac{K_1 t}{2.303}$	log cumulative remaining vs time
Hixson-Crowell	$M_0^{1/3} - M_t^{1/3} = K_{HX} t$	Cumulative remaining$^{1/3}$ vs time
Higuchi	$Q_t = K_H t^{1/2}$	Cumulative release vs time$^{1/2}$
Korsmeyer-Peppas	$\log Q_t = n \log t + \log K_{KP}$	log cumulative release vs log time

Q_t is the cumulative amount of drug release at time (t), Q_0 is the initial amount of drug release at (t_0), M_t is the cumulative amount of drug remaining at time (t), M_0 is the initial amount of drug remaining at (t_0), t is time, n is the released exponent of Korsmeyer-Peppas, and K_0, K_1, K_{HX}, K_H, and K_{KP} are the zero-order, first-order, Hixson-Crowell, Higuchi, and Korsmeyer-Peppas constants, respectively.

Table 1.
Mathematical models of drug release [6].

of release mechanisms (**Figure 6**). The first type is the mechanism of Fickian diffusion, where the rate of diffusion of drug release is considerably greater than the rate of polymeric chain relaxation. The second mechanism is anomalous transportation via diffusion and swelling/erosion via slow rearrangement of polymeric chains. The final type is only the swelling/erosion mechanism. The release mechanisms of swelling and erosion are affected by an expansion in porosity and polymeric chain cleavage, respectively. Thus, the anomalous transportation and swelling/erosion mechanisms are both non-Fickian diffusion [36].

Using equations to predict release mechanisms can be confusing. Therefore, we proposed the flowchart sequence of use steps for these equations to describe drug release from PLGA nanoparticles [6]. The initial step investigates whether the rate of drug release is independent or dependent on the various concentrations by comparing R^2 values between the *zero-order* and *first-order* models. Next, the *Hixson-Crowell equation* and *Higuchi equation* were compared to determine whether the release rate depends on the probability of matrix dissolution or is diffusion controlled. Finally, the mechanism of drug release was investigated via the *Korsmeyer-Peppas equation* to determine the exponential n-value, as proposed in **Figure 6.**

3.5 Estimation of the formulation parameters for the polymeric nanoparticle system

Nanoparticles are one of the best choices of novel delivery systems because of their ease of preparation and long shelf life. Nanoparticle systems have fascinating physical properties that have been recognized over a wide range of utilizations. The characterization of different formulation parameters of nanoparticles is considered in the following sections.

3.5.1 Physical appearance

The physical appearance of nanoparticles can be examined visually for optical clarity, homogeneity, and fluidity, and also microscopically using a scanning electron microscope [37]. **Figure 7** illustrates digital photographs of PLGA nanoparticles [6] compared to PLGA microparticles [7] prepared via an emulsion process. Due to the optical transparency, the nanoparticles appeared as more transparent dispersions than the microparticles, which appeared white.

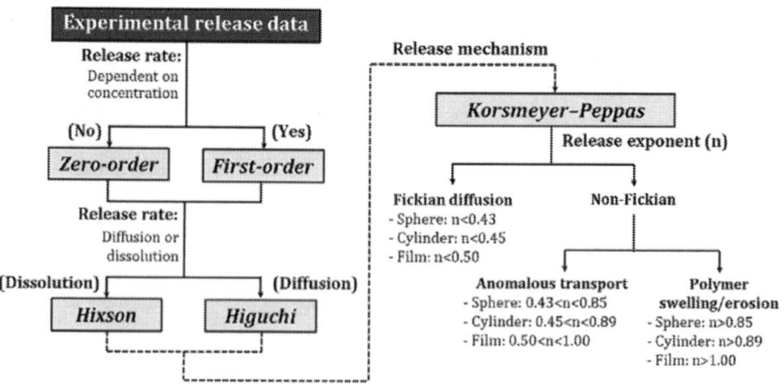

Figure 6.
Flowchart sequence of the steps used for the equations that predict drug release.

3.5.2 Rheology

Nanoparticles have high surface energy, resulting in agglomeration. In particular, aliphatic polyester-based nanoparticles rapidly agglomerate due to the strong interactions between the hydroxyl, carboxylic acid, and ester groups of the polymeric structures interacting with other nanoparticles. This behavior promotes the nanoparticles to be dispersed in media, affecting the rheological properties, such as viscosity and yield stress, of the suspension. Rheological characteristics can be examined with a Brookfield viscometer. The rheological properties show the nanoparticle region and its separation from other regions and play a principal role in stability [37, 38].

3.5.3 Particle size, polydispersity, and zeta potential

Dynamic light scattering is used to investigate particle size, zeta potential, and fluctuations in the intensities of scattering of particles due to Brownian motion. This technique also analyzes the polydispersity index to measure the wideness of the size distribution and quality of the dispersion [39, 40].

3.5.4 Drug stability

The stability of nanoparticles can be measured via visual inspection in closed tubes at both room temperature and elevated temperatures. Each month, the nanoparticles can be evaluated based on their phase separation, % transmittance, and globule size [7, 41]. Examples include PLGA nanoparticle dispersions [6] compared to PLGA microparticle dispersions [7] in phosphate-buffered saline (pH 7.4 at 37°C) to mimic the physiological environment. The nanoparticle suspension presented no phase separation, suggesting that these nanoparticles did not precipitate (**Figure 7a**). The microparticles could have a higher gravitational force relative to the nanoparticles, leading to their easy precipitation, which can be observed from the phase separation of the microparticle solution (**Figure 7b**). Therefore, drug administration of these microparticles needs to carry a "*shake well before use*" label [22].

3.5.5 Drug solubility

Excess drug was added to the nanoparticles to optimize the formulation, similar to the optimization of the other ingredients. The nanoparticles were continuously stirred

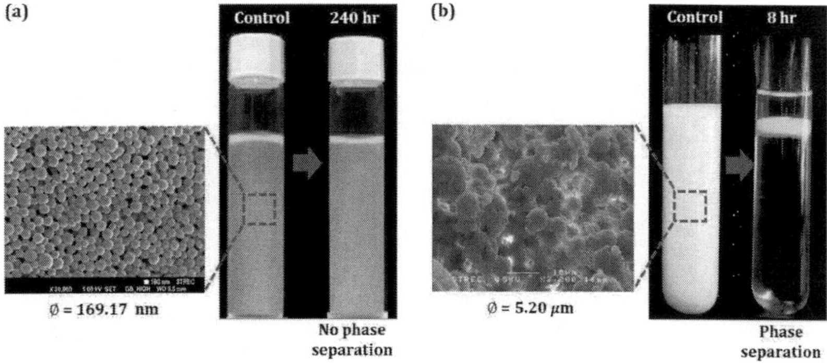

Figure 7.
SEM micrographs and digital photographs of PLGA nanoparticles (a) and PLGA microparticles (b) prepared via an emulsion process [6, 7].

for 24 h at room temperature, and samples were removed and centrifuged at 600 rpm for 10 min at predetermined time points. The quantity of soluble drugs in the optimized nanoparticles was determined by calculating the amount of drug present in the residue and comparing it with the total amount of added drug. The individual ingredients were used for comparison of the solubility of the drug in the nanoparticles [7, 42].

3.5.6 In vitro, ex vivo, *and* in vivo *drug release*

In vitro and *in vivo* studies provide extrapolated data to reflect the bioavailability of drug formulations. The *in vitro* drug release profile of nanoparticles can be determined with a Franz diffusion cell. The donor compartment has a cellophane membrane as a barrier, comprising the encapsulated drug in the nanoparticles. The receptor compartment is filled with buffer solution, usually phosphate-buffered saline (pH 7.4), and the system is stirred with a magnetic stirrer at 100 rpm and 37°C. At predetermined time intervals, samples of the dispersion are withdrawn from the medium of the receptor compartment and an equal amount of medium is returned to the system at this same time. The withdrawn sample is filtered using a 0.22–50 μm filter (e.g., Millipore, USA) and analyzed for drug release using UV-visible spectrophotometry at the specific wavelength that shows peak absorption of the drug [39, 43, 44].

An *ex vivo* drug release study profile of nanoparticles can be performed with a diffusion cell. Suitable skin and the underlying cartilage removed from ears can be cut up and placed on the diffusion cell filled with receptor solution. Vesicular process samples are placed on the dorsal surface of the skin. At predetermined time intervals, samples of the dispersion are withdrawn from the medium of the receptor compartment and an equivalent amount of the medium is returned at the same time. The withdrawn sample is then analyzed for the amount of drug released using high-performance liquid chromatography (HPLC) or UV-visible spectrophotometry at a specific wavelength [44].

In vivo, drug release study profiles of nanoparticles can be carried out by administering the nanoparticles to living animals. At predetermined time intervals, blood samples are withdrawn, followed by centrifugation and analysis of drug release using HPLC.

3.6 Applications of polymeric nanoparticle systems

Nanoparticle systems have been used as delivery vehicles in a variety of drug delivery systems for controlled release because of their potential to solubilize active agents. Aliphatic polyester nanoparticles have various goals, which are accomplished in different ways, as outlined in the following sections.

3.6.1 Oral delivery

Nanoparticle formulations have many benefits over conventional oral delivery methods, including increased absorption, minimized drug toxicity, enhanced oral bioavailability, and excellent clinical potency. Hence, nanoparticle systems have been modified for use in drug delivery systems for compounds such as oral drugs, steroids, hormones, diuretics, and antibiotics [40, 45, 46].

3.6.2 Parenteral delivery

Parenteral delivery via the intravenous route has been used for controlled drug delivery and drug targeting to particular sites. Aliphatic polyester nanoparticles significant in the parenteral delivery system since they can improve drug solubility, long-term stability in the body, biocompatibility, and ease of development for delivery to a targeted site. Nanoparticle formulations have prominent advantages over other systems. Additionally, fine nanoparticles are cleared more slowly than coarse particles [47, 48].

3.6.3 Topical delivery

Hydrophilic and lipophilic drugs poorly penetrate the skin due to the limitations of their solubility in both the lipid phase and aqueous solution. The topical delivery of drugs via nanoparticle formulations has several advantages over other conventional topical methods for the treatment of skin disorders while showing minimal side effects. Nanoparticles can incorporate both lipophilic and hydrophilic drugs. Additionally, drug degradation, salivary degradation, and hepatic first-pass metabolism in the stomach can be avoided, while benefiting from sustained drug delivery, long-term stability, enhanced permeability, and reduced toxicity [49, 50].

3.6.4 Pulmonary drug delivery

The treatment of lower respiratory infections is difficult due to the presence of microbes deep in the respiratory system. Nanoparticles as a targeted drug delivery system to the site of infection have been actively applied to enhance antimicrobial drug resistance, sustain drug release, and increase bioavailability. Importantly, nanoparticle systems that contain multiple antimicrobial substances can be used [51, 52].

3.6.5 Vaccine delivery

Recently, there have been many research topics related to nanoparticles as carriers for vaccines. The main idea is to use the nanoparticle as an effective carrier to deliver an inactivated organism to the membrane to stimulate the immune system. One study found that it is possible to generate genital mucosa immunity from vaccines that are added to the nasal mucosa. The synthesized proteins passed into the mucosal membrane surface by using nanoparticles to absorb the antigen using adjuvant facilitation [53–55].

There are several mechanisms to load antigens into the nanoparticles, such as encapsulation, encapsulation with coating, encapsulation with targeting, physical adsorption, chemical conjugation, and conjugation with a targeting mechanism. Hydrophobic interactions are known to be effective ways to load antigens into nanoparticles by physical adsorption processes, which apply weak interactions to dissociate antigens and nanoparticles in the body. During protein synthesis, the encapsulated antigens are mixed with nanoparticle precursors, which is a consequence of the release of the encapsulated antigen when the nanoparticle degrades *in vivo*.

The first clinical trial application received was for the use of nanoparticles for influenza and human immunodeficiency virus (HIV) proteins. A recombinant HIV glycoprotein 120 (HIV-gp120) antigen mix in nanoparticles was studied in mice and guinea pigs by intranasal immunization and demonstrated a robust serum anti-gp120 immunoglobulin G (IgG) response [53]. The constituent of Prepandrix® has been approved for the use of the flu vaccine AS03 (an adjuvant system containing α-tocopherol and squalene in an oil-in-water emulsion) during the influenza pandemic. AS03 has been used as a reference for other vaccines, such as Arepanrix®, to control influenza infection caused by H1N1 and H5N1 [54].

The balance between immunogenic benefits and safety needs to be considered and is achieved by selecting the correct adjuvant, antigen, and emulsion composition. These factors are considered the main factors of concern during vaccine development, as they directly affect the benefit-risk balance. Vaccine efficiency is vital, and this factor is the major element controlling pandemics through the selection of the correct oil composition, adjuvant, surfactant, and antigen for the specific disease.

Aliphatic polyester-based nanoparticles could be delivered as adjuvants for vaccines during the coronavirus disease 2019 (COVID-19) pandemic [56, 57]. Polymers are the main material for vaccine delivery. For example, the most popular aliphatic polyesters have been used in vaccine adjuvants for lymph nodes targeting HIV, *Bacillus anthracis*, *Chlamydia trachomatis*, and malaria [58]. Moreover, the addition of a poly(ethylene glycol) (PEG) coating around PLA (PEG-PLA) nanoparticles has been found to facilitate the transport of the antigen of tetanus toxoid to the rat nasal epithelium for nasal vaccine delivery [59].

Acknowledgements

The authors would like to thank (a) the Chuan Ratanarak Foundation; (b) the Neurosurgery Unit, Surgery Department, Faculty of Medicine Ramathibodi Hospital Mahidol University, Thailand; and (c) the Industrial Chemistry Department, Faculty of Applied Science, King Mongkut's University of Technology North Bangkok, Thailand for financial support (in-house grant no. 5841103 and KMUTNB-62-DRIVE-036).

References

[1] Chumnanvej S, Sarnvivad P. Retrospective 5-year clinical outcome of interdisciplinary treatment for ruptured cerebral arteriovenous malformation: The lesson learned. Archives of Medicine. 2015;7(44):1-7

[2] Alahamd Y, Swehli H, Rahhal A, Sardar S, Elhassan M, Alsamel A, et al. Calcium channel blockers. In: Ambrosi P, Ahmad R, Abdullahi A, Agrawal A, editors. New Insight into Cerebrovascular Diseases—An Updated Comprehensive Review. London: IntechOpen; 2020. pp. 216-233

[3] Kasuya H. Development of nicardipine prolonged-release implants after clipping for preventing cerebral vasospasm: From laboratory to clinical trial. Acta Neurochirurgica Supplement. 2013;**115**:41-44

[4] Barth M, Pena P, Seiz M, Thomé C, Muench E, Weidauer S, et al. Feasibility of intraventricular nicardipine prolonged release implants in patients following aneurysmal subarachnoid haemorrhage. British Journal of Neurosurgery. 2011;**25**(6):677-683

[5] Thomé C, Seiz M, Schubert GA, Barth M, Vajkoczy P, Kasuya H, et al. Nicardipine pellets for the prevention of cerebral vasospasm. Acta Neuro chirurgica Supplement. 2011;**110**(Pt 2): 209-211

[6] Soomherun N, Kreua-ongarjnukool N, Niyomthai ST, Chumnanvej S. kinetics of drug release via nicardipine hydrochloride-loaded carboxymethyl cellulose/poly(D,L-lactic-co-glycolic acid) nanocarriers using a contemporary emulsion process. ChemNanoMat. 2020;**6**(12):1754-1769

[7] Soomherun N, Kreua-ongarjnukool N, Chumnanvej S, Thumsing S. Encapsulation of nicardipine hydrochloride and release from biodegradable poly(D,L-lactic-co-glycolic acid) microparticles by double emulsion process: Effect of emulsion stability and different parameters on drug entrapment. International Journal of Biomaterials. 2017;**2017**:1743765

[8] Urbánek T, Jäger E, Jäger A, Hrubý M. Selectively biodegradable polyesters: Nature-inspired construction materials for future biomedical applications. Polymers. 2019;**11**(6): 1061

[9] Silvers AL, Chang C-C, Parrish B, Emrick T. Strategies in aliphatic polyester synthesis for biomaterial and drug delivery applications. In: Degradable Polymers and Materials: Principles and Practice. 2nd ed. Washington, DC: American Chemical Society; 2012. pp. 237-254

[10] Mochizuki M, Hirami M. Structural effects on the biodegradation of aliphatic polyesters. Polymers for Advanced Technologies. 1997;**8**(4): 203-209

[11] Jacquel N, Freyermouth F, Fenouillot F, Rousseau A, Pascault J-P, Fuertes P, et al. Synthesis and properties of poly(butylene succinate): Efficiency of different transesterification catalysts. Journal of Polymer Science Part A Polymer Chemistry. 2011;**49**:5301

[12] Ginjupalli K, Shavi GV, Averineni RK, Bhat M, Udupa N, Nagaraja UP. Poly(α-hydroxy acid) based polymers: A review on material and degradation aspects. Polymer Degradation and Stability. 2017;**144**:520-535

[13] Burg K. Chapter 6—Poly(α-ester)s. In: Kumbar SG, Laurencin CT, Deng M, editors. Natural and Synthetic Biomedical Polymers. Oxford: Elsevier; 2014. pp. 115-121

[14] Panyachanakul T, Sorachart B, Lumyong S, Lorliam W,

Kitpreechavanich V, Krajangsang S. Development of biodegradation process for poly(DL-lactic acid) degradation by crude enzyme produced by *Actinomadura keratinilytica* strain T16-1. Electronic Journal of Biotechnology. 2019;**40**:52-57

[15] Netti PA, Biondi M, Frigione M. Experimental studies and modeling of the degradation process of poly(lactic-co-glycolic acid) microspheres for sustained protein release. Polymers (Basel). 2020;**12**(9):2042

[16] Casalini T. 3—Bioresorbability of polymers: Chemistry, mechanisms, and modeling. In: Perale G, Hilborn J, editors. Bioresorbable Polymers for Biomedical Applications. Cambridge: Woodhead Publishing; 2017. pp. 65-83

[17] Ali M, Walboomers XF, Jansen JA, Yang F. Influence of formulation parameters on encapsulation of doxycycline in PLGA microspheres prepared by double emulsion technique for the treatment of periodontitis. Journal of Drug Delivery Science and Technology. 2019;**52**:263-271

[18] Vey E, Rodger C, Booth J, Claybourn M, Miller AF, Saiani A. Degradation kinetics of poly(lactic-co-glycolic) acid block copolymer cast films in phosphate buffer solution as revealed by infrared and Raman spectroscopies. Polymer Degradation and Stability. 2011;**96**(10):1882-1889

[19] Makadia HK, Siegel SJ. Poly lactic-co-glycolic acid (PLGA) as biodegradable controlled drug delivery carrier. Polymers (Basel). 2011;**3**(3): 1377-1397

[20] Gorrasi G, Pantani R. Hydrolysis and biodegradation of poly(lactic acid). In: Di Lorenzo ML, Androsch R, editors. Synthesis, Structure and Properties of Poly(Lactic Acid). Cham: Springer International Publishing; 2018. p. 119-151.

[21] Soonklang C, Tassanarangsan C, Soomherun N, Kreua-ongarjnukool N, Niyomthai ST. Study kinetics models of clindamycin hydrochloride from poly(D,L-lactic-co-glycolic acid) particles. International Journal of Pharma Medicine and Biological Sciences. 2021;**10**(2):68-74

[22] Soomherun N, Kreua-ongarjnukool N, Niyomthai ST, Chumnanvej S. Enhancement vehicles of cardene loading poly(D,L-lactic-co-glycolic acid) nanoparticles in vitro controlled release for biomedical application. International Journal of Pharma Medicine and Biological Sciences. 2021;**10**(1):1-7

[23] Park K, Otte A, Sharifi F, Garner J, Skidmore S, Park H, et al. Potential roles of the glass transition temperature of PLGA microparticles in drug release kinetics. Molecular Pharmaceutics. 2021;**18**(1):18-32

[24] De Jong WH, Borm PJA. Drug delivery and nanoparticles: Applications and hazards. International Journal of Nanomedicine. 2008;**3**(2):133-149

[25] Garg A, Garg S, Swarnakar NK. Chapter 11—Nanoparticles and prostate cancer. In: Yadav AK, Gupta U, Sharma R, editors. Nano Drug Delivery Strategies for the Treatment of Cancers. Cambridge: Academic Press; 2021. pp. 275-318

[26] Wilkosz N, Łazarski G, Kovacik L, Gargas P, Nowakowska M, Jamróz D, et al. Molecular insight into drug-loading capacity of PEG–PLGA nanoparticles for itraconazole. The Journal of Physical Chemistry B. 2018;**122**(28):7080-7090

[27] Metheeparakornchai C, Kreua-ongarjnukool N, Thumsing S, Pavasant P, Limjeerajarus C. Development of amoxicillin-loaded modified polycaprolactone microparticles in medical application.

International Journal of Pharma Medicine and Biological Sciences. 2021;**10**(2):88-93

[28] Zheng Y, Zheng M, Ma Z, Xin B, Guo R, Xu X. 8—Sugar fatty acid esters. In: Ahmad MU, Xu X, editors. Polar Lipids. Cambridge: Academic Press and AOCS Press; 2015. pp. 215-243

[29] Björkegren S, Karimi RF, Martinelli A, Jayakumar NS, Hashim MA. A new emulsion liquid membrane based on a palm oil for the extraction of heavy metals. Membranes. 2015;**5**(2):168-179

[30] Rescignano N, Fortunati E, Armentano I, Hernandez R, Mijangos C, Pasquino R, et al. Use of alginate, chitosan and cellulose nanocrystals as emulsion stabilizers in the synthesis of biodegradable polymeric nanoparticles. Journal of Colloid and Interface Science. 2015;**445**:31-39

[31] Shi J. Steric Stabilization, Literature Review, Center for Industrial Sensors and Measurements. Department of Materials science & Engineering Group Inorganic Materials Science. 2002:1-42

[32] Murakami H, Kobayashi M, Takeuchi H, Kawashima Y. Preparation of poly(DL-lactide-co-glycolide) nanoparticles by modified spontaneous emulsification solvent diffusion method. International Journal of Pharmaceutics. 1999;**187**(2):143-152

[33] Tham CY, Abdul Hamid Z, Ismail H, Ahmad Z. Poly(vinyl alcohol) in fabrication of PLA micro- and nanoparticles using emulsion and solvent evaporation technique. Advanced Materials Research. 2014; **1024**:296-299

[34] Hixson AW, Crowell JH. Dependence of reaction velocity upon surface and agitation. Industrial & Engineering Chemistry. 1931;**23**(8): 923-931

[35] Higuchi T. Mechanism of sustained-action medication. Theoretical analysis of rate of release of solid drugs dispersed in solid matrices. Journal of Pharmaceutical Sciences. 1963;**52**(12): 1145-1149

[36] Korsmeyer RW, Gurny R, Doelker E, Buri P, Peppas NA. Mechanisms of solute release from porous hydrophilic polymers. International Journal of Pharmaceutics. 1983;**15**(1):25-35

[37] Basheer HS, Noordin MI, Ghareeb M. Characterization of microemulsions prepared using isopropyl palmitate with various surfactants and cosurfactants. Tropical Journal of Pharmaceutical Research. 2013;**12**(3):305-310

[38] Thakker KD, Chern WH. Development and validation of in vitro release tests for semisolid dosage forms-case study. Dissolution Technologies. 2003;**10**(2):10-16

[39] Thumsing S, Israsena N, Boonkrai C, Supaphol P. Preparation of bioactive glycosylated glial cell-line derived neurotrophic factor-loaded microspheres for medical applications. Journal of Applied Polymer Science. 2014;**131**(8):40168

[40] Sonthirak P, Kreua-ongarjnukool N, Thumsing S. Fabrication of PLGA/GELATIN micro particles for control release bio-substances. International Journal of Advances in Science, Engineering and Technology. 2018;**6**(4): 81-85

[41] Jadhav K, Shetye S, Kadam V. Design and evaluation of microemulsion based drug delivery system. International Journal of Advances in Pharmacological Science. 2010;**1**:156-166

[42] Tomšič M, Podlogar F, Gašperlin M, Bešter-Rogač M, Jamnik A. Water–Tween 40®/Imwitor 308®–isopropyl

myristate microemulsions as delivery systems for ketoprofen: Small-angle X-ray scattering study. International Journal of Pharmaceutics. 2006;**327**(1): 170-177

[43] Bendas ER, Tadros MI. Enhanced transdermal delivery of salbutamol sulfate via ethosomes. AAPS PharmSciTech. 2007;**8**(4):214-220

[44] Touitou E, Dayan N, Bergelson L, Godin B, Eliaz M. Ethosomes—novel vesicular carriers for enhanced delivery: characterization and skin penetration properties. Journal of Controlled Release. 2000;**65**(3):403-418

[45] Metheeparakornchai C, Kreua-ongarjnukool N, Thumsing S, editors. Encapsulation of biological substance in polycaprolactone-graft-chitosan microparticles by layer-by-layer technique in dental application. In: Proceedings of the Pure and Applied Chemistry International Conference (PACCON'19). 2019: p. PO47-PO52. 7-8 February 2019. Bangkok, Thailand: Mahidol University and Chemical Society of Thailand.

[46] Limjeerajarus CN, Sonntana S, Pajaree L, Kansurang C, Pitt S, Saowapa T, et al. Prolonged release of iloprost enhances pulpal blood flow and dentin bridge formation in a rat model of mechanical tooth pulp exposure. Journal of Oral Science. 2019;**61**(1): 73-81

[47] Araújo FA, Kelmann RG, Araújo BV, Finatto RB, Teixeira HF, Koester LS. Development and characterization of parenteral nanoemulsions containing thalidomide. European Journal of Pharmaceutical Sciences. 2011;**42**(3): 238-245

[48] Patel R, Patel K. Advances in novel parentral drug delivery systems. Asian Journal of Pharmaceutics. 2010;**4**: 193-199

[49] Aggarwal N, Goindi S, Khurana R. Formulation, characterization and evaluation of an optimized microemulsion formulation of griseofulvin for topical application. Colloids and Surfaces B: Biointerfaces. 2013;**105**:158-166

[50] Bakshi P, Jiang Y, Nakata T, Akaki J, Matsuoka N, Banga A. Formulation development and characterization of nanoemulsion-based formulation for topical delivery of heparinoid. Journal of Pharmaceutical Sciences. 2018; **107**:2883-2890

[51] Mansour HM, Rhee Y-S, Wu X. Nanomedicine in pulmonary delivery. International Journal of Nanomedicine. 2009;**4**:299-319

[52] Bivas-Benita M, Oudshoorn M, Romeijn S, van Meijgaarden K, Koerten H, van der Meulen H, et al. Cationic submicron emulsions for pulmonary DNA immunization. Journal of Controlled Release. 2004;**100**(1): 145-155

[53] Zhao L, Seth A, Wibowo N, Zhao C-X, Mitter N, Yu C, et al. Nanoparticle vaccines. Vaccine. 2014;**32**(3):327-337

[54] Reed SG, Bertholet S, Coler RN, Friede M. New horizons in adjuvants for vaccine development. Trends in Immunology. 2009;**30**(1):23-32

[55] Akhter S, Jain G, Ahmad F, Khar R, Jain N, Iqbal Z, et al. Investigation of nanoemulsion system for transdermal delivery of domperidone: ex-vivo and in vivo studies. Current Nanoscience. 2008;**4**:381-390

[56] Gadhave RV, Vineeth SK, Gadekar PT. Polymers and polymeric materials in COVID-19 pandemic: A review. Open Journal of Polymer Chemistry. 2020;**10**:66-75

[57] Stojanowski J, Gołębiowski T. Focus on COVID-19: Antiviral polymers in

drugs and vaccines. Polymers in Medicine. 2020;**50**(2):75-78

[58] Gutjahr A, Phelip C, Coolen A-L, Monge C, Boisgard A-S, Paul S, et al. Biodegradable polymeric nanoparticles-based vaccine adjuvants for lymph nodes targeting. Vaccines. 2016;**4**(4):34

[59] Vila A, Evora C, Soriano I, Jato JL, Alonso M. PEG-PLA nanoparticles as carriers for nasal vaccine delivery. Journal of Aerosol Medicine. 2004; **17**:174-185

Chapter 6

Strategies to Develop Cyclodextrin-Based Nanosponges for Smart Drug Delivery

Abstract

In recent years, the development of various cyclodextrin (CD)-based nanosponges (NSs) has gained great importance in the controlled and-or targeted release of drugs due to their versatility and simple preparation. In this chapter, an introduction of different administration routes is explained. Further, different ways to obtain CD-NSs and their classification are shown with a brief explanation of the characterization of the inclusion complexes. Finally, illustrative examples in diverse processes or diseases will be reviewed and explained to demonstrate the potential of CD-NSs. Therefore, this division will serve to compile information on CD-NSs in recent years and to illustrate to readers how to generate and apply different derivatives of interest.

Keywords: Cyclodextrin nanosponges, drug delivery, synthesis, nanocarrier, release

1. Introduction

Society demands better treatments for each disease and therefore the industry tries to obtain them. Novel drugs with better bioactivity are researched to achieve the best result in our bodies. However, several novel drugs present problems related to their chemical properties that prevent them from being used as a pharma or nutraceutical product. The molecule can be unstable in water solution, and/or easily oxidized, and presents poor bioavailability. Different strategies might improve the current therapy. One possibility is to find a good formulation, which stabilizes the drug or carries it to the desired tissue. Moreover, the adverse effect due to the dosage can also be reduced. For this reason, a great number of carriers are been proposed to challenge the previous problems.

One of them is called cyclodextrin (CD), truncated cone-shaped oligosaccharides made up of α-(1→4) linked glucopyranoside units with six, seven and eight glucose units, α, β and γ-CD, respectively [1, 2]. A derivative called 2-Hydroxypropyl-βCD (HPβ-CD) is used as an orphan drug for Niemann Pick disease type C [3, 4]. Complexes formed of molecules and cyclodextrins (CDs) are called "inclusion complexes". Generally, CDs encapsulate poorly water-soluble compounds and hydrophobic moieties of amphiphilic molecules. Nevertheless, the solubility of these complexes not only depends on the CD used but also on different factors such as pH or guess molecule [5–8]. The capacity of CDs to increase solubility and protect several molecules has increased their use in the pharmaceutical and food industries [1, 9, 10].

However, the improvement achieved by adding CDs is sometimes insufficient. Then, researchers developed a novel material based on these excipients baptized as Cyclodextrin-based Nanosponge (CD-NS), innovative cross-linked polymer structures with a three-dimensional network, and with a crystalline and amorphous structure, spherical and possessing good swelling properties [11]. Recent reviews [12–14] point to their wide potential and minimal toxicity [15, 16]. Some applications of these polymers include i) increasing the apparent solubility of poorly soluble drugs, ii) modulating drug release and activity, iii) protecting drugs against several agents, iv) enhancing bioactivities, v) absorbing contaminants ability, vi) delivering the drug, etc.

Cross-linking CDs brings significant benefits to CD-NSs compared with the respective native CDs. In general, CD-NSs can form complexes with a series of different molecules due to their structure. They achieve a hindered diffusion of loaded guest molecules, thus promoting slower release kinetics [17, 18]. Another important property of CD-NSs is that they can be easily recovered from aqueous media and recycled. Although they are insoluble, soluble hyperbranched NS can also be synthesized [19]. Finally, one of their principal disadvantages has been recently solved, they have been tested as a good carrier not only for small molecules but also for higher ones like proteins [20, 21].

This chapter tends to be a first step for the researcher who starts with CD-NSs: i) an introduction of the routes of administration, including advantages and disadvantages is explained, ii) an explanation about the various types of CD-NSs, including its synthesis and classification is written, iii) the different ways to characterize the inclusion complexes are reported and iv) examples of smart delivery are displayed as an encourage study to demonstrate their potential.

2. Routes of administration, advantages, and disadvantages

The choice of the route of administration is crucial as it dramatically affects drug bioavailability and thus requires specific delivery strategies. Parenteral routes include intravenous, intramuscular, and subcutaneous routes, whereas the enteral routes are the oral, sublingual, and rectal routes [22]. Others are inhalation, intranasal, etc. [23]. In this section, each route will be described briefly and special attention will be paid to the oral route, which is the most desired but, at the same time, the most challenging.

When administered via intravenous injection (IV), the drug reaches the systemic circulation directly bypassing absorption and carrying out its effect rapidly. This route is ideal for unstable or scarcely absorbed drugs (e.g. blood products), and irritating drug formulations, the administration of which via subcutaneous and intramuscular routes will be painful. It is also intended for patients who are not able to take the formulations orally, due to mental disorders, nausea, or vomiting.

Intramuscular injection (IM) can involve various muscles, including the gluteal muscle to which up to 5 ml of the formulation can be administered. Via this route, aqueous or oil-based solutions, suspensions, and emulsions are accepted. Aqueous solutions are generally absorbed in 10–30 minutes, whereas drugs insoluble at interstitial pH or suspended in oil-based solutions present a long time of absorption. Vascularisation of the muscle, the volume, and the osmolarity of the injected formulations also affect the absorption time. A depot preparation of the drug can be given via this route with a sustained release of the drug into the bloodstream. IM injection is selected when the drug has a low oral bioavailability or when the patient is not compliant. Vaccines are also administered via this route.

Subcutaneous injections can be given in the forearm or abdomen. Up to 2 ml of the formulation can be administered. Together with aqueous solutions and suspensions, adrenalin can be added to induce vasoconstriction and therefore increase the residence time of drugs (e.g. local anesthetics) or hyaluronidase to make the extracellular matrix more fluid, thus improving the absorption rate.

The absorption rate is extremely variable as it is influenced by the blood flow. Subcutaneous injections are also used for depot formulations. It is easy to administer and requires minimal skills, thus allowing self-administration. Insulin and heparin are given via this route.

Among all, oral delivery has been recognized as the most attractive route, as it is cheap, simple, accepted by patients, requires fewer sterility restrictions, and offers more possibilities in the design of the formulation (including sustained and controlled delivery) [24]. It is used for drugs with topical action in the gut and systemic effects when they reach the bloodstream. However, it is not suitable for emergencies in which an immediate effect is fundamental.

Over the past few years, many efforts have been made to develop oral delivery systems able to overcome the obstacles in the gastrointestinal tract (GI) in which the mechanism of absorption is complex with multiple levels of barriers [24].

There is a long list of variables that influence the GI absorption of drugs, which are grouped in technical challenges, physicochemical properties of the drug, and environmental factors [25].

The technical challenges concern the pharmaceutical form, i.e. liquid or solid. In solid forms, *the rate* and extent of disintegration, and dissolution of the formulation are important to a drug, and to carry out its effect, needs to be in a solution for developing the absorption.

Most drugs are absorbed in the small intestine, characterized by a large surface area of absorption and having a crucial influence on bioavailability.

The walls of the GI tract are characterized by the presence of mucus, which has been a target for drug delivery systems (DDS) capable of mucopenetration or mucoadhesion [24]. Mucopenetration consists in regulating the hydrophobicity/hydrophilicity of the carrier's matrix or combining mucolytic enzymes to promote drug penetration. On the contrary, mucoadhesive carriers, which have attracted significant attention [26–28], can adhere to mucus, thus increasing the residence time. CD NSs have proven to possess this property, making them particularly promising for oral delivery [20].

Last but not least, the first-pass effect should be borne in mind when dealing with the oral route as it is certainly a limiting factor. It refers to the metabolism (mainly in the liver) of the drug before it reaches the systemic circulation, which may lead to a drop in bioavailability [29]. For this reason, several drugs are administered via other enteral routes (e.g. rectal and sublingual).

The sublingual route offers the benefit of bypassing the first-pass effect due to the passive diffusion through the highly permeable mucosa underneath the tongue. It is simple with a low risk of infection and the effect is rapid. Nitroglycerin is administered via this route.

The rectal route exploits the highly vascularized rectal mucosa for drug absorption. The first-pass effect is partially avoided. It is indicated for patients with gastrointestinal motility problems, nausea, vomiting, and children.

Inhalation is used to obtain a rapid effect as the drug crosses the large surface area of the respiratory tract epithelium and reaches the systemic circulation. It avoids the first-pass metabolism. The particle size and morphology of the

Route of administration	Advantages	Disadvantages
Oral	• easy • safe • cheap	• not Emergency therapy • not for GI-sensitive drugs (unless they are encapsulated • first pass effect • risk of interaction with food and drugs
Sublingual	• rapid effect • suitable for emergency therapy	• uncertain dosage
Rectal	• for pediatric use • for patients with impaired GI function	• risk of irritation • unpredictable absorption
Inhalation	• rapid absorption • suitable for general anesthesia and emergency therapy	• risk of irritation • specific equipment is needed
Intravenous	• suitable for emergency therapy • adjustable • accurate dosage	• complications due to rapid onset • allergic reactions
Intramuscular	• rapid absorption • systemic administration of hydrophilic drugs • administration of sustained-release formulations	• small volumes • painful • care must be taken to avoid veins and arteries • risk of infections and abscesses
Subcutaneous	• rapid absorption • administration of sustained-release formulations	• administration of very small volumes

Table 1.
Advantages and disadvantages of the main routes of administration.

formulation inhaled are crucial. It is mainly used for the treatment of respiratory diseases. The intranasal route enables the drug to be absorbed via passive diffusion across the highly-vascularised respiratory epithelium directly into the systemic circulation. Nasal decongestants and anti-allergic drugs are administered via this route (**Table 1**).

3. Synthesis and classification of CD-NSs

The choice of appropriate synthetic conditions, allowed to obtain both water-soluble and water-insoluble polymer products, known also as CD-NSs or insoluble, and branched or soluble polymer [30–32]. The latter case allowed to overcome the limits of pristine CDs in terms of solubility in water and specific organic solvent, while the resulting formation of a three-dimensional cross-linked network was related to the presence of interstitial spaces among the monomers [33]. In this regard, the nature of the cross-linker and its amount in respect to the CD, ratio which defines the so-called cross-linking density, are presented to have a great impact on the properties and structure of the final material [34]. Also, being said interstices wider and more hydrophilic in respect to the cavities of CDs, a wider hosting capability was observed as a result.

3.1 General synthesis protocol

The most common method announced for the synthesis of CD based polymers, is characterized by employing a suitable solvent which could be either organic solvent or, in specific cases water, for the dissolution of the CDs. Afterwards, under continuous stirring, the chosen linking agent is added to the solution. Nevertheless, when required, the introduction of a catalyst occurs before the linking agent, and in specific cases, an increase in temperature is necessary to start the cross-linking reactions. The use of an ultrasound bath instead of stirring was also considered [35]. Eventually, either a sol–gel process or a precipitation polymerization can be observed, leading to the formation of a monolithic block or a precipitate, respectively. Also, in those cases in which the cross-linker is in the liquid form, and able to solubilize the CD, a melt polymerization can be performed [36, 37].

Once the synthesis is completed, the solvent, the catalyst, eventual unreacted monomers, and by-products are removed from the synthesized product by purification with water or other volatile solvents. In the end, a dry solid powder is collected [37–39]. Another well-known approach to synthesize CD-NSs is achieved through simple dehydration reactions. In this case, the CDs and the cross-linker, which is usually an acid bearing two or more carboxylic groups, are solubilized in water. After the addition of a suitable catalyst, the solution is heated to remove the water introduced as solvent as well as the water released as a by-product of the cross-linking condensation reaction. Moreover, the use of vacuum together with the temperature allows to shift the equilibrium of the reaction toward the products [40, 41]. Besides, less used synthetic routes report the use of interfacial or radical polymerization. In the first case, two immiscible phases such as a water solution of CD and a chlorinated solvent solution containing the chosen cross-linker, are mixed and stirred vigorously. The cross-linking occurs rapidly at the interface of the immiscible phases, and a precipitate is obtained [39]. While in the second case, a multistep procedure involving also preliminary derivatization of CD was displayed [42].

3.2 General classification

In general, based on the technological evolution of these materials, CD-NSs can be classified into four generations, considering their chemical composition and properties [19]. The first generation comprises all those NSs synthesized by a simple one-step reaction of CDs with a cross-linker. This generation was further divided into sub-categories according to the chemical nature of the linking molecules adopted for the synthesis. In this frame, carbonate, ester, ether, and urethane types are the most reported. These specific types of NSs will be described in more detail in the following paragraphs. Subsequently, the introduction of specific functions such as charge or luminescence to the final polymer structure defined the second generation of NSs. These materials displayed more complex polymer architectures achieved either via pre- or post-synthesis functionalization. In the first case, the introduced functions were limited to the surface of the polymer, whereas in the second case a more homogeneous distribution was observed. Referring to the division into generations, the 3rd generation deals with stimuli-responsive NSs, able to modulate their behavior (for example increasing/decreasing a drug release) according to the external environment.

3.2.1 CD-based polyurethane NSs

Urethane, or carbamate, CD-NSs are synthesized by reacting CDs (or a different dextrin) with a suitable diisocyanate as, for example, hexamethylene diisocyanate (HDI), toluene–2,4-diisocyanate (TDI). The reaction scheme is reported below

(**Figure 1**, inset a). The resulting NSs are usually characterized by a rigid structure and a negligible swelling in water (in comparison with other CD-NSs), and organic solvent and high resistance to chemical degradation. Carbamate CD-NSs, were originally developed by Li and Ma for the treatment of wastewaters, as an alternative for activated carbon. They demonstrated with NSs remarkable performances in the removal of organic molecules such as p-nitrophenol reducing concentration of waste from 10^{-7}–10^{-9} M to ppt level. The surface area was usually lower than activated carbon, (1–2 m^2/g, two orders of magnitude) but it is supposed that organic molecules can be adsorbed, diffuse through the surface, and be absorbed inside the bulk of NSs [43].

The good affinity of organic molecules showed for pollutants [44], is also demonstrated by the application of urethane NSs in the complexation with biologically relevant compounds, such as bilirubin or amino acids. In 2006, Tang et al. evaluated the difference in absorption of aromatic amino acids and branched-chain amino acids: the absorption of branched-chain amino acids was negligible whereas NSs absorbed 24% of the aromatic amino acids.

In previous works the same polymer was tested for the absorption of bilirubin, reducing the initial concentration of bilirubin (40 mg/l) up to 92.6% after the addition of the NS [45].

3.2.2 CD-based polycarbonate NSs

Polycarbonate CD-NSs are usually synthesized using active difunctional carbonyl compounds such as 1,1′-carbonyldiimidazole, triphosgene, and diphenylcarbonate (**Figure 1**, inset b). Since the resulting CD NSs present carbonate bonds between CD monomers, these NSs present short cross-linking bridges and, consequentially, a reduced swelling ability (if compared to CD- based polyesters NSs, for example) and good stability to acidic solutions. The affinity to organic molecules and the surface area are comparable to carbamate NS [46]. The ability of β-CD carbonate NS to remove from wastewater chlorinated persistent organic pollutants (also known as POP) was investigated by Trotta and Cavalli in 2009 [47]: the absorption efficiency was higher than the average of activated carbon. For the specific case of hexachlorobenzene the NS was capable of removing around 99.5% of the pollutant.

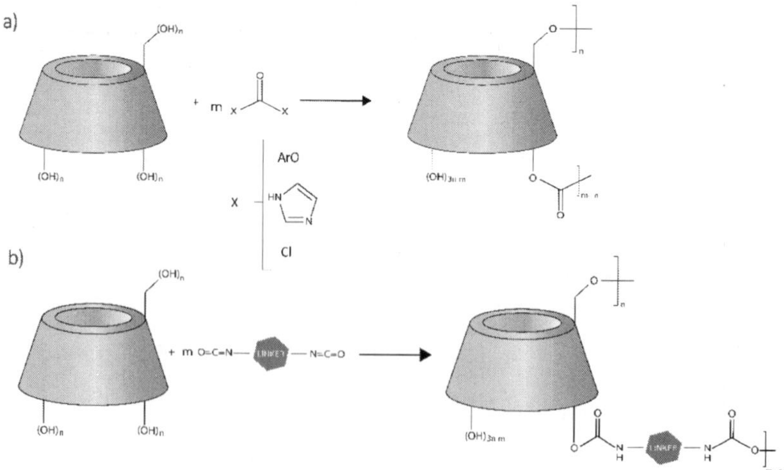

Figure 1.
Schematic synthesis of a) CD-based polyurethane NSs and b) CD-based polycarbonate NSs.

An interesting method to evaluate the degree of cross-linking of carbonate β-CD NSs, employing infrared and Raman spectroscopy, was described by Castiglione et al. [48]. Data from spectroscopic analysis and chemical computation demonstrated a correlation between the intensity of carbonyl absorption peak and the degree of cross-linking: the degree of cross-linking increased with the amount of cross-linker, in total agreement with the stoichiometry. Dealing with sugar-based predominantly amorphous materials, the reported method represents a valid and advantageous alternative to x-ray. The crosslinking density or the amount of crosslinker, strongly influences the stiffness and elastic properties of the NSs. Rossi et al. demonstrated in their study that the mechanical features of the NSs can be easily tuned by changing the molar ratio CD/cross-linker, on the other hand, the CD used for the synthesis does not affect the mechanical properties of the final NS [34, 49].

3.2.3 CD-based polyester NSs

Ester CD-based NSs are synthesized using dianhydrides or di/polycarboxylic acids, such as pyromellitic dianhydride (PMDA), ethylenediamine- tetraacetic dianhydride (EDTA dianhydride), butanetetracarboxylic dianhydride, citric acid [46, 50].

Dissimilarly from polycarbonate and polyurethane NSs, polyester NSs are generally able to absorb remarkable amounts of water (up to 25 times/g dry sample), and form stable hydrogels. Similarly as seen before with mechanical properties, the swelling capability of the CD-NSs is generally dependent on the degree of cross-linking. The swelling capability is usually inversely proportional to the density of cross-linking: the lower the degree of cross-linking, the higher the water uptake. The structure of the material dramatically influences chemical stability. Ester NSs are subjected to hydrolysis in aqueous media more easily than polycarbonate and polyurethane NSs. The structure is remarkably interesting because of the presence of free carboxyl groups in their chemical structure, moieties that can be exploited for the absorption of cations, using the material as an ionic exchange resin.

There are in literature many examples of the formation of complexes with a metal cation. The metal ions complexation ability of pyromellitic NSs is studied by Berto et al. in for different metal cations, such as Al^{3+}, Mn^{2+}, Co^{2+}, Ni^{2+}, Cu^{2+}, Zn^{2+}, Cd^{2+} and Pd^{2+}.

In most cases, pyromellitic NSs were found to be capable of absorbing more than 70% of the tested cation [51].

A similar test of removing heavy metals from wastewaters, crosslinking also CDs with citric acid, is performed by Rubin Pedrazzo et al. in 2019 [52]. At a metal concentration of 500 ppm, the pyromellitic NSs (substituted before absorption with Na^{+}) exhibited a higher retention capacity than the citrate NSs. At lower metal concentrations ($\leq$ 50 ppm) both the citrate and the pyromellitic NSs showed high retention capacities (up to 94% of the total amount of metal). While in the presence of interfering sea water salts, the citrate NSs were able to selectively adsorb a significantly higher amount of heavy metals than the pyromellitic NSs.

For ester NSs, similar studies of the correlation of cross-linking degree with properties are performed. Surprisingly, the highest cross-linking degree was observed in the sample prepared using the molar ratio 1: 6, CD: PMDA [53].

Higher contents of cross-linker, molar ratios like 1:8 and 1:10, led to a decrease of the degree of cross-linking; this is possibly related to the steric hindrance generated by the pyromellitic units linked to CDs. Interestingly, by working under limited dilution conditions during the reaction and with an even lower CD/cross-linker ratio (e.g., 1:2 molar ratio), it is possible to obtain a hyperbranched water-soluble polymer [54]. As already described for carbonate NSs,

Raman and Brillouin scattering experiments permitted Rossi et al. to evaluate a relationship between the mechanical characteristics of the polyester pyromellitic β-CD NS and the molar ratios CD/cross-linker: as seen before, stiffness and elasticity of the polymeric structure can be tuned by varying the amount of cross-linker [49].

4. Inclusion complex preparation and analysis

4.1 Preparation of inclusion complexes

Once the CD-NS is ready, the inclusion complex can be obtained by several procedures [55] as its summarized in **Figure 2**. Firstly, it is performed the classical mixing of drug and CD-NS in a solvent, commonly water for 24 h to form the complexes. In this procedure, we should consider the insoluble or soluble nature of our complexes. Depending on this, the desire fraction is purified. Using kneading, the drug and the CD-NS are mixed in a mortar with an appropriate quantity of water or another solvent to form the complexes. At this point, other additional techniques are used to form the powder: The solvent can be removed using lyophilization, co-evaporation, or spray-drying procedures.

4.2 Analysis of inclusion complexes

Different techniques can be employed to characterize not only inclusion complexes but also CD-NS. For information purposes, we will name some of them and briefly explain their possibilities [56, 57]:

4.2.1 Ultraviolet/visible spectroscopy

UV–vis is a simple, easy, and fast method for studying the host-guest complexation when its formation changes any particularity of the spectrum of a guest molecule or to check the solubilization efficacy [14, 16, 58, 59].

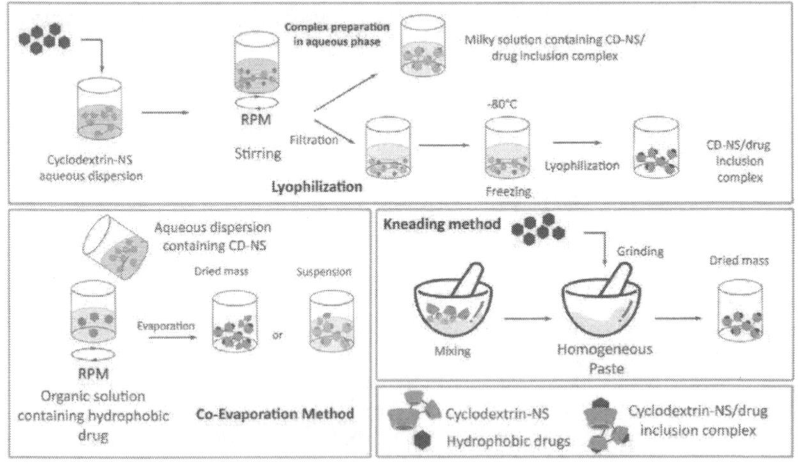

Figure 2.
Different methods to prepare inclusion complexes.

4.2.2 Fourier-transform infra-red (FTIR)

This technique is usually used in solid complexes, generally in the range of 400–4000 cm^{-1}, although it depends on the studied drug [58, 60]. Changes in the characteristics bands of the guest molecule or shifts in the wavenumber can indicate the formation of the complex. In addition, the same principle can be used to follow the CD-NS synthesis.

4.2.3 Nuclear magnetic resonance (NMR) spectroscopy

NMR is one of the most useful procedures to obtain complete analytical information of the CD-NS and the complex formed. An alteration in the chemical shift of the protons occurs when the drug enters the CD-NS providing specific information about the orientation of the guest molecule inside the cavity.

4.2.4 Thermogravimetric analysis (TGA)

TGA determines the changes of weight to temperature increases. The comparison of the weight loss profile of pure components, physical mixture, and the complex shows differences correlatives to the complex formation. A stage on TGA around 300°C is found in CD-NS due to CD decomposition [59].

4.2.5 Differential scanning calorimetry (DSC)

It can provide detailed information about their physical and energetic properties. The comparison of the thermal curves of single components, their physical mixture, and the presumed inclusion compound ought to provide insight into modifications and interactions due to the formation of the inclusion complex. The change that occurs in the fusion point of the guest molecule is usually hiding by the complex formation, while it remains in the physical mixture. This, and several modifications in the shape and temperature peak of the CD dehydration and/or with the disappearance of the drug melting peak among others, are proves of the complexation.

5. Applications in smart drug delivery

5.1 Improving solubility and controlled release of drugs

5.1.1 CD-based polyurethane NSs

Another study showed the capability of CD polyurethane to reduce the levels of natural product contaminants, particularly, Ochratoxin A (OTA) from spiked solutions between 1 and 10 µgL-1 [61]. Following the attracted considerable interest that these polymers have shown in their use for water purification systems [62] and drug delivery [63], there were further done several chemical modifications on the CD NSs. Even though the modified CD NSs were used to enhance the properties and usefulness of CD NSs, their characterization at the molecular level remained a challenge. Therefore, a study described the structural characterization at the molecular level of both, native CD nanosponge polyurethanes and bionanosponge polyurethane cyclodextrin nanocomposite (pMWCNT-CD/Ag-TiO2) showing a great antibacterial and antifungal activity. The greatest antimicrobial activities were in the case of the developed polyurethane nanocomposite (pMWCNT-CD/

Ag-TiO2). Consequently, it was concluded that this developed synthesis can be considered an active antimicrobial compound [64]. Another potential application of CD polyurethane polymer is as immobilization supports in enzyme catalysis. The lipase was immobilized into the aforementioned polymers via physisorption. It is observed an improvement in the stability and catalytic activity of lipase, knowing that the enzymes are generally unstable, insoluble in organic solvents, and sensitive. Accordingly, this study presented the chance to prepare immobilized biocatalysts with tunable catalytic activities attributed to the alteration of reaction conditions [65]. Further research was focused on the novel polyurethanes containing simultaneously β-cyclodextrin (β-CD), β-glycerophosphate groups, and hexamethylene-diisocyanate (HDI). This polymer developed was used to complex the delivering therapeutic agents such as antibiotic ciprofloxacin. It was observed an improvement of the drug release in the case of the drug-polymers complexation than that of the free drug [63].

5.1.2 CD-based polycarbonate NSs

CD-based polycarbonate NSs synthesized using carbonyldiimidazole (CDI) showed antimicrobial activity against various microorganisms such as *E. coli*, *S. aureus*, *P. aeruginosa*, *S. typhi*, *C. albicans*, and Clostridia, when compared with Ciprofloxacin that was used as a standard drug. The formulations were prepared by polymer condensation, and interfacial phenomenon, and were effective for 6 months at a condition of 40°C and 75% of relative humidity [66]. This type of CD NSs was further used to deliver and increase the activity of several anticancer drugs such as paclitaxel [67], bortezomib [68], flutamide [69], tamoxifen [70], etc. Following their high potential to entrap a variety of molecules, the β-CD/CDI NSs were also used to deliver and improve the solubility and dissolution of paliperidone, an antipsychotic drug for the treatment of schizophrenia [71]. Further, rilpivirine is used for the treatment of HIV infection but has low aqueous solubility. Therefore, the β-CD/CDI NSs presented a strategy to improve this drawback and also the bioavailability and dissolution rate [72]. The antioxidant activity of kynurenic acid, an endogenous substance, was improved by loading it in β-CD/CDI NSs. The higher antioxidant activity was observed because of the increment in solubilization of kynurenic acid [60]. CD-based polycarbonate NSs synthesized using diphenyl carbonate (DPC) were used to overcome the poor solubility and stability of Babchi oil that is known for possessing numerous activities such as antifungal, antibacterial, antiviral, antitumor, antioxidant, etc. [73]. Further, the bioactive properties of the piperine, an alkaloid with anti-microbial, anti-inflammatory, anti-cancer properties, etc., were protected by the β-CD/DPC NSs [74]. This type of NSs exhibited complexing ability toward nifedipine, as an oral calcium channel blocking agent that is used to treat angina pectoris and hypertension. It was observed an improvement in the oral solubility of nifedipine after its incorporation into NSs [75].

5.1.3 CD-based polyester NSs

CD-based Ester NSs synthesized with pyromellitic dianhydride (PMDA) are well known for delivering, enhancing solubility, and preventing the degradation of various drugs such as Curcumin [76], Insulin [20], Resveratrol [77], Erlotinib hydrochloride [78], among others. Ethylenediaminetetraacetic dianhydride (EDTA) is another cross-linker to synthesize ester CD NSs. Based on HRMAS probe-heads in a high-resolution NMR spectrometer on the transport properties of Ibuprofen sodium salt (IP), it was found that these NSs can be utilized for the rational design of smart systems for drug delivery and controlled release [79]. The various applications of CD-based polyester NSs ranging from the environment to pharmacy, chemistry, agriculture, gene delivery, cosmetics, biocatalysis, brought to a detailed study on their cross-linking density. Being a very challenging task, it presented the effect of cross-linking density on β-CD NSs physicochemical properties. Flory-Rehner theory and rheology enabled the authors to understand the correlation between the structural features of NSs and their physicochemical properties, which is a key requirement for future applications [34].

5.2 Last generations of NSs for selected target drug delivery

Stimuli-responsive NSs represent the third generation, polymers that have been designed to modulate their behavior according to the surrounding environment. In this case, changes in the chemical structure of the material were reported to be triggered by pH, temperature gradients, or oxidative/reducing conditions. This feature was exploited for studying the targeted release of drugs, changes in color, and permeability. The use of glutathione (GSH) bioresponsive CD-NS was proposed as the system to deliver anticancer drugs or bioactive compounds [80–83]. This is because GSH is 100 to 1000 times higher inside cells than that in the extracellular fluids and circulation. Indeed, in cancer cells, this concentration is almost higher being a good system for target drug delivery [84]. Different drugs such as doxorubicin [81] or bioactive compounds such as resveratrol [82] were tested showing a well-targeted drug delivery, and therefore is considered a promising therapy. In addition, the linkage of cholesterol was proposed as a good procedure for increase the targeted drug delivery of doxorubicin-loaded CD-NS [85].

Lastly, molecularly imprinted cyclodextrin-based polymers (**Figure 3**) define the fourth generation of NSs. Molecular imprinting represents a specific approach of inducing molecular recognition features to a three-dimensional polymer. This property can be achieved as a result of the presence of a template molecule introduced during synthesis. The template molecule after being removed from the polymer matrix leaves size-complementary vacancies, enabling the network to display high selectivity and affinity toward the chosen template. Eventually, molecularly

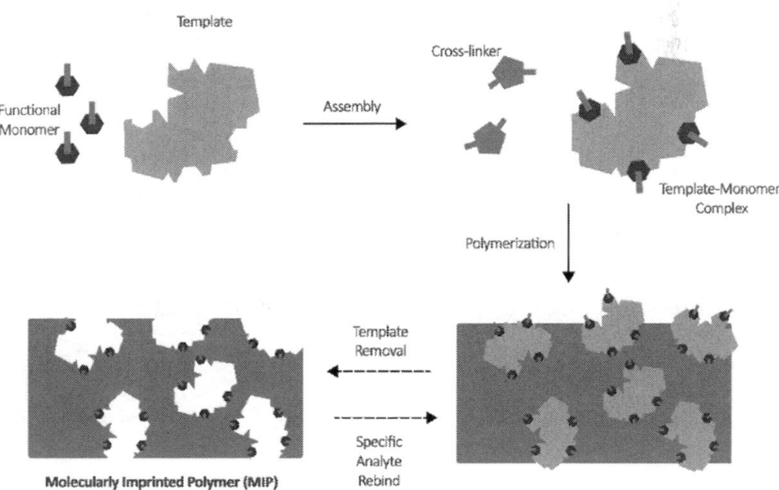

Figure 3.
Schematic synthesis of molecularly imprinted NSs.

Drug	Nanocarrier prepared	Outcome	References
Controlled Drug Delivery			
CD-based Polyurethane NSs			
Erythromycin, vancomycin, and rifampicin	βCD/HDI	*Long-term sustained release of antibiotics.*	[89]
Mitomycin C	ϒCD/HDI	*Prolonged anti-proliferative drug release.*	[90]
CD-based Polycarbonate NSs			
Curcumin	βCD/DMC	*Increased anti-cancer drug solubility, and prolonged release.*	[91]
Norfloxacin	βCD/DPC	*Enhanced anti-bacterial drug permeability.*	[92]
Tamoxifen	βCD/CDI	*Increased anti-cancer drug solubility, and bioavailability.*	[93]
Resveratrol	βCD/CDI	*Increased the permeation, stability, and cytotoxicity against cancer*	[94]
Camptothecin	βCD/DPC	*Increased anti-cancer drug stability, and prolonged release.*	[95]
Acyclovir	βCD/CDI	*Enhanced anti-viral drug loading, and prolonged release.*	[96]
Telmisartan	βCD/DPC	*Enhanced anti-hypertensive drug solubility, improved bioavailability, and prolonged release.*	[97]
Babchi Oil	βCD/DPC	*Enhanced anti-bacterial essential oil solubility, photo-stability, and safety.*	[98]
Rilpivirine	βCD/CDI; PMDA; DPC	*Enhanced anti-viral drug solubility, and bioavailability.*	[99, 100]
Paclitaxel	βCD/CDI	*Enhanced anti-cancer drug solubility, and pharmacological effect.*	[101]
Sulfamethoxazole	βCD/CDI	*Enhanced anti-bacterial drug solubility.*	[102]
Quercetin	βCD/DPC	*Enhanced anti-oxidative drug dissolution, and prolonged release.*	[103]
Melatonin	βCD/CDI	*Controlled drug release through skin.*	[104]
Kynurenic acid	βCD/CDI	*Enhanced anti-oxidant potential of kynurenic acid.*	[105]
D-Limonene	βCD/DPC	*Enhanced anti-bacterial potential of the drug.*	[106]
Azelaic acid	βCD/DPC	*Enhanced drug solubility, and its depigmenting action on the skin via antioxidant, and antityrosinase effect.*	[107]
Chrysin	βCD/DPC	*Enhanced drug solubility, in-vitro antioxidant, and antitumoral activity.*	[108]
Paliperidone	βCD/CDI	*Enhanced antipsychotic drug solubility.*	[109]

Drug	Nanocarrier prepared	Outcome	References
Ferulic acid	βCD/DPC	*Enhanced drug solubility, and bioavailability for the local therapy of vessels wall.*	[110]
Flutamide	βCD/CDI	*Enhanced anti-cancer drug dissolution rate.*	[111]
Griseofulvin	βCD/DPC	*Enhanced antifungal oral drug bioavailability, and improved dissolution rate.*	[112]
CD-based Polyester NSs			
Insulin	βCD/PMDA	*Enhanced anti-diabetic drug stability, and prolonged release.*	[113]
Imiquimod	βCD/PMDA	*Enhanced drug aqueous solubility, and skin permeation capability.*	[114]
Acetyl salicylic acid	βCD/PMDA	*Enhanced anti-inflammatory drug stability, and prolonged release.*	[115]
Doxorubicin	βCD/PMDA	*Improved anti-cancer effectiveness.*	[116]
Meloxicam	βCD/PMDA	*Increased anti-inflammatory drug solubility, and wettability.*	[117]
Targeted Drug Delivery			
DB103 - [2-(3, 4-dimethoxyphenyl)-3-phenyl-4H-pyrido]	βCD/DPC	*Enhanced drug solubility, and bioavailability for the local therapy of vessels wall.*	[118]
L-DOPA	βCD/CDI; PMDA (Molecularly imprinted cyclodextrin-based polymers)	*Enhanced drug solubility, and prolonged release.*	[119]
Doxorubicin	Tripeptide glutathione (GSH) nanosponge (NS)	*Enhanced antioxidant potential, and it is useful in targeting chemo-resistant tumors.*	[120]
Strigolactones	GSH/pH-NS	*Enhanced anticancer activity.*	[121]
Erlotinib hydrochloride (ETB)	GSH-NS	*Exhibited excellent drug uptake, extended drug release, in-vivo antitumor efficacy, and biodistribution.*	[122]

βCD, Beta Cyclodextrin; ϒCD, Gama Cyclodextrin; HDI, Hexamethylene diisocyanate; CDI, Carbonyldiimidazole; DMC, Dimethyl Carbonate; DPC, Diphenyl carbonate; PMDA, Pyromellitic Dianhydride.

Table 2.
The use of cyclodextrin based nanosponges in drug delivery.

imprinted CD-NSs are studied as suitable material to develop biosensors, drug delivery systems, catalysts, or synthetic antibody mimics [86–88]. A good example of this application is the L-Dopa as a novel possibility to treat Parkinson's Disease. The molecularly imprinted CD-NSs showed a slower and more prolonged release profile than the non-imprinted NSs, indicating the good capacity to better complex L-Dopa than non-imprinted NS. The use of CDs in controlled and targeted drug delivery is shown in **Table 2**.

6. Conclusions

CD-NSs are demonstrated to be safe, cheap, and biocompatible polymers. Consequently, several authors are focused on this field recently achieving novel applications. This chapter summarized the general information that will guide the advanced research to investigate the CD-NSs. Information about the routes of administration, synthesis protocols, recommendations, classifications, and applications of the novel synthesized materials, with special attention to targeted drug delivery, are mostly collected. It is shown the ability of CD-NSs to entrap drugs and to control their release from the matrix which can be modulated by different physicochemical agents.

As a remark, CD-NS is a good promise to improve the current problems in drug formulations and open novel strategies for drug delivery that identify the light in the future.

Acknowledgements

This work is the result of aid to postdoctoral training and improvement abroad (for Adrián Matencio, number 21229/PD/19) financed by the Fundación Séneca (Región de Murcia, Spain).

Conflict of interest

The authors declare no conflict of interest.

References

[1] Matencio A, Navarro-Orcajada S, García-Carmona F, López-Nicolás JM. Applications of cyclodextrins in food science. A review. Trends Food Sci Technol 2020.

[2] Szente L, Szejtli J. Cyclodextrins as food ingredients. Trends in Food Science & Technology 2004; **15**: 137-142.

[3] Matencio A, Alcaráz-Gómez MA, García-Carmona F, Arias B, López-Nicolás JM. Application of a simple methodology to analyze Hydroxypropyl-β-Cyclodextrin in urine using HPLC–LS in early Niemann–Pick disease type C patient. Journal of Chromatography B 2018; **1093-1094**: 47-51.

[4] Matencio A, Navarro-Orcajada S, González-Ramón A, García-Carmona F, López-Nicolás JM. Recent advances in the treatment of Niemann pick disease type C: A mini-review. International Journal of Pharmaceutics 2020; **584**: 119440.

[5] Matencio A, García-Carmona F, López-Nicolás JM. The inclusion complex of oxyresveratrol in modified cyclodextrins: A thermodynamic, structural, physicochemical, fluorescent and computational study. Food Chemistry 2017; **232**: 177-184.

[6] Matencio A, Bermejo-Gimeno MJ, García-Carmona F, López-Nicolás JM. Separating and Identifying the Four Stereoisomers of Methyl Jasmonate by RP-HPLC and using Cyclodextrins in a Novel Way. Phytochemical Analysis 2017; **28**: 151-158.

[7] Matencio A, Navarro-Orcajada S, García-Carmona F, Manuel López-Nicolás J. Ellagic acid–borax fluorescence interaction: application for novel cyclodextrin-borax nanosensors for analyzing ellagic acid in food samples. Food & Function 2018; **9**: 3683-3687.

[8] Matencio A, Caldera F, Rubin Pedrazzo A, Khazaei Monfared Y, K. Dhakar N, Trotta F. A physicochemical, thermodynamical, structural and computational evaluation of kynurenic acid/cyclodextrin complexes. Food Chemistry 2021; **356**: 129639.

[9] Jansook P, Ogawa N, Loftsson T. Cyclodextrins: structure, physicochemical properties and pharmaceutical applications. International Journal of Pharmaceutics 2018; **535**: 272-284.

[10] Matencio A, Caldera F, Cecone C, López-Nicolás JM, Trotta F. Cyclic Oligosaccharides as Active Drugs, an Updated Review. Pharmaceuticals 2020; **13**: 281.

[11] Cavalli R, Trotta F, Tumiatti W. Cyclodextrin-based Nanosponges for Drug Delivery. J Incl Phenom Macrocycl Chem 2006; **56**: 209-213.

[12] Sherje AP, Dravyakar BR, Kadam D, Jadhav M. Cyclodextrin-based nanosponges: A critical review. Carbohydrate Polymers 2017; **173**: 37-49.

[13] Swaminathan S, Cavalli R, Trotta F. Cyclodextrin-based nanosponges: a versatile platform for cancer nanotherapeutics development. WIREs Nanomed Nanobiotechnol 2016; **8**: 579-601.

[14] Krabicová I, Appleton SL, Tannous M, *et al.* History of Cyclodextrin Nanosponges. Polymers (Basel) 2020; **12**.

[15] Shende P, Kulkarni YA, Gaud RS, *et al.* Acute and Repeated Dose Toxicity Studies of Different β-Cyclodextrin-Based Nanosponge Formulations. Journal of Pharmaceutical Sciences 2015; **104**: 1856-1863.

[16] Matencio A, Guerrero-Rubio MA, Caldera F, *et al.* Lifespan extension in Caenorhabditis elegans by oxyresveratrol supplementation in hyper-branched cyclodextrin-based nanosponges. International Journal of Pharmaceutics 2020; **589**: 119862.

[17] Caldera F, Tannous M, Cavalli R, Zanetti M, Trotta F. Evolution of Cyclodextrin Nanosponges. International Journal of Pharmaceutics 2017; **531**: 470-479.

[18] Trotta F, Caldera F, Cavalli R, *et al.* Synthesis and characterization of a hyper-branched water-soluble β-cyclodextrin polymer. Beilstein Journal of Organic Chemistry 2014; **10**: 2586-2593.

[19] Trotta F, Caldera F, Cavalli R, *et al.* Synthesis and characterization of a hyper-branched water-soluble β-cyclodextrin polymer. Beilstein Journal of Organic Chemistry 2014; **10**: 2586-2593.

[20] Appleton SL, Tannous M, Argenziano M, *et al.* Nanosponges as protein delivery systems: Insulin, a case study. Int J Pharm 2020; **590**: 119888.

[21] Deshmukh K, Tanwar YS, Sharma S, Shende P, Cavalli R. Functionalized nanosponges for controlled antibacterial and antihypocalcemic actions. Biomedicine & Pharmacotherapy 2016; **84**: 485-494.

[22] Paoletti R, Nicosia S, Clementi F, Fumagalli G. *Farmacologia Generale e Molecolare*. (UTET, ed.)., 2004.

[23] Kim J, De Jesus O. *Medication Routes of Administration*. (StatPearls, ed.). StatPearls Publishing, 2021.

[24] Homayun B, Lin X, Choi HJ. Challenges and recent progress in oral drug delivery systems for biopharmaceuticals. Pharmaceutics 2019; **11**.

[25] Fuccella LM, Perucca E, Sirtori C. *Farmacologia clinica*. (Mediche US, ed.)., 2006.

[26] Boddupalli BM, Mohammed ZNK, Ravinder Nath A.1 DB. Mucoadhesive drug delivery system: An overview. J Adv Pharm Tech Res 2010.

[27] Ahuja A, Khar RK, Ali J. Mucoadhesive drug delivery systems. Drug Development and Industrial Pharmacy 1997; **23**: 489-515.

[28] Gatti THH, Eloy JO, Ferreira LMB, *et al.* Insulin-loaded polymeric mucoadhesive nanoparticles: Development, characterization and cytotoxicity evaluation. Brazilian Journal of Pharmaceutical Sciences 2018; **54**: 1-10.

[29] Rowland M, Tozer TN. *Clinical Pharmacokineticsand Pharmacodynamics Concepts and Applications*. (Wilkins LW&, ed.)., 2011.

[30] Sherje AP, Dravyakar BR, Kadam D, Jadhav M. Cyclodextrin-based nanosponges: A critical review. Carbohydrate Polymers 2017; **173**: 37-49.

[31] Chilajwar S V., Pednekar PP, Jadhav KR, Gupta GJC, Kadam VJ. Cyclodextrin-based nanosponges: A propitious platform for enhancing drug delivery. Expert Opinion on Drug Delivery 2014; **11**: 111-120.

[32] Tejashri G, Amrita B, Darshana J. Cyclodextrin based nanosponges for pharmaceutical use: A review. Acta Pharmaceutica 2013; **63**: 335-358.

[33] Kumar S, Dalal P, Rao R. Cyclodextrin Nanosponges: A Promising Approach for Modulating Drug Delivery. Colloid Science in Pharmaceutical Nanotechnology 2020.

[34] Hoti G, Caldera F, Cecone C, *et al.* Effect of the cross-linking density on the swelling and rheological behavior of ester-bridged β-cyclodextrin nanosponges. Materials 2021; **14**: 1-20.

[35] Trotta F, Cavalli R, Tumiatti W, Zerbinati O, Roggero C, Vallero R. Ultrasound synthesis of nanosponges. pdf. 2006.

[36] Trotta F, Cavalli R. Characterization and applications of new hyper-cross-linked cyclodextrins. Composite Interfaces 2009; **16**: 39-48.

[37] Cecone C, Hoti G, Krabicova I, *et al.* Sustainable synthesis of cyclodextrin-based polymers exploiting natural deep eutectic solvents. Green Chemistry 2020; **22**: 5806-5814.

[38] Trotta F. Cyclodextrin nanosponges and their applications. In: *Cyclodextrins in Pharmaceutics, Cosmetics, and Biomedicine: Current and Future Industrial Applications*. First., 2011, 323-42.

[39] Trotta F, Zanetti M, Cavalli R. Cyclodextrin-based nanosponges as drug carriers. Beilstein Journal of Organic Chemistry 2012; **8**: 2091-2099.

[40] Martel B, Ruffin D, Weltrowski M, Lekchiri Y, Morcellet M. Water-soluble polymers and gels from the polycondensation between cyclodextrins and poly(carboxylic acid) s: A study of the preparation parameters. Journal of Applied Polymer Science 2005; **97**: 433-442.

[41] Zhao D, Zhao L, Zhu C-S, Huang W, Hu J. Water-insoluble b-cyclodextrin polymer crosslinked by citric acid : synthesis and adsorption properties toward phenol and methylene blue. J Incl Phenom Macrocycl Chem 2009; **63**: 195-201.

[42] Lu D, Yang L, Zhou T, Lei Z. Synthesis, characterization and properties of biodegradable polylactic acid-β-cyclodextrin cross-linked copolymer microgels. European Polymer Journal 2008; **44**: 2140-2145.

[43] B. B. Mamba, Krause RW, Malefetse TJ, Gericke G, S. P. Sithole. Nanosponges for water purification. Clean Products and Processes 2. 2000; **2**: 112-6.

[44] B. B. Mamba, R. W. Krause, T. J. Malefetse GG e SPS. Cyclodextrin nanosponges in the removal of organic matter to produce water for power generation. 2008; **34**: 657-60.

[45] Zheng C, Huang X, Kong L, Li X, Zou H. Cross-linked beta-cyclodextrin polymer used for bilirubin removal. Chinese journal of chromatography, 2004; **22**: 128-130.

[46] Trotta F. Cyclodextrin Nanosponges and their Applications. Cyclodextrins in Pharmaceutics, Cosmetics, and Biomedicine: Current and Future Industrial Applications 2011: 323-342.

[47] Trotta F, Cavalli R. Characterization and application of new hyper-cross-linked cyclodextrins. Compos Interf 2009; **16**: 39-48.

[48] Castiglione F, Crupi V, Majolino D, *et al.* Inside new materials: An experimental numerical approach for the structural elucidation of nanoporous cross-linked polymers. Journal of Physical Chemistry B 2012; **116**: 13133-13140.

[49] Rossi B, Caponi S, Castiglione F, *et al.* Networking properties of cyclodextrin-based cross-linked polymers probed by inelastic light-scattering experiments. Journal of Physical Chemistry B 2012; **116**: 5323-5327.

[50] Caldera F, Tannous M, Cavalli R, Zanetti M, Trotta F. Evolution of Cyclodextrin Nanosponges. International Journal of Pharmaceutics 2017; **531**: 470-479.

[51] Berto S, Bruzzoniti MC, Cavalli R, *et al.* Synthesis of new ionic β-cyclodextrin polymers and characterization of their heavy metals retention. Journal of

Inclusion Phenomena and Macrocyclic Chemistry 2007; **57**: 631-636.

[52] Rubin Pedrazzo A, Smarra A, Caldera F, *et al.* Eco-Friendly β -cyclodextrin and Linecaps Polymers for the Removal of Heavy Metals. Polymers 2019: 1-15.

[53] Crupi V, Fontana A, Giarola M, *et al.* Connection between the vibrational dynamics and the cross-linking properties in cyclodextrins-based polymers. Journal of Raman Spectroscopy 2013; **44**: 1457-1462.

[54] Trotta F, Caldera F, Cavalli R, *et al.* Synthesis and characterization of a hyper-branched water-soluble β-cyclodextrin polymer. Beilstein Journal of Organic Chemistry 2014; **10**: 2586-2593.

[55] Gharib R, Greige-Gerges H, Fourmentin S, Charcosset C, Auezova L. Liposomes incorporating cyclodextrin–drug inclusion complexes: Current state of knowledge. Carbohydrate Polymers 2015; **129**: 175-186.

[56] Mura P. Analytical techniques for characterization of cyclodextrin complexes in aqueous solution: A review. Journal of Pharmaceutical and Biomedical Analysis 2014; **101**: 238-250.

[57] Mura P. Analytical techniques for characterization of cyclodextrin complexes in the solid state: A review. Journal of Pharmaceutical and Biomedical Analysis 2015; **113**: 226-238.

[58] Dhakar NK, Matencio A, Caldera F, *et al.* Comparative Evaluation of Solubility, Cytotoxicity and Photostability Studies of Resveratrol and Oxyresveratrol Loaded Nanosponges. Pharmaceutics 2019; **11**: 545.

[59] Matencio A, Dhakar NK, Bessone F, *et al.* Study of oxyresveratrol complexes with insoluble cyclodextrin based nanosponges: Developing a novel way to obtain their complexation constants and application in an anticancer study. Carbohydrate Polymers 2020; **231**: 115763.

[60] Dhakar NK, Caldera F, Bessone F, *et al.* Evaluation of solubility enhancement, antioxidant activity, and cytotoxicity studies of kynurenic acid loaded cyclodextrin nanosponge. Carbohydrate Polymers 2019; **224**: 115168.

[61] Appell M, Jackson MA. Sorption of Ochratoxin A from Aqueous Solutions Using β-Cyclodextrin-Polyurethane Polymer. Toxins 2012; **4**: 98-109.

[62] Leudjo Taka A, Pillay K, Yangkou Mbianda X. Nanosponge cyclodextrin polyurethanes and their modification with nanomaterials for the removal of pollutants from waste water: A review. Carbohydrate Polymers 2017; **159**: 94-107.

[63] Moreira MP, Andrade GRS, De Araujo MVG, Kubota T, Gimenez IF. Ternary cyclodextrin polyurethanes containing phosphate groups: Synthesis and complexation of ciprofloxacin. Carbohydrate Polymers 2016; **151**: 557-564.

[64] Taka AL, Doyle BP, Carleschi E, *et al.* Spectroscopic characterization and antimicrobial activity of nanoparticle doped cyclodextrin polyurethane bionanosponge. Materials Science& Engineering C 2020: 1-15.

[65] Dhake KP, Karoyo AH, Mohamed MH, Wilson LD, Bhanage BM. Enzymatic activity studies of Pseudomonas cepacia lipase adsorbed onto copolymer supports containing β-cyclodextrin. Journal of Molecular Catalysis B: Enzymatic 2013; **87**: 105-112.

[66] Desai D, Shende P. Drug-Free Cyclodextrin-Based Nanosponges for Antimicrobial Activity. Journal of Pharmaceutical Innovation 2020: 11.

[67] Mognetti B, Barberis A, Marino S, *et al.* In vitro enhancement of anticancer activity of paclitaxel by a Cremophor free cyclodextrin-based nanosponge formulation. Journal of Inclusion Phenomena and Macrocyclic Chemistry 2012; **74**: 201-210.

[68] Allahyari S, Valizadeh H, Roshangar L, *et al.* Preparation and characterization of cyclodextrin nanosponges for bortezomib delivery. Expert Opinion on Drug Delivery 2020; **17**: 10.

[69] Allahyari S, Esmailnezhad N, Valizadeh H, *et al.* In-vitro characterization and cytotoxicity study of flutamide loaded cyclodextrin nanosponges. Journal of Drug Delivery Science and Technology 2021; **61**: 1-7.

[70] Torne S, Darandale S, Vavia P, Trotta F, Cavalli R. Cyclodextrin-based nanosponges: effective nanocarrier for Tamoxifen delivery. Pharmaceutical Development and Technology 2013; **18**: 619-625.

[71] Sherje AP, Surve A, Shende P. CDI cross-linked β -cyclodextrin nanosponges of paliperidone : synthesis and physicochemical characterization. Journal 2019.

[72] Rao MRP, Chaudhari J, Trotta F, Caldera F. Investigation of Cyclodextrin-Based Nanosponges for Solubility and Bioavailability Enhancement of Rilpivirine. AAPS PharmSciTech 2018; **19**: 2358-2369.

[73] Kumar S, Pooja, Trotta F, Rao R. Encapsulation of Babchi Oil in Cyclodextrin-Based Nanosponges: Physicochemical Characterization, Photodegradation, and In Vitro Cytotoxicity Studies. Pharmaceutics 2018; **10**:1-18

[74] Garrido B, González S, Hermosilla J, *et al.* Carbonate-β-Cyclodextrin-Based Nanosponge as a Nanoencapsulation System for Piperine: Physicochemical Characterization. Journal of Soil Science and Plant Nutrition 2019; **19**: 620-630.

[75] Shringirishi M, Mahor A, Gupta R, Prajapati SK, Bansal K, Kesharwani P. Fabrication and characterization of nifedipine loaded β-cyclodextrin nanosponges: An in vitro and in vivo evaluation. Journal of Drug Delivery Science and Technology 2017; **41**: 344-350.

[76] Pushpalatha R, Selvamuthukumar S, Kilimozhi D. Cross-linked, cyclodextrin-based nanosponges for curcumin delivery - Physicochemical characterization, drug release, stability and cytotoxicity. Journal of Drug Delivery Science and Technology 2018; **45**: 45-53.

[77] Pushpalatha R, Selvamuthukumar S, Kilimozhi D. Carbonyl and carboxylate crosslinked cyclodextrin as a nanocarrier for resveratrol: in silico, in vitro and in vivo evaluation. Journal of Inclusion Phenomena and Macrocyclic Chemistry 2018; **92**: 261-272.

[78] Momin MM, Zaheer Z, Zainuddin R, Sangshetti JN. Extended release delivery of erlotinib glutathione nanosponge for targeting lung cancer. Artificial Cells, Nanomedicine and Biotechnology 2018; **46**: 1064-1075.

[79] Ferro M, Castiglione F, Punta C, *et al.* Anomalous diffusion of Ibuprofen in cyclodextrin nanosponge hydrogels: an HRMAS NMR study. Beilstein Journal of Organic Chemistry 2014; **10**: 2715-2723.

[80] Rossi B, Venuti V, D'Amico F, *et al.* Toward an understanding of the thermosensitive behaviour of pH-responsive hydrogels based on cyclodextrins. Soft Matter 2015; **11**: 5862-5871.

[81] Daga M, Ullio C, Argenziano M, *et al.* GSH-targeted nanosponges increase doxorubicin-induced toxicity "in vitro" and "in vivo" in cancer cells with high antioxidant defenses. Free Radical Biology and Medicine 2016; **97**: 24-37.

[82] Palminteri M, Dhakar NK, Ferraresi A, *et al.* Cyclodextrin nanosponge for the GSH-mediated delivery of Resveratrol in human cancer cells. Nanotheranostics 2021; **5**: 197-212.

[83] Argenziano M, Lombardi C, Ferrara B, *et al.* Glutathione/pH-responsive nanosponges enhance strigolactone delivery to prostate cancer cells. Oncotarget 2018; **9**: 35813-35829.

[84] Traverso N, Ricciarelli R, Nitti M, *et al.* Role of glutathione in cancer progression and chemoresistance. Oxid Med Cell Longev 2013; **2013**: 972913.

[85] Singh P, Ren X, Guo T, *et al.* Biofunctionalization of β-cyclodextrin nanosponges using cholesterol. Carbohydr Polym 2018; **190**: 23-30.

[86] Shende P, Kulkarni YA, Gaud RS, *et al.* Acute and repeated dose toxicity studies of different β-cyclodextrin-based nanosponge formulations. Journal of Pharmaceutical Sciences 2015; **104**: 1856-1863.

[87] Kyzas GZ, Lazaridis NK, Bikiaris DN. Optimization of chitosan and β-cyclodextrin molecularly imprinted polymer synthesis for dye adsorption. Carbohydrate Polymers 2013; **91**: 198-208.

[88] Deshmukh K, Tanwar YS, Shende P, Cavalli R. Biomimetic estimation of glucose using non-molecular and molecular imprinted polymer nanosponges. International Journal of Pharmaceutics 2015; **494**: 244-248.

[89] T. R. Thatiparti and H. A. Von Recum, "Cyclodextrin Complexation for Affinity-Based Antibiotic Delivery," Macromol. Biosci., vol. 10, pp. 82-90, 2010.

[90] S. R. Merritt, G. Velasquez, and H. A. Von Recum, "Adjustable release of mitomycin C for inhibition of scar tissue formation after filtration surgery," Exp. Eye Res., vol. 116, pp. 9-16, 2013.

[91] S. S. Darandale and P. R. Vavia, "Cyclodextrin-based nanosponges of curcumin: Formulation and physicochemical characterization," in *Journal of Inclusion Phenomena and Macrocyclic Chemistry*, 2013, vol. 75, no. 3-4, pp. 315-322.

[92] C. Mendes, G. C. Meirelles, C. G. Barp, J. Assreuy, M. A. S. Silva, and G. Ponchel, "Cyclodextrin based nanosponge of norfloxacin: Intestinal permeation enhancement and improved antibacterial activity," Carbohydr. Polym., vol. 195, pp. 586-592, 2018.

[93] S. Torne, S. Darandale, P. Vavia, F. Trotta, and R. Cavalli, "Cyclodextrin-based nanosponges: effective nanocarrier for tamoxifen delivery," Pharmaceutical development and technology, vol. 18, no. 3. pp. 619-625, 2013.

[94] K. A. Ansari, P. R. Vavia, F. Trotta, and R. Cavalli, "Cyclodextrin-Based Nanosponges for Delivery of Resveratrol: In vitro Characterisation, Stability, Cytotoxicity and Permeation Study," AAPS PharmSciTech, vol. 12, no. 1, pp. 279-286, Mar. 2011.

[95] S. Swaminathan *et al.*, "Cyclodextrin-based nanosponges encapsulating camptothecin: Physicochemical characterization, stability and cytotoxicity," Eur. J. Pharm. Biopharm., vol. 74, pp. 193-201, 2010.

[96] D. Lembo *et al.*, "Encapsulation of Acyclovir in new carboxylated cyclodextrin-based nanosponges improves the agent's antiviral efficacy,"

Int. J. Pharm., vol. 443, pp. 262-272, Feb. 2013.

[97] M. Rao, A. Bajaj, I. Khole, G. Munjapara, and F. Trotta, "In vitro and in vivo evaluation of β-cyclodextrin-based nanosponges of telmisartan," J. Incl. Phenom. Macrocycl. Chem., vol. 77, pp. 135-145, Dec. 2013.

[98] S. Kumar, Pooja, F. Trotta, and R. Rao, "Encapsulation of Babchi Oil in Cyclodextrin-Based Nanosponges: Physicochemical Characterization, Photodegradation, and In Vitro Cytotoxicity Studies," *Pharmaceutics*, vol. 10, p. 169, Sep. 2018.

[99] R. Zainuddin, Z. Zaheer, J. N. Sangshetti, and M. Momin, "Enhancement of oral bioavailability of anti- HIV drug rilpivirine HCl through nanosponge formulation," Drug Dev. Ind. Pharm., vol. 43, no. 12, pp. 2076-2084, 2017.

[100] M. R. P. Rao, J. Chaudhari, F. Trotta, and F. Caldera, "Investigation of Cyclodextrin-Based Nanosponges for Solubility and Bioavailability Enhancement of Rilpivirine," AAPS PharmSciTech, pp. 2358-2368, 2018.

[101] B. Mognetti *et al.*, "In vitro enhancement of anticancer activity of paclitaxel by a Cremophor free cyclodextrin-based nanosponge formulation," J. Incl. Phenom. Macrocycl. Chem., vol. 74, pp. 201-210, Dec. 2012.

[102] G. Yaşayan, B. Şatıroğlu Sert, E. Tatar, and İ. Küçükgüzel, "Fabrication and characterisation studies of cyclodextrin-based nanosponges for sulfamethoxazole delivery," J. Incl. Phenom. Macrocycl. Chem., vol. 97, pp. 175-186, 2020.

[103] S. Anandam and S. Selvamuthukumar, "Fabrication of cyclodextrin nanosponges for quercetin delivery: physicochemical characterization, photostability, and antioxidant effects," J. Mater. Sci., vol. 49, pp. 8140-8153, 2014.

[104] M. Mihailiasa, F. Caldera, J. Li, R. Peila, A. Ferri, and F. Trotta, "Preparation of functionalized cotton fabrics by means of melatonin loaded β-cyclodextrin nanosponges," Carbohydr. Polym., vol. 142, pp. 24-30, 2016.

[105] N. K. Dhakar *et al.*, "Evaluation of solubility enhancement, antioxidant activity, and cytotoxicity studies of kynurenic acid loaded cyclodextrin nanosponge," Carbohydr. Polym., vol. 224, pp. 1-9, 2019.

[106] O. Salehi, S. Masoud, and A. Rezaei, "Limonene loaded cyclodextrin nanosponge: Preparation, characterization, antibacterial activity and controlled release," Food Biosci., vol. 42, pp. 1-9, 2021.

[107] A. Kumar and R. Rao, "Enhancing efficacy and safety of azelaic acid via encapsulation in cyclodextrin nanosponges: development, characterization and evaluation," Polym. Bull., vol. 78, pp. 5275-5302, 2021.

[108] M. Sundararajan, P. A. Thomas, K. Venkadeswaran, K. Jeganathan, and P. Geraldine, "Synthesis and Characterization of Chrysin-Loaded β-Cyclodextrin-Based Nanosponges to Enhance In-Vitro Solubility, Photostability, Drug Release, Antioxidant Effects and Antitumorous Efficacy," J. Nanosci. Nanotechnol., vol. 17, p. 10, 2017.

[109] A. P. Sherje, A. Surve, and P. Shende, "CDI cross-linked β -cyclodextrin nanosponges of paliperidone : synthesis and physicochemical characterization," *Journal*, 2019.

[110] A. Rezaei, J. Varshosaz, M. Fesharaki, A. Farhang, and S. M. Jafari,

"Improving the solubility and in vitro cytotoxicity (anticancer activity) of ferulic acid by loading it into cyclodextrin nanosponges," pp. 4589-4599, 2019.

[111] S. Allahyari *et al.*, "In-vitro characterization and cytotoxicity study of flutamide loaded cyclodextrin nanosponges," J. Drug Deliv. Sci. Technol., vol. 61, pp. 1-7, 2021.

[112] S. M. Omar, F. Ibrahim, and A. Ismail, "Formulation and evaluation of cyclodextrin-based nanosponges of griseofulvin as pediatric oral liquid dosage form for enhancing bioavailability and masking bitter taste," Saudi Pharm. J., vol. 28, pp. 349-361, 2020.

[113] S. Lucia Appleton *et al.*, "Nanosponges as protein delivery systems : Insulin, a case study," Int. J. Pharm., vol. 590, pp. 1-11, 2020.

[114] M. Argenziano *et al.*, "In Vitro Enhanced Skin Permeation and Retention of Imiquimod Loaded in β -Cyclodextrin Nanosponge Hydrogel," Pharmaceutics, vol. 11, no. 138, pp. 1-17, 2019.

[115] P. K. Shende, F. Trotta, R. S. Gaud, K. Deshmukh, R. Cavalli, and M. Biasizzo, "Influence of different techniques on formulation and comparative characterization of inclusion complexes of ASA with β-cyclodextrin and inclusion complexes of ASA with PMDA cross-linked β-cyclodextrin nanosponges," J. Incl. Phenom. Macrocycl. Chem., vol. 74, pp. 447-454, 2012.

[116] M. Argenziano *et al.*, "Improvement in the Anti-Tumor Efficacy of Doxorubicin Nanosponges in In Vitro and in Mice Bearing Breast Tumor Models," Cancers (Basel)., vol. 12, no. 162, pp. 1-19, 2020.

[117] P. K. Shende, R. S. Gaud, R. Bakal, and D. Patil, "Effect of inclusion complexation of meloxicam with β-cyclodextrin-and β-cyclodextrin-based nanosponges on solubility, in vitro release and stability studies," Colloids Surfaces B Biointerfaces, vol. 136, pp. 105-110, 2015.

[118] V. Coviello, S. Sartini, L. Quattrini, C. Baraldi, M. C. Gamberini, and C. La Motta, "Cyclodextrin-based nanosponges for the targeted delivery of the anti-restenotic agent DB103: A novel opportunity for the local therapy of vessels wall subjected to percutaneous intervention," Eur. J. Pharm. Biopharm., vol. 117, pp. 276-285, 2017.

[119] F. Trotta *et al.*, "Molecularly imprinted cyclodextrin nanosponges for the controlled delivery of L-DOPA: perspectives for the treatment of Parkinson's disease," Expert Opin. Drug Deliv., vol. 13, no. 12, pp. 1671-1680, 2016.

[120] M. Daga *et al.*, "GSH-targeted nanosponges increase doxorubicin-induced toxicity 'in vitro' and 'in vivo' in cancer cells with high antioxidant defenses," Free Radic. Biol. Med., vol. 97, pp. 24-37, 2016.

[121] M. Argenziano *et al.*, "Glutathione/pH-responsive nanosponges enhance strigolactone delivery to prostate cancer cells," Oncotarget, vol. 9, no. 88, pp. 35813-35829, 2018.

[122] M. M. Momin, Z. Zaheer, R. Zainuddin, and J. N. Sangshetti, "Extended release delivery of erlotinib glutathione nanosponge for targeting lung cancer," Artificial Cells, Nanomedicine and Biotechnology, vol. 46, no. 5. pp. 1064-1075, 2018.

Chapter 7

Targeted Nano-Drug Delivery System to Colon Cancer

Abstract

Cancer has been considered as the most cause of death in world. Employing of nanocarriers as drug delivery systems provide a platform for delivering drugs with increasing the anti-cancer efficacy, enhancing bioavailability of drugs, reducing side effects, enhancing the circulation half-life of drugs, improving the distribution of drugs and overcoming drug resistance. A number of nanocarriers have been studied as drug delivery systems for improving the treatment of cancer including liposomes, micelle, polymeric nanoparticles, carbon nanotubes, dendrimers, solid lipid nanoparticle (SLN) and nanostructure lipid carrier (NLC). In order to enhance recognition and internalization of nanocarriers by the target tissues, their surfaces can be modified with targeting ligands such as integrins, transferrin, folic acid, polysaccharides and antibodies. In this chapter, we are going to introduce the targeted nanocarriers for improving the cytotoxic action of drugs with further attempt of decreasing dose to achieve higher anticancer activity. Targeted nanocarriers would provide a promising therapeutic approach for cancer.

Keywords: Colon cancer, Nanoparticles, Drug delivery

1. Introduction

Colon cancer is one of the most commonly causing death in the world [1]. The conventional chemotherapy for colon cancer has a poor efficacy due to side effects on normal cells [2, 3]. Moreover, development of *multidrug resistance* (*MDR*) remains a major obstacle in the cancer treatment [4]. Using of nanocarriers as drug delivery systems provide a platform for delivering of drugs with increasing the anti-cancer efficacy, reducing side effects, improving therapeutic index, increasing the solubility of drugs, increasing bioavailability of drugs, enhancing the circulation half-life of drugs, improving the distribution of drugs and overcoming drug resistance [5, 6].

A number of nanocarriers have been employed as drug delivery systems for improving cancer treatment including dendrimer [7], chitosan [8], liposome [4], polymeric NPs [9], micelle [10] and exosomes [11]. Decorated nanocarriers with targeted ligands can identify receptors on cell surface which lead to enhance cellular uptake, reduce adverse effects and provide effective release of drugs [12, 13].

2. Nanocarries for colon cancer drug delivery

Sodium alginate, as natural polysaccharide is widely considered as a polymer for drug delivery due to hydrophilic, biodegradability, biocompatibility and negatively charged. Stable micelles of sodium alginate-curcumin bioconjugate were developed for anti-cancer applications. Sodium alginate-curcumin bioconjugate rapidly internalized in colon cancer cells; however, normal cells were less sensitive to this bioconjugate. Moreover, these micelles did not induce hemolysis and red cells aggregation [10].

Dendrimers are widely considered as nanocarrier for drug delivery due to biocompatibility, high drug loading and high surface functionality [7]. PAMAM G5 dendrimers encapsulated with curcumin and gold NPs (AuNPs) and decorated with MUC-1 aptamer were developed for targeted delivery to the colon cancer. AuNPs improve the contrast and resolution in the computed tomography (CT). MUC-1 receptors are overexpressed in the colorectal cancer; therefore, they can be considered as target for active targeting drug delivery. Targeted PAMAM dendrimers exhibited higher cellular cytotoxicity than non-targeted nanocarriers due to the higher affinity between MUC1 aptamer and MUC-1 receptor in cancer cells which increases the internalization of nanocarriers through receptor-mediated endocytosis. *In vivo* studies also illustrated the capability of targeted dendrimer as an effective theranostic system for colon cancer [13].

Employing of pH-controlled drug delivery systems lead to release of drug under acidic condition and not under neutral condition. CuS@Cu2S@Au nanoparticles (NPs), as a pH-sensitive carrier developed for delivery of doxorubicin (DOX) to colon cancer cells. The drug loaded NPs exhibited pH sensitive release and higher toxicity than free drug on cancer cells. Furthermore, these NPs showed good biocompatibility which make them as promising carrier for drug delivery [5].

Chitosan (CS) as biocompatible polymer is mostly considered as drug delivery system due to *low* toxicity, *low immunogenicity*, *bioadhesion* and *biodegradability* [8]. In addition, CS increases the permeability of drugs by regulating the tightness between cells [2]. CS NPs were prepared for oral co-delivery of 5-Aminolevulinic acid (5-ALA) and photothermal agent (IR780). Results showed that co-delivery system increased photodynamic effects against colon cancer cells *via* enhancing oxidative stress, ROS, superoxide and $^1O_2$ production [14].

Luteolin is found in numerous plants that is showed remarkable anti-cancer activity against skin, breast, liver, prostate and colon cancer. However, its clinical application is limited due to poor solubility and low bioavailability. A liposomal formulation was designed for improving the anti-tumor activity of luteolin. Liposomal luteolin significantly displayed anti-cancer activity against colon cancer cells than free luteolin *in vitro* and *in vivo*. These findings indicated that liposome formulation improved solubility and bioavailability of luteolin [15]. Mannose receptors are overexpressed in the drug resistant human colon tumor cell lines. Dihydroartemisinin (DHA, a derivative of artemisinin) and DOX were co-loaded into mannosylated liposomes for targeted delivery to colon cancer cells. These targeted liposomes increased the accumulation of both drugs in cancer cells which led to inhibit the growth of cancer cells through enhancing apoptosis, low expression of Bcl-xl and induction of autophagy [4].

5-Fluorouracil (5FU) has been commonly used for treatment of colon cancer. However, its medical application is restricted due to *multidrug resistance*, short half-life, side effects and low therapeutic index [16, 17]. Folic acid-decorated liposomal drug delivery system was designed for tumor targeting of 5FU. Targeted liposomes displayed higher cellular uptake and more activated apoptotic pathway than free drug on cancer cells. Results of hemolysis assay indicated the blood biocompatibility of the liposomes. Furthermore, folate targeted liposomes exhibited better tumor inhibition than free drug [18, 19]. Transferrin targeted liposomal 5FU also triggered apoptosis through mitochondria signaling pathway in cancer cells [20].

Cell differentiation 44 (CD44) is also frequently overexpressed on colon cancer cells. CD44 is the major receptor of hyaluronic acid (HA) in cancer cells. A smart micelle formulation was prepared using tocopherol succinate (TOS) conjugated HA by redox-responsive disulfide bond as a linker. According to the results, the micelle could specifically attach to CD44 receptors overexpressed tumor cells and responded selectively to high level of glutathione (GSH) in cells which led to inducing disulfide bond breakage and the release of paclitaxel (PTX) and triggered apoptosis in cancer cells [21].

A biocompatible pH-sensitive copolymer methoxy poly (ethylene glycol)-b-poly[(hydroxypropyl methacrylamide)-g-α-tocopheryl succinate-g-histidine)] (PTH) was synthesized for co-delivery of DOX and α-TOS. Results of *in vivo* biodistribution showed that micelles considerably accumulated in the cancer tissues. Moreover, these formulations exhibited higher cytotoxicity on cancer cells than normal cells [22].

PLGA, a synthetic copolymer is widely employed as nanocarrier for drug delivery system due to biodegradable, biocompatible and non-immunogenic [23]. DOTAP-PLGA hybrid NPs were prepared for delivery of 17-allylaminogeldanamycin (17AAG) as a HSP90 inhibitor and NPs were decorated with HA. Findings showed that internalization of HA-NPs in colon cancer cells was through CD44 receptor mediated endocytosis. HA-NPs-17AAG induced apoptosis more than free 17AAG in cancer cells. Additionally, HA-NPs-17AAG significantly inhibited tumor growth than free 17AAG in mice [12]. Poly (3-hydroxybutyrate-co-3-hydroxyvalerate acid) (PHBV)/PLGA NPs were developed for co-delivery of 5FU and oxaliplatin for colon cancer treatment. Co-loaded NPs showed significantly higher cytotoxicity and anti-tumor efficiency compared to free drugs combination, indicating that PHBV/PLGA NPs can be employed as a platform for co-delivery of 5FU and oxaliplatin [23].

Nanogels are nanosized particles that are formed by chemically or physically crosslinked polymer networks [24]. Folic acid functionalized amylopectin-albumin core-shell nanogels were designed for improving colon cancer cell targeted delivery of curcumin. The curcumin loaded in nanogels exhibited stability against physiological degradation and efficiently triggered apoptosis than free curcumin in HT29 cells.

Exosomes are natural membrane vesicles that are secreted into the extracellular environment and can be exploited as drug delivery. Exosomes contain bioactive molecules such as lipids, DNA, mRNAs and proteins [11]. Engineered exosomes were designed for co-delivery of 5FU and miR-21i (miR-21 inhibitor oligonucleotide) to colon cancer cells. The engineered exosome efficiently facilitated cellular uptake of drugs and significantly inhibited miR-21 expression in 5FU resistant colon cell lines and increased apoptosis. Moreover, systematic administration of 5FU and miR-21i encapsulated exosomes significantly showed anti-cancer effect in mice [16].

References

[1] Song Q, Jia J, Niu X, Zheng C, Zhao H, Sun L, Zhang H, Wang L, Zhang Z, Zhang Y: An oral drug delivery system with programmed drug release and imaging properties for orthotopic colon cancer therapy. Nanoscale 2019, 11:15958-15970.

[2] Zheng Y, Wang W, Zhao J, Wu C, Ye C, Huang M, Wang S: Preparation of injectable temperature-sensitive chitosan-based hydrogel for combined hyperthermia and chemotherapy of colon cancer. Carbohydrate Polymers 2019, 222:115039.

[3] Ge P, Niu B, Wu Y, Xu W, Li M, Sun H, Zhou H, Zhang X, Xie J: Enhanced cancer therapy of celastrol in vitro and in vivo by smart dendrimers delivery with specificity and biosafety. Chemical Engineering Journal 2020, 383:123228.

[4] Kang X-J, Wang H-Y, Peng H-G, Chen B-F, Zhang W-Y, Wu A-H, Xu Q, Huang Y-Z: Codelivery of dihydroartemisinin and doxorubicin in mannosylated liposomes for drug-resistant colon cancer therapy. Acta Pharmacologica Sinica 2017, 38:885-896.

[5] Yan E, Zhang Z: pH-sensitive CuS@ Cu2S@ Au nanoparticles as a drug delivery system for the chemotherapy against colon cancer. Biochemical and Biophysical Research Communications 2020, 525:204-207.

[6] Sunoqrot S, Abujamous L: pH-sensitive polymeric nanoparticles of quercetin as a potential colon cancer-targeted nanomedicine. Journal of Drug Delivery Science and Technology 2019, 52:670-676.

[7] Pooja D, Reddy TS, Kulhari H, Kadari A, Adams DJ, Bansal V, Sistla R: N-acetyl-d-glucosamine-conjugated PAMAM dendrimers as dual receptor-targeting nanocarriers for anticancer drug delivery. European Journal of Pharmaceutics and Biopharmaceutics 2020, 154:377-386.

[8] Tan LS, Tan HL, Deekonda K, Wong YY, Muniyandy S, Hashim K, Pushpamalar J: Fabrication of radiation cross-linked diclofenac sodium loaded carboxymethyl sago pulp/chitosan hydrogel for enteric and sustained drug delivery. Carbohydrate Polymer Technologies and Applications 2021, 2:100084.

[9] Handali S, Moghimipour E, Rezaei M, Ramezani Z, Dorkoosh FA: PHBV/PLGA nanoparticles for enhanced delivery of 5-fluorouracil as promising treatment of colon cancer. Pharmaceutical Development and Technology 2020, 25:206-218.

[10] Lachowicz D, Karabasz A, Bzowska M, Szuwarzyński M, Karewicz A, Nowakowska M: Blood-compatible, stable micelles of sodium alginate–Curcumin bioconjugate for anti-cancer applications. European Polymer Journal 2019, 113:208-219.

[11] Gao T, Wen T, Ge Y, Liu J, Yang L, Jiang Y, Dong X, Liu H, Yao J, An G: Disruption of core 1-mediated O-glycosylation oppositely regulates CD44 expression in human colon cancer cells and tumor-derived exosomes. Biochemical and biophysical research communications 2020, 521:514-520.

[12] Pan C, Zhang T, Li S, Xu Z, Pan B, Xu S, Jin S, Lu G, Yang S, Xue Z: Hybrid nanoparticles modified by hyaluronic acid loading an HSP90 inhibitor as a novel delivery system for subcutaneous and orthotopic colon cancer therapy. International Journal of Nanomedicine 2021, 16:1743.

[13] Alibolandi M, Hoseini F, Mohammadi M, Ramezani P, Einafshar E, Taghdisi SM, Ramezani M,

Abnous K: Curcumin-entrapped MUC-1 aptamer targeted dendrimer-gold hybrid nanostructure as a theranostic system for colon adenocarcinoma. International Journal of Pharmaceutics 2018, 549:67-75.

[14] Chen G, Zhao Y, Xu Y, Zhu C, Liu T, Wang K: Chitosan nanoparticles for oral photothermally enhanced photodynamic therapy of colon cancer. International Journal of Pharmaceutics 2020, 589:119763.

[15] Wu G, Li J, Yue J, Zhang S, Yunusi K: Liposome encapsulated luteolin showed enhanced antitumor efficacy to colorectal carcinoma. Molecular Medicine Reports 2018, 17:2456-2464.

[16] Liang G, Zhu Y, Ali DJ, Tian T, Xu H, Si K, Sun B, Chen B, Xiao Z: Engineered exosomes for targeted co-delivery of miR-21 inhibitor and chemotherapeutics to reverse drug resistance in colon cancer. Journal of Nanobiotechnology 2020, 18:1-15.

[17] Karan S, Choudhury H, Chakra BK, Chatterjee TK: Polymeric microsphere formulation for colon targeted delivery of 5-fluorouracil using biocompatible natural gum Katira. Asian Pacific Journal of Cancer Prevention: APJCP 2019, 20:2181.

[18] Moghimipour E, Rezaei M, Ramezani Z, Kouchak M, Amini M, Angali KA, Dorkoosh FA, Handali S: Folic acid-modified liposomal drug delivery strategy for tumor targeting of 5-fluorouracil. European Journal of Pharmaceutical Sciences 2018, 114:166-174.

[19] Handali S, Moghimipour E, Rezaei M, Ramezani Z, Kouchak M, Amini M, Angali KA, Saremy S, Dorkoosh FA: A novel 5-fluorouracil targeted delivery to colon cancer using folic acid conjugated liposomes. Biomedicine & Pharmacotherapy 2018, 108:1259-1273.

[20] Moghimipour E, Rezaei M, Kouchak M, Ramezani Z, Amini M, Ahmadi Angali K, Saremy S, Abedin Dorkoosh F, Handali S: A mechanistic study of the effect of transferrin conjugation on cytotoxicity of targeted liposomes. Journal of Micro encapsulation 2018, 35:548-558.

[21] Zhu C, Zhang H, Li W, Luo L, Guo X, Wang Z, Kong F, Li Q, Yang J, Du Y: Suppress orthotopic colon cancer and its metastasis through exact targeting and highly selective drug release by a smart nanomicelle. Biomaterials 2018, 161:144-153.

[22] Debele TA, Lee K-Y, Hsu N-Y, Chiang Y-T, Yu L-Y, Shen Y-A, Lo C-L: A pH sensitive polymeric micelle for co-delivery of doxorubicin and α-TOS for colon cancer therapy. Journal of Materials Chemistry B 2017, 5:5870-5880.

[23] Handali S, Moghimipour E, Rezaei M, Saremy S, Dorkoosh FA: Co-delivery of 5-fluorouracil and oxaliplatin in novel poly (3-hydroxybutyrate-co-3-hydroxy valerate acid)/poly (lactic-co-glycolic acid) nanoparticles for colon cancer therapy. International Journal of Biological Macromolecules 2019, 124:1299-1311.

[24] Samah NA, Williams N, Heard CM: Nanogel particulates located within diffusion cell receptor phases following topical application demonstrates uptake into and migration across skin. International Journal of Pharmaceutics 2010, 401:72-78.

Section 2

Novel Tools and Techniques in Drug Delivery System

Chapter 8

Artificial Intelligence in Healthcare: An Overview

Abstract

The healthcare industry is advancing ahead swiftly. For many healthcare organizations, being able to forecast which treatment techniques are likely to be successful with patients based on their makeup and treatment framework is a big step forward. Artificial intelligence has the potential to help healthcare providers in a variety of ways, including patient care and administrative tasks. The technology aims to mimic human cognitive functions, as it offers numerous advantages over traditional analytics and other clinical decision-making tools. Data becomes more precise and accurate, allowing the healthcare industry to have more insights into the theranostic processes and patient outcomes. This chapter is an overview of the use of artificial intelligence in radiology, cardiology, ophthalmology, and drug discovery process.

Keywords: artificial intelligence, algorithms, healthcare, radiology, cardiology, drug discovery

1. Introduction

In the field of healthcare, Artificial Intelligence (AI) is the privilege to breathe. It's a maneuver of the algorithm for the purpose of diagnosis, prognosis, or treatment of certain diseases. AI is the convergence of human and machine learning. John McCarthy, one of the founding fathers of AI, defined it as "the science and engineering of making intelligent machines" [1]. In this current era, intelligent machines pertain in various domains like financial, automatic driving, smart home, etc. In healthcare, machine learning is widely used to build automated clinical decision systems and in the treatment of different diseases [2]. AI utilizes advanced algorithms to learn from healthcare data and assist healthcare professionals in clinical practice. It has self-correcting and learning capabilities to cope with its exactness based on analysis [3]. AI can detect the spread of endemics by tracking animals and plant diseases and by accessing global airline ticketing data that are when and where the infected residents are moving and detect when an endemic can become a pandemic. The advancement in AI and its caliber to imitate human intelligence is heading towards the passing of Turing test [4] and AI will have a major impact on the forthcoming industrial revolution [5].

1.1 History/evolution

AI is the ray of computer science that deals with counterfeit intelligent human behavior. Using an electric circuit, Dr. Warren Mculloch and Dr. Walter Pitts [6] described neuronal activity and their modeling and explained the notion of neural networks. AI was first coined at Dartmouth college conference in 1956 [7] and the primitive work of AI was recorded in the 1970s after 15 years of existence of AI. The dendral experiment was the early employment of AI in life science [8]. The interpretation of electrocardiogram (ECG) stepped from 1970 to 1990 is considered as a major development in the field of AI [9]. A clinical decision support system was developed during the 20th century [10, 11]. However, the eagerness about AI was at its peak during the 1980s, but the phenomena of "AI winter" occurred due to groundless forecasting by the observers led to a lack of funding and interest [12]. There was continuous progress in building artificial intelligence in mid-20s by improving the algorithm and feeding the huge data of healthcare and its intelligence makes it cognizance of assisting the clinical cases of patients with the support of healthcare professionals. The renaissance of AI happened in 2012 after the evolution of image classifiers [13] and incorporation of AI in patients treatment needs to be trained on the basis of large data of clinical case studies so that it can examine the patient condition on the basis of history and the data which it has and results in diagnosis and in treatment methodology. The devices which favors in the department of healthcare are trained through machine learning. Basically, machine learning makes computer learn by the provided data i.e. algorithm in great measure [14, 15]. Supervised and unsupervised machine learning are two paradigms of machine learning [16]. Supervised machine learning classified the large data result and separate it into different categories and also predicts the result i.e. regression. In unsupervised machine learning there is no result prediction and it conglomerates the results [17].

The proof of AI and its concept has been demonstrated since older times. The history has been recorded with such minds related to the AI and executed their intellections and till today there are a new development, researches, and inventions going on in the field of AI and its application in different branches of healthcare.

2. Applications in healthcare industry

AI has proliferated its roots in the noble profession of healthcare. There is a boom in the use of AI, from detection of pulse rate to cancer detection and therapy consultation, from complete medical history to health monitoring to maintain and analyze the healthcare system. It is a helping hand in drug discovery and drug creation database and all this is implemented by the use of the algorithm and deep neural network.

Currently, AI is being used in various healthcare departments like radiology, cardiology, hematology, ophthalmology, and also in the management of various diseases.

2.1 AI in cardiology

AI in cardiology assists healthcare professionals in detecting the changes in normal heart functioning and helping in making a clinical decision. ECG is also a contribution of AI. There are various devices that are used in the monitoring of heart rate, blood pressure, tachycardia, bradycardia, stroke, and atrial fibrillation which works on the algorithm and deep neural network. These devices are

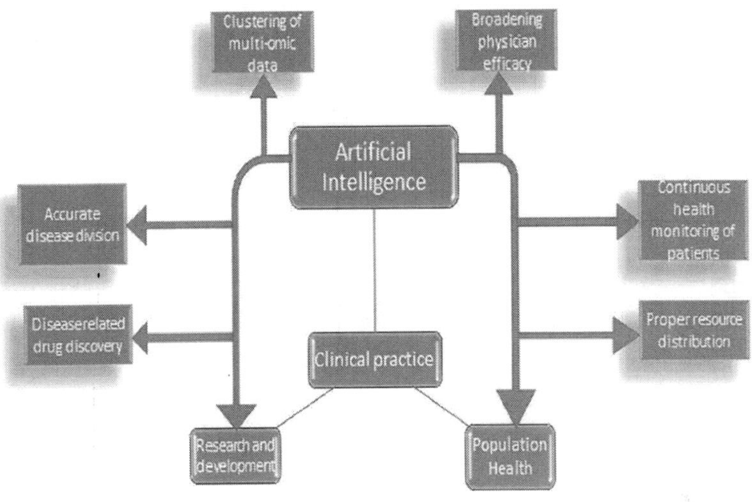

Figure 1.
Use of artificial intelligence in cardiology.

user-friendly and alarm the individual who is using them. Wearables that detect biological activity also work on the same principle [18]. A schematic representation of the use of AI in cardiology is given in **Figure 1**.

2.2 AI in radiology

AI and radiology together have brought a drastic change in the field of healthcare. The dawn of the application of AI in radiology was since 1960s [19]. Medical imaging in the detection and diagnosis of diseases is the widest use of machine learning in the field of healthcare [20]. CT scans, MRI, tomography, X-Ray are used algorithms in radiodiagnosis. The machines detect and pinpoint the changes on the basis of large data by which the neural network has been trained. The AI in radiology is applied for the detection of breast cancer at an early stage by mammography scans [21, 22] and tumors, tuberculosis, or diseases related to lungs with chest radiography [23–27]. A schematic representation of clinical radiology workflow is given in **Figure 2**.

2.3 AI in ophthalmology

In ophthalmology AI is tremendously used in detection and monitoring of diabetic retinopathy [28–33], glaucoma [29, 34, 35], age-related macular degeneration (AMD) [29, 36, 37], retinopathy of prematurity (ROP) [38] with the help of retinal cameras of fundus photography [16]. The diagnosis of ocular diseases is based on the deep learning system that is trained on the numerous images of each disease. A study of the population with diabetes from US, Australia, Europe, and Asia in the years between 1980 to 2008 shows the frequency of diabetic retinopathy of 34.6% and 7% vision-threatening diabetic retinopathy [39]. Thus, continuous monitoring along

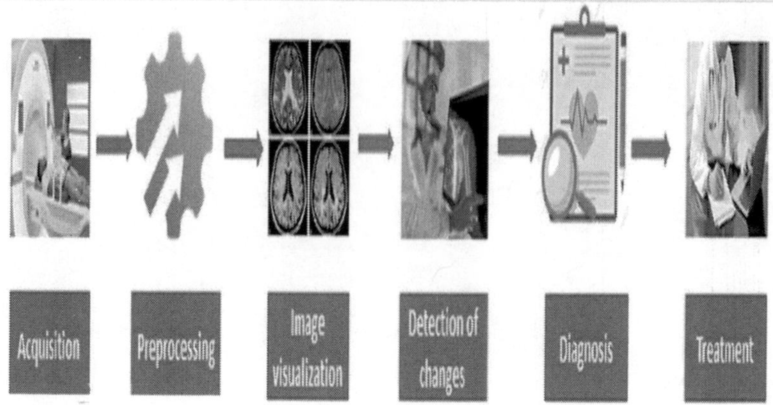

Figure 2.
Clinical radiology workflow.

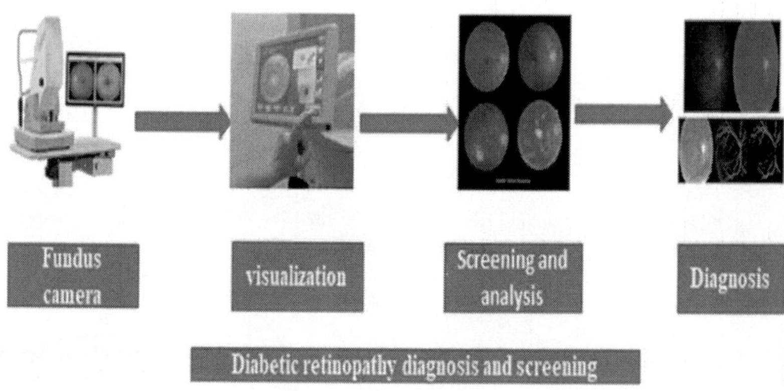

Figure 3.
Use of AI in diabetic retinopathy diagnosis and treatment.

with the treatment can prevent vision loss. A schematic representation of the use of AI in ophthalmology is depicted in **Figure 3** [40].

Machine learning models such as visual fields, optical coherence tomography (OCT), and optic disc characters are used for the diagnosis of glaucoma [41]. Glaucoma is a medical condition in which the intraocular pressure inside the eye rises up. Age-related macular degeneration (AMD) is a condition in which there is degeneration in the center of the retina and is responsible for vision loss. Spectral OCT is used in the diagnosis of AMD [42]. Retinopathy of Prematurity (ROP) is a disease that occurs in premature born babies and the leading cause of childhood blindness due to abnormal growth of blood vessels towards the edge of retina. Wide-angle retinal images with machine learning [43] and i-ROP DL system which works on the basis of convolutional neural network (CNN) was trained on the images more than 5000 in number with a single standard reference diagnosis (RSD) [44] for the diagnosis of ROP.

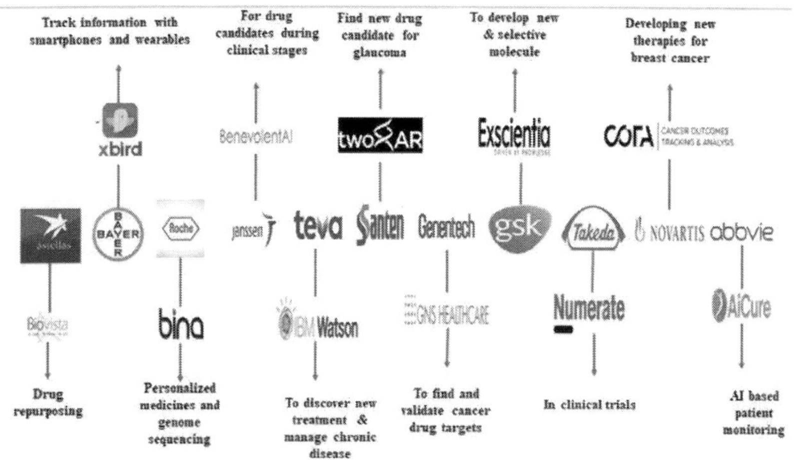

Figure 4.
Biopharmaceutical companies using AI technology in drug discovery.

2.4 AI in drug discovery

In this modern era, AI is used for drug discovery and drug design on the basis of artificial neural network (ANN), algorithm, and deep learning. In drug discovery, inaugural employment of ANN was in 1970 to detect whether the 1,3-dioxane is physiologically active or not [45]. The application of ANN in Quantity Structure Activity Relationship (QSAR) is the next stage in the field of drug discovery [46]. QSAR studies were involved in drug design since 1960 by involving the simple structures to know the activity of the combination of compounds [47]. Currently the biological and physicochemical activity i.e. ADMET (Absorption, distribution, metabolism, excretion, and toxicity), binding constants according to their binding sites are also vaticinated using ANN which is trained on various sets of compounds in the field of drug discovery [48]. The application of AI is at every step of the drug discovery process, from identification of drug targets to new drug molecule research following its volunteer election for clinical trials [49–51] also its pharmacological property [52], its binding effect with protein, potency and synergistic effect with other drugs [53, 54]. Docking software which is used to find the perfect binding molecule for the particular receptor and its activity also works on the algorithm. AI has simplified the process of drug discovery by saving time and money expenditure of US$2.5 billion on R&D [55]. Thus, AI has routed the drug discovery process into simpler, quicker, and cost-effective, an example of drug discovery is by BenevolentBio which has its own AI platform and was asked to suggest the treatment of amyotrophic lateral sclerosis (ALS) also called as motor neuron diseases (MND) and has displayed nearly 100 of drugs, five drugs were selected out of which four of them were effective and one was showing delayed neurological symptoms on mice [56]. The top multinational biopharmaceutical companies have started using AI technology in their drug discovery (**Figure 4**) [57].

3. Conclusion

Artificial intelligence is an important and valuable technology that offers promising solutions to healthcare industry needs. It opens up gateways to individualized treatment approaches tailored to the needs of individual patients. It offers multiple advantages over traditional analytics and other clinical decision-making tools. Data becomes more precise and accurate allowing the healthcare industry to have more insights into the diagnosis and treatment processes thereby improving patient outcomes.

References

[1] Reddy S, Fox J, Purohit MP. Artificial intelligence-enabled healthcare delivery. Journal of the Royal Society of Medicine. 2019;**112**(1):22-28

[2] Koprowski R and Foster KR. Machine Learning and Medicine: Book Review and Commentary. 2018

[3] Pearson T. How to Replicate Watson Hardware and Systems Design for your Own Use in your Basement. Watson, MN, USA: IBM; 2011

[4] Alan M. Turing. Computing machinery and intelligence. Mind. 1950;**59**(236):433-460

[5] Monostori L. Cyber-physical production systems: Roots, expectations and R&D challenges. Procedia CIRP. 2014;**17**:9-13

[6] Palm G. Warren mcculloch and walter Pitts: A logical calculus of the ideas immanent in nervous activity. In: Brain Theory. Berlin, Heidelberg: Springer; 1986. pp. 229-230

[7] History of Artificial Intelligence. Available from: http://en.wikipedia.org/wiki/History_of_artificial_intelligence [Accessed: June 1, 2020]

[8] Lindsay R, Buchanan B, Feigenbaum E and Lederberg J. Applications of Artificial Intelligence for Organic Chemistry. 1980

[9] Kundu M, Nasipuri M, Basu DK. Knowledge-based ECG interpretation: A critical review. Pattern Recognition. 2000;**33**(3):351-373

[10] Miller RA. Medical diagnostic decision support systems—Past, present, and future: A threaded bibliography and brief commentary. Journal of the American Medical Informatics Association. 1994;**1**(1): 8-27

[11] Musen MA, Middleton B, Greenes RA. Clinical decision-support systems. In: Biomedical Informatics. London: Springer; 2014. pp. 643-674

[12] Shortliffe EH. Artificial intelligence in medicine: Weighing the accomplishments, hype, and promise. Yearbook of Medical Informatics. 2019;**28**(01):257-262

[13] Krizhevsky A, Sutskever I, Hinton GE. Imagenet classification with deep convolutional neural networks. In: Advances in Neural Information Processing Systems. 2012. pp. 1097-1105

[14] Hastie T, Tibshirani R, Friedman J. The Elements of Statistical Learning: Data Mining, Inference, and Prediction. Springer Science & Business Media; 2009

[15] Abu-Mostafa YS, Magdon-Ismail M and Lin HT. Learning from Data. 2012. *AMLbook. Com*. 2008

[16] Yu KH, Beam AL, Kohane IS. Artificial intelligence in healthcare. Nature Biomedical Engineering. 2018;**2**(10):719-731

[17] Deo RC. Machine learning in medicine. Circulation. 2015;**132**(20): 1920-1930

[18] Krittanawong C, Johnson KW, Hershman SG, Tang WW. Big data, artificial intelligence, and cardiovascular precision medicine. Expert Review of Precision Medicine and Drug Development. 2018;**3**(5): 305-317

[19] Lodwick GS, Haun CL, Smith WE, Keller RF, Robertson ED. Computer diagnosis of primary bone tumors: A preliminary report. Radiology. 1963;**80**(2):273-275

[20] Yu KH, Beam AL, Kohane IS. Artificial intelligence in healthcare.

Nature Biomedical Engineering. 2018;*2*(10):719-731

[21] Samala RK, Chan HP, Hadjiiski L, Helvie MA, Wei J, Cha K. Mass detection in digital breast tomosynthesis: Deep convolutional neural network with transfer learning from mammography. Medical Physics. 2016;*43*(12):6654-6666

[22] Arevalo J, González FA, Ramos-Pollán R, Oliveira JL, Lopez MAG. Convolutional neural networks for mammography mass lesion classification. In: 2015 37th Annual International Conference of the IEEE Engineering in Medicine and Biology Society (EMBC). IEEE; 2015. pp. 797-800

[23] Lakhani P, Sundaram B. Deep learning at chest radiography: Automated classification of pulmonary tuberculosis by using convolutional neural networks. Radiology. 2017;**284**(2):574-582

[24] Wang X, Peng Y, Lu L, Lu Z, Bagheri M, Summers RM. Chestx-ray8: Hospital-scale chest x-ray database and benchmarks on weakly-supervised classification and localization of common thorax diseases. In: Proceedings of the IEEE Conference on Computer Vision and Pattern Recognition. 2017. pp. 2097-2106

[25] Yao L, Poblenz E, Dagunts D, Covington B, Bernard D, Lyman K. Learning to diagnose from scratch by exploiting dependencies among labels. arXiv preprint arXiv:1710.10501. 2017

[26] Rajpurkar P, Irvin J, Zhu K, Yang B, Mehta H, Duan T, et al. Chexnet: Radiologist-level pneumonia detection on chest x-rays with deep learning. arXiv preprint arXiv:1711.05225. 2017

[27] Hosny A, Parmar C, Quackenbush J, Schwartz LH, Aerts HJ. Artificial intelligence in radiology. Nature Reviews Cancer. 2018;**18**(8):500-510

[28] Varma R. How AI Benefits Patients and Physicians. 2018

[29] Ting DSW, Cheung CYL, Lim G, Tan GSW, Quang ND, Gan A, et al. Development and validation of a deep learning system for diabetic retinopathy and related eye diseases using retinal images from multiethnic populations with diabetes. JAMA. 2017;**318**(22): 2211-2223

[30] Gulshan V, Peng L, Coram M, Stumpe MC, Wu D, Narayanaswamy A, et al. Development and validation of a deep learning algorithm for detection of diabetic retinopathy in retinal fundus photographs. JAMA. 2016;**316**(22): 2402-2410

[31] Lee CS, Tyring AJ, Deruyter NP, Wu Y, Rokem A, Lee AY. Deep-learning based, automated segmentation of macular edema in optical coherence tomography. Biomedical Optics Express. 2017;**8**(7):3440-3448

[32] Abràmoff MD, Lou Y, Erginay A, Clarida W, Amelon R, Folk JC, et al. Improved automated detection of diabetic retinopathy on a publicly available dataset through integration of deep learning. Investigative Ophthalmology & Visual Science. 2016;**57**(13):5200-5206

[33] Gargeya R, Leng T. Automated identification of diabetic retinopathy using deep learning. Ophthalmology. 2017;**124**(7):962-969

[34] Li Z, He Y, Keel S, Meng W, Chang RT, He M. Efficacy of a deep learning system for detecting glaucomatous optic neuropathy based on color fundus photographs. Ophthalmology. 2018;**125**(8): 1199-1206

[35] Zheng C, Johnson TV, Garg A, Boland MV. Artificial intelligence in glaucoma. Current Opinion in Ophthalmology. 2019;**30**(2):97-103

[36] Burlina PM, Joshi N, Pekala M, Pacheco KD, Freund DE, Bressler NM. Automated grading of age-related macular degeneration from color fundus images using deep convolutional neural networks. JAMA Ophthalmology. 2017;**135**(11):1170-1176

[37] Grassmann F, Mengelkamp J, Brandl C, Harsch S, Zimmermann ME, Linkohr B, et al. A deep learning algorithm for prediction of age-related eye disease study severity scale for age-related macular degeneration from color fundus photography. Ophthalmology. 2018;**125**(9):1410-1420

[38] Brown JM, Campbell JP, Beers A, Chang K, Ostmo S, Chan RP, et al. Automated diagnosis of plus disease in retinopathy of prematurity using deep convolutional neural networks. JAMA Ophthalmology. 2018;**136**(7): 803-810

[39] Yau JW, Rogers SL, Kawasaki R, Lamoureux EL, Kowalski JW, Bek T, et al. Global prevalence and major risk factors of diabetic retinopathy. Diabetes Care. 2012;**35**(3):556-564

[40] Du XL, Li WB, Hu BJ. Application of artificial intelligence in ophthalmology. International Journal of Ophthalmology. 2018;**11**(9):1555

[41] Kapoor R, Walters SP, Al-Aswad LA. The current state of artificial intelligence in ophthalmology. Survey of Ophthalmology. 2019;**64**(2):233-240

[42] Treder M, Lauermann JL, Eter N. Automated detection of exudative age-related macular degeneration in spectral domain optical coherence tomography using deep learning. Graefe's Archive for Clinical and Experimental Ophthalmology. 2018;**256**(2):259-265

[43] Ataer-Cansizoglu E, Bolon-Canedo V, Campbell JP, Bozkurt A, Erdogmus D, Kalpathy-Cramer J, et al. Computer-based image analysis for plus disease diagnosis in retinopathy of prematurity: Performance of the "i-ROP" system and image features associated with expert diagnosis. Translational Vision Science & Technology. 2015;**4**(6):5-5

[44] Brown JM, Campbell JP, Beers A, Chang K, Ostmo S, Chan RP, et al. Automated diagnosis of plus disease in retinopathy of prematurity using deep convolutional neural networks. JAMA Ophthalmology. 2018;**136**(7):803-810

[45] Hiller SA, Golender VE, Rosenblit AB, Rastrigin LA, Glaz AB. Cybernetic methods of drug design. I. Statement of the problem—The perceptron approach. Computers and Biomedical Research. 1973;**6**(5):411-421

[46] Aoyama T, Suzuki Y, Ichikawa H. Neural networks applied to structure-activity relationships. Journal of Medicinal Chemistry. 1990;**33**(3): 905-908

[47] Duch W, Swaminathan K, Meller J. Artificial intelligence approaches for rational drug design and discovery. Current Pharmaceutical Design. 2007;**13**(14):1497-1508

[48] Baskin II, Winkler D, Tetko IV. A renaissance of neural networks in drug discovery. Expert Opinion on Drug Discovery. 2016;**11**(8):785-795

[49] Huang Z, Juarez JM, Li X. Data mining for biomedicine and healthcare. Journal of Healthcare Engineering. 2017;**2017**

[50] Zhang Y, Zhang G, Shang Q. Computer-aided clinical trial recruitment based on domain-specific language translation: A case study of retinopathy of prematurity. Journal of Healthcare Engineering. 2017;**2017**

[51] Mamoshina P, Vieira A, Putin E, Zhavoronkov A. Applications of deep

learning in biomedicine. Molecular Pharmaceutics. 2016;**13**(5):1445-1454

[52] Klopman G, Chakravarti SK, Zhu H, Ivanov JM, Saiakhov RD. ESP: A method to predict toxicity and pharmacological properties of chemicals using multiple MCASE databases. Journal of Chemical Information and Computer Sciences. 2004;**44**(2):704-715

[53] Menden MP, Iorio F, Garnett M, McDermott U, Benes CH, Ballester PJ, et al. Machine learning prediction of cancer cell sensitivity to drugs based on genomic and chemical properties. PLoS One. 2013;**8**(4)

[54] Nascimento AC, Prudêncio RB, Costa IG. A multiple kernel learning algorithm for drug-target interaction prediction. BMC Bioinformatics. 2016;**17**(1):46

[55] Mohs RC, Greig NH. Drug discovery and development: Role of basic biological research. Alzheimer's & Dementia: Translational Research & Clinical Interventions. 2017;**3**(4): 651-657

[56] Fleming N. How artificial intelligence is changing drug discovery. Nature. 2018;**557**(7706):S55-S55

[57] Mak KK, Pichika MR. Artificial intelligence in drug development: Present status and future prospects. Drug Discovery Today. 2019;**24**(3): 773-780

Chapter 9

Applications of Statistical Tools for Optimization and Development of Smart Drug Delivery System

Abstract

In the novel dosage form development, quality is the key criterion in pharmaceutical industry. The quality by design tools used for development of the quality products with tight specification and rigid process. The specifications of statistical tools are essentially based upon critical process parameters (CPPs), critical material attributes (CMAs), and critical quality attributes (CQAs) for the development of quality products. The application of quality by design in pharmaceutical dosage form development is systematic, requiring multivariate experiments employing process analytical technology (PAT) and other experiments to recognize critical quality attributes depend upon risk assessments (RAs). The quality by design is a modern technique to stabilize the quality of pharmaceutical dosage form. The elements of quality by design such as process analytical techniques, risk assessment, and design of experiment support for assurance of the strategy control for every dosage form with a choice of regular monitoring and enhancement for a quality dosage form. This chapter represents the concepts and applications of the most common screening of designs/experiments, comparative experiments, response surface methodology, and regression analysis. The data collected from the dosage form designing during laboratory experiments, provide the substructure for pivotal or pilot scale development. Statistical tools help not only in understanding and identifying CMAs and CPPs in product designing, but also in comprehension of the role and relationship between these in attaining a target quality. Although, the implementation of statistical approaches in the development of dosage form is strongly recommended.

Keywords: Quality by design, Critical quality attributes, Critical process attributes, Critical material attributes, Design of experiments, Smart drug delivery

1. Introduction

In an endeavour to fight various pathological manifestations, medicaments have been administered via various possible routes [1]. Experimental designs techniques have long been used for the optimization of various processes and the development of smart drug delivery system such as the factorial designs since 1926 [2], the designs for screening since 1946 [3], the central composite designs since 1951 [4], and the mixture designs since 1958 [5]. According to Joseph Juran, most of the quality problems are associated with the way by which a pharmaceutical smart drug delivery was designed. A poorly designed pharmaceutical dosage form will show poor efficacy and safety, no matter how many analyses or tests have been done to check its quality.

The quality by design (QbD) is a systemic approach for the development of pharmaceutical formulations that starts with predefined objectives and emphasizes process and product comprehension and process control, based on quality risk management and sound science [6]. The food and drug administration guidance, such as pharmaceutical product development (ICH Q8), quality risk evaluation (ICH Q9), pharmaceutical quality systems (ICH Q10), the briefly highlighted ICH approach to the achieve quality of product through QbD [7], and development and manufacture of drug substances (ICH Q11) [8]. The QbD based approach will provide scientific understanding and knowledge to support smart drug delivery system development [9]. The prime goals of QbD for pharmaceuticals may include: (a) to attain meaningful product and quality specification; (b) to enhance process ability and reduce product variability; (c) to enhance smart dosage form development and manufacturing efficiencies, and (d) to increase cause-effect investigation and regulatory flexibility [6]. The QbD is used to establish the relationship of product performance with the process and product attributes [7, 10]. The applications of QbD in pharmaceutical smart drug delivery system development is systematic, requiring multivariate experiments employing process analytical technology (PAT) and other experiments to recognize critical quality attributes (CQAs) depend upon risk assessments (RAs) [7].

The smart dosage form design and process development cannot be distinguished since dosage form cannot become a product unaccompanied by a defined process. The production process needs to produce a desired standard product typically requires multiple units operating conditions and operations [11]. The outline has to contain all the factors that require to be contemplated for the design of the process. The process factors which cause a vital impact on the quality of the product if changes are contemplated as the critical process attribute (CPAs). The process factor variability, which causes a vital impact on the critical quality of the ingredients should be controlled and monitored, at all times to make sure the process for the targeted quality [6, 11].

2. Basic elements of quality by design

2.1 Set the standard profile for the target smart dosage form

A target standard profile for smart dosage form describes how a smart dosage form will be utilized by the end-user. A systematically developed standard profile can ensure the arrangement of objectives across departments of the company, advance development of timelines, reduction of risks, and finally lead to an optimal smart dosage form. A targeted standard product profile is very important for smart drug delivery development due to the variety of administrations and the variety of possible end-user (patients, nurses, physicians, and pharmacists) [12].

2.2 Recognition of the critical quality attributes (CQAs)

The next step in QbD for smart dosage form development is recognition of the critical quality attributes (CQAs). CQAs are physical, chemical, biological, or microbiological characteristics or properties of the pharmaceutical smart drug delivery system (in-process or finished) that must be within specified standards to ensure quality. CQAs may include identification, content, assay, uniformity, solvents, degradation, products, dissolution or drug release, moisture content, moisture uptake, microbial limits, and other properties such as color, size, shape, etc. [9, 13].

2.3 Smart dosage form design and development

The physic-chemical and pharmacological properties of the medicaments determine the critical attributes for novel dosage form development. The objectives of the novel dosage form development by using QbD for identification of attributes and to achieve desired patient requirements that the resultant product should possess to exhibit intended therapeutic response. The smart dosage form development must invariably be scientific, systemic, and with basic risk management facilitation to achieve these predefined objectives. The CQAs identification is strongly and thoroughly based on the understanding of product and manufacturing process. These CQAs must be controlled to get reproducible and desired results. **Table 1** summarizes the different CQAs for medicaments, additives, in-process

Attribute (CMAs, CQAs & CPAs)	Comments
Drug-related	
Indication	Note if target patients may have limitations (e.g., sodium hydrochloride and hypertension)
Types of the route of administration	May impact the acceptability of drug product (e.g., the tablet is more preferred than parenteral)
Range of dose, frequency of dosing, duration of therapy	The concentration, duration of therapy, and frequency of dosing may affect the use of some additives (are these outside the statutory use levels?)
Pharmacokinetic properties (in-vitro/in-vivo)	Is activity associated or toleration with total exposure or the plasma concentration? For novel drug delivery formulations, what is the required profile?
Drug combination which may be designed or mixed for the formulation	Are there possible incompatibilities?
Dosage form-related	
pH, tonicity, site of application etc. Administration ante/post cibum (oral), need to reconstitute/dilute and with what? Packaging types (single/multi-dose packaging)	If more than a single, will be available at the initial stage? Does existing machinery work for packaging? Will the packaging be a kit (with a device, diluent, etc.)? Are there any considerations for disposal (may differ for various regions)? Is functional labelling required (e.g., anti-counterfeiting measures, freeze indicators, etc.)?
Storage conditions	Include in-use constraints and stability requirements (e.g., requirement of secondary packaging to protect from light, "do not freeze")
Requirements for shipping	Are there any limitations (susceptibility to shaking, temperature excursion, etc.)?
Legitimate-related	
Liberty to operate	Does the process or product contravene any patents, copyright, and applications?
Manufacturing-related	
Cost of the product	It should cover any royalties as appropriate
The machinery required for manufacture	Will the process according to existing machinery?
Processing time for the dosage form	Required to consider sterility. Also, may be a matter for some processes (e.g., freeze-drying).

Table 1.
Different critical attributes to formulate a novel dosage form [12].

materials, and dosage form [14, 15]. On the basis of suitable statistical methods such as DoE (design of experiments), proper risk assessment, and management tools can escort to a good and knowledge-based smart dosage form development. Further, understanding of CQAs helps to set up flexible and meaningful regulatory product specifications. Knowledge of smart drug delivery development can facilitates QbD and increase the manufacturing capability (**Figure 1**) [16].

2.4 Critical process attributes (CPAs)

To develop an optimal manufacturing procedure, all the critical process attributes including facilities, equipment, manufacturing variables, and material transfer

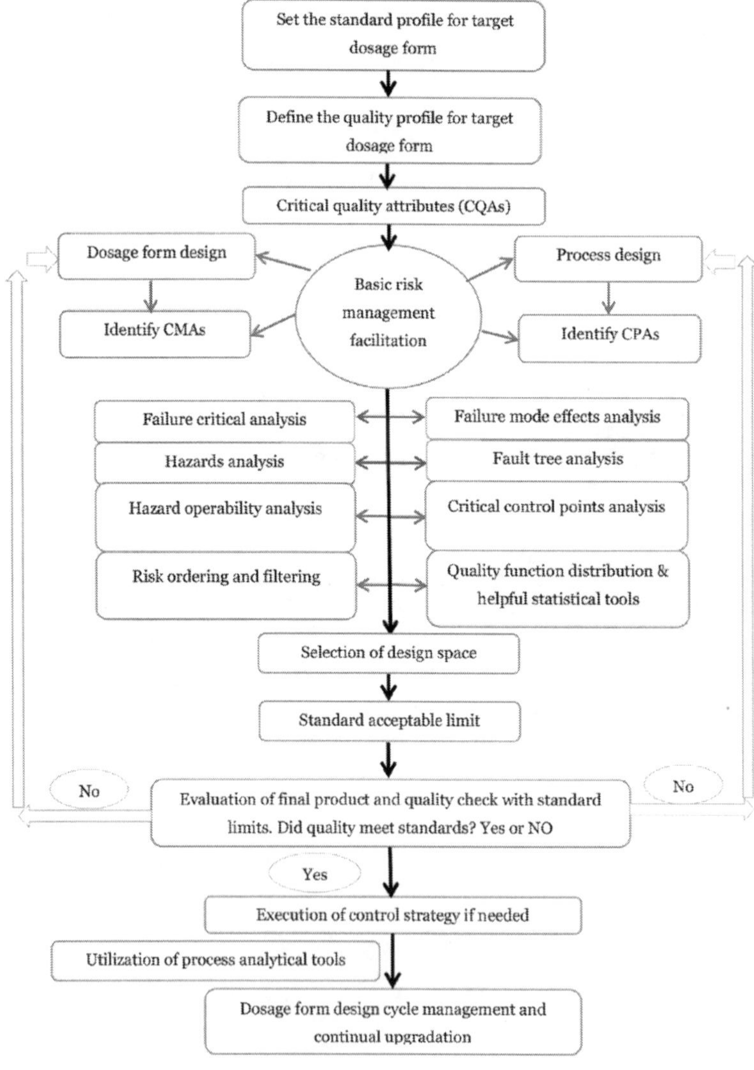

Figure 1.
The fundamental approach of QbD for designing of a pharmaceutical dosage form.

should be considered. Pulverization, homogenization time/mixing, type of mixer, and energy input are the major critical attributes in the manufacturing of novel dosage form. The process attributes using these associated factors require be identifying and carefully controlling to formulate batches with reproducible quality [17].

Size reduction of the material may be affected by the types of mill used. Different types of material need a special type of mill for pulverization such as lignocellulosic biomass material (like wood) required 'fine grinding' (less than 100 μm) [18] but in other studies, the 'fine grinding' has been used for particle sizes up to 1 mm [19–21]. The excess temperature during processing can increase the degradation of ingredients [22, 23], while less temperature can cause the failure of the process due to drug solubility issues [24]. Mixing speed and time is a critical attribute to develop a smart dosage form. For optimizing the mixing speed and time, the minimum needed time to dissolve the components and the maximum time of mixing can affect the viscosity of the product (causing product failure) and it should be identified [22, 25, 26].

2.5 Critical material attributes (CMAs)

The quantitative and qualitative information of active pharmaceutical ingredients (API) is prime attributes as material attributes [11]. Although an API is mostly incorporated at low concentrations and occupies a negligible part in the final formulation, the additives (inactive ingredients) usually elucidate the physical properties of a formulation [11, 27]. A number of researches have shown that additive(s) can influence the fate of an API in dosage form [28, 29]. Different grades of additives show a substantial effect on quality attributes of the final product as well as the API stability in the product [30]. Impurities in a raw material may show a detrimental impact on the stability of API/additives. Another prime challenge during the design and development of a novel dosage form is the compatibility of additives and API.

2.6 Design of experiments (DOEs)

The DOEs is not a replacement for experience, intelligence, or expertise; it is a precious element for choosing experiments systematically and efficiently to give dependable and coherent information [31]. DOEs are defined as "an organized, structured technique for deciding the relationship between attributes influencing a process and the output of the process" [32]. The DOEs can be applied for the screening of designs/experiments, comparative experiments, response surface methodology, and regression analysis [33].

2.6.1 Common experimental designs

In order to provide a logical relationship among the dependent variables and independent variables, experimental designs may be classified into four classes: a) screening designs, b) optimization designs [34–36] c) comparative experiments, and d) regression modelling.

2.6.1.1 Screening of designs/experiments

Screening of designs involves the selection of prime factors affecting a response. For the selection of experiments; fractionate factorial designs, the full factorial designs, and Placket-Burman designs are mostly used for screening because these designs have cost-effective advantages. These screening designs permit one to study various input factors with minimum numbers of experiments. However, these designs also show some limitations that should be contemplated in order to impart a better interpretation of the effects of input elements on output responses [34–36]. Only the linear responses are supported by screening designs. Thus, if a nonlinear response is observed, or a more accurate phenomenon of the response surface is required or more complex design may be applied [37].

2.6.1.2 The factorial approach

The full factorial and fractional factorial designs are generally used by the most of the researchers as an alternative methodological technique to standard relative randomized controlled trials (RCTs) and module designs, which has supremacy over both for determining the active elements of formulations. The factorial designs are employed to explore the prime impacts of critical factors and interactions among factors [38–42].

The common and simple full factorial design is the 2^2 factorial designs, where 2^2 is indicating two factors at two levels means the total run of experiments is four, which are located in 2-dimensional factor space at the rectangle's corners. If there are 2^3 factorial designs is applied then total eight experiments are mandatory which are located at the corners of an orthogonal hexahedron on a 3-dimensional space. If large numbers of factors are used at large numbers of levels then the number of runs needed to finish the task. To minimize the number of runs, the fractional factorial design should be used (i.e., ½ or ¼ of the real number of runs of full factorial design) [43–45].

Table 2 shows the three factors at two coded levels 0 and 1, where 0 represents a low level and 1 represents a high level. In **Table 2**, the last column shows the response values of random variables. The main effect of any factor (A, B, C) or interaction (AB, AC, BC, ABC) is the difference of two means, the means of the responses corresponding to high levels and the means of responses corresponding to low levels.

When we compare the suggestions of **Table 2** with the suggestions of fractionate factorial design shown in **Table 3**. In **Table 3**, every-even numbered test experiment eliminated from **Table 2**. Again, factor effects are differences in mean responses. Even though, the prime effect for factor A is absolutely similar and opposite in sign from the interaction AB; i.e., A is aliased with -AB. Each result in **Table 3** is aliased with another result, having the prime result for B which is aliased with the evaluation of the overall average response. Therefore, every difference in means measures the difference of two results; e.g., A-AB. Had the half-fraction accompanied the odd-numbered test experiments been removed, every difference of means for a result would be evaluating the sum of two results; e.g., A + AB.

Experiment	A	B	C	AB	AC	BC	ABC	Response
1	0	0	0	1	1	1	0	R_1
2	0	0	1	1	0	0	1	R_2
3	0	1	0	0	1	0	1	R_3
4	0	1	1	0	0	1	0	R_4
5	1	0	0	0	0	1	1	R_5
6	1	0	1	0	1	0	0	R_6
7	1	1	0	1	0	0	0	R_7
8	1	1	1	1	1	1	1	R_8

Table 2.
Full factorial design with three factors at two levels.

Experiment	A	B	C	AB	AC	BC	ABC	Response
1	0	0	0	1	1	1	0	R_1
3	0	1	0	0	1	0	1	R_3
5	1	0	0	0	0	1	1	R_5
7	1	1	0	1	0	0	0	R_7

Table 3.
Fractional factorial design of a full factorial design with three factors.

Every fractional factorial design needs the aliasing of all or some of the factor effects. Many times the selection of fractional factorial designs is the unscientific that can lead to ambiguity, even wrong, conclusions about factor effects. Inversely, it is precisely the attentive selection of which fraction is applied that can increase the experimentation efficiently without the aliasing of main effects. **Table 4** shows another half-fraction of the full factorial design.

2.6.1.3 Plackett-Burman designs or Hadamard designs

This design is special two-level full factorial design and generally employed for the screening of factors. Plackett-Burman designs are mainly applicable for screening a large number of factors if we want to test the effect of 7 factors then we have to put some dummy factors. The results of full factorial designs, Plackett-Burman design, and Taguchi design are interpreted by using a half-normal plot and Pareto chart. By using these designs we can detect all prime effects economically and all other interactions assumed as negligible when compared with few prime effects [46–48].

2.6.1.4 Response surface methodology (RSM)

Response surface methodology is used after the identification of the critical variables affecting a response. Response surface methods such as central composite design, Box–Behnken design, and three-level factorial designs can recognize the optimum/suitable processing parameters or conditions [49, 50]. The primary advantages of response surface methodology are as hitting a target, minimizing or maximizing a response, minimizing variations, setting a robust process, and finding multiple objectives.

2.6.1.5 Central composite designs or Box-Wilson design

This is one of the most commonly employed optimization design because this is used for 5 levels of each loaded factor with a less number of runs required when compared with 3 levels full factorial designs. Central composite designs are

Experiment	A	B	C	AB	AC	BC	ABC	Response
2	0	0	1	1	0	0	1	R_2
4	0	1	1	0	0	1	0	R_4
6	1	0	0	0	0	1	1	R_6
8	1	1	1	1	1	1	1	R_8

Table 4.
Fractional factorial design of a full factorial design, prime results can be estimated.

generally used for nonlinear responses. In this model, a two-factor central composite design is similar to a 32 factorial design by using the experimental domain at $\alpha = \pm 1$. Dash RN et al. successfully developed a glipizide-loaded formulation by using central composite designs [51].

2.6.1.6 Box–Behnken design

This is a specially made design, which needs only three levels for each factor and it is widely employed in response surface methodology for fitting second-order models for all responses. In this method, 15 experiments are run three levels for each factor. Box–Behnken designs are a combination of incomplete block designs with two-level factorial designs and these are almost rotatable. This design has the benefits that there are no runs where three levels for each factor and that there are no corner points run. Runs at the corner points may be expensive or inconvenient [52].

2.6.1.7 Three level factorial designs

This design is mainly used only for two-three factors because the large numbers of runs are needed. The required number of runs may be calculated as 3 K, where K is selected factor for study.

2.6.1.8 Comparative experiments

Comparative studies are performed for selecting a suitable one between two/more alternatives. From a sample of data, the mean results are generated and compared for suitable selection from each alternative. For example, the selection of a vendor for a medicament from two/more vendors can be a relative experiment. The narrow scoped comparative designs are good for an initial comparison and broad scope design is appropriate for a confirmatory comparison [53].

2.6.1.9 Regression modelling

Regression modelling is an essential statistical component for the analysis of the data. It is employed for the identification and depiction of relationships among various factors. It is also used for the identification of prognostically pertinent risk elements and the determination of risk results for each prognostication [54]. The most commonly used regression techniques are the following: Linear regression, Cox regression, and Logistics regression. Regression modelling is used for the statistical evaluation of the data by enabling three things: (a) Description analysis shows the relationship among the independent variables and the dependent variables and it can be statistically defined. (b) Estimation of the data for the dependent variables can be estimated from defined data of the independent variables. (c) Prediction of risk elements that influence the results can be identified, and individual prediction can be determined [55].

3. Conclusion

The ever-rising cost of novel dosage form development projects have not provided assurance of increased efficiency for delivering new drugs. In recent times, quality by design has shown great attention and is being spotlighted more than previously among pharmaceutical producers. Although consideration about its nomenclature and concepts remains indistinct, that may result in a lack of confidence in applying the smart dosage form development. Knowing the disadvantages of quality by design on the one hand and in the other hand, getting a comprehensive understanding of quality by design can enable pharmaceutical manufacturers for employing the concepts of quality by design in utilization.

Robust manufacturing of smart pharmaceutical dosage forms, with their numerous complex formulations and the necessity for rigid similarity with the commercial formulations, essential for the understanding of CPPs and CMAs. The details collected from the development of novel dosage form overtime at laboratory scale provide the substructure for pivotal or pilot scale development. Statistical tools help not only in understanding and identifying CMAs and CPPs in dosage form development, but also in comprehension of the role and relationship between these in attaining a target quality. Although, the implementation of statistical approaches in the development of dosage form is strongly recommended. From a commercial point of view, at all stages of product development, the implementation of quality by design reduces the costs and accelerates the process of product commercialization.

Authors' contributions

I declare that this work was done by the author named in this article. PS conceived, designed the study, carried out the literature collection of the data, writing, and corrected the manuscript. The author read and approved the final manuscript.

Consent for publication

Not applicable.

Competing interests

The authors declare no competing interest.

Availability of data and materials

All the information in the manuscript has been referred from the included references and is available upon request from the corresponding author.

Abbreviations

QbD	Quality by design
ICH	International conference on harmonization
PAT	Process analytical technology
CQAs	Critical quality attributes
RAs	Risk assessments
CPAs	Critical process attributes
CMAs	Critical material attributes
API	Active pharmaceutical ingredients
DOEs	Design of experiments
RCTs	Randomized controlled trials
RSM	Response surface methodology

References

[1] Singh B, Pahuja S, Kapil R, Ahuja N. Formulation development of oral controlled release tablets of hydralazine: optimization of drug release and bioadhesive characteristics. Acta Pharm. 2009;59(1):1-13. DOI: 10.2478/v10007-009-0005-z.

[2] Fısher RA. Handbook of The design of experiments. 1st ed. Oliver and Boyd: Edinburgh;1935. 39 p.

[3] Plackett RL, Burman JP. The design of optimum multifactorial experiments. Biometrika. 1946; 33:305-325. DOI: https://doi.org/10.1093/biomet/33.4.305.

[4] Box GEP, Wilson KB. On the experimental attainment of optimum conditions. J Royal Stat Soc Ser B. 1951; 13:1-45.

[5] Scheffe H. Experiments with mixtures. J Royal Stat Soc Ser B. 1958;20:344-360.

[6] Yu LX, Amidon G, Khan MA, Hoag SW, Polli J, Raju GK, Woodcock J. Understanding pharmaceutical quality by design. AAPS J. 2014;16(4):771-783.

[7] Lionberger RA, Lee SL, Lee L, Raw A, Yu LX. Quality by design: concepts for ANDAs. AAPSJ. 2008;10(2):268-276.

[8] International conference on harmonization (ICH). ICH guideline Q11 on development and manufacture of drug substances (chemical entities and biotechnological/biological entities) EMA/CHMP/ICH/425213/2011 [Internet]. 2011. Available from: https://www.ema.europa.eu/en/documents/scientific-guideline/draft-ich-guideline-q11-development-manufacture-drug-substances-chemical-entities-biotechnological/biological-entities_en.pdf. [Accessed: 2021-02- 20].

[9] Sangshetti JN, Deshpande M, Zaherr Z, Shinde DB, Arote R. Quality by design approach: regulatory need. Arab J Chem. 2017;10(2):S3412-S3425.

[10] Peri P. Quality by design (qbd) approaches for orally inhaled and nasal drug products (OINDPs) in the USA [Internet]. 2007. Available from: http://www.fda.gov/downloads/AboutFDA/CentersOffices/CDER/ucm103526.pdf. [Accessed: 2021-02-18].

[11] Yu LX. Pharmaceutical quality by design: product and process development, understanding, and control. Pharm Res. 2008;25(4):781-791.

[12] William JL. Considerations in developing a target product profile for parenteral pharmaceutical products. AAPS Pharm Sci Tech. 2010;11(3): 1476-1481.

[13] Zhang L, Mao S. Application of quality by design in the current drug development. Asian J Pharm Sci. 2017; 12(1):1-8.

[14] International conference on harmonization (ICH). The international conference on harmonization of technical requirements for registration of pharmaceuticals for human use, quality guideline Q6A specifications: Test procedures and acceptance criteria for new drug substances and new drug products: chemical substances [Internet]. 1999. Available from: http://www.ich.org/fileadmin/Public_Web_Site/ICH_Products/Guidelines/Quality/Q6A/Step4/Q6Astep4.pdf. [Accessed: 2021-02-17].

[15] International conference on harmonization (ICH). The international conference on harmonization of technical requirements for registration of pharmaceuticals for human use, quality guideline Q6B specifications: Test procedures and acceptance criteria for biotechnological/biological products [Internet]. 1999. Available from: http://www.ich.org/fileadmin/Public_Web_Site/ICH_Products/Guidelines/Quality/Q6B/Step4/Q6B_Guideline.pdf. [Accessed: 2021-02-17].

[16] Somma R. Development knowledge can increase manufacturing capability and facilitate quality by design. J Pharm Innov. 2007;2:87-92.

[17] Chang RK, Raw A, Lionberger R, Yu L. Generic development of topical dermatologic products, Part II: quality by design for topical semisolid products. AAPS J. 2013;15:674-683.

[18] Barakat A, Vries H, Rouau X. **Dry fractionation process as an important step in current and future ligno-cellulose biorefineries: a review.** Bioresour Technol. 2013;134:362-373.

[19] Repellin V, Govin A, Rolland M, Guyonnet R. **Energy requirement for fine grinding of torrefied wood.** Biomass Bioenerg. 2010;34:923-930.

[20] Kokko L, Tolvanen H, Hamalainen K, Raiko R . **Comparing the energy required for fine grinding torrefied and fast heat treated pine** Biomass Bioenerg. 2012;42:219-223.

[21] Kobayashi N, Guilin P, Kobayashi J, Hatano S, Itaya Y, Mori S. **A new pulverized biomass utilization technology.** Powder Technol. 2008;180: 272-283.

[22] Maqbool A, Mishra MK, Pathak S, Kesharwani A, Kesharwani A. Semisolid dosage forms manufacturing: Tools, critical process parameters, strategies, optimization, and recent advances. Indo Am J Pharm Res. 2017;7:882-893.

[23] Anju G, Pandey P. Process validation of pharmaceutical dosages form: a review. Biomed J. 2017;1:1467-1475.

[24] Gramaglia D, Conway BR, Kett VL, Malcolm RK, Batchelor HK. High speed DSC (hyper-DSC) as a tool to measure the solubility of a drug within a solid or semi-solid matrix. Int J Pharm. 2005; 301:1-5.

[25] Kimball M. Manufacturing topical formulations: Scale-up from lab to pilot production. In: Dayan N, editor. Handbook of formulating dermal applications: A definitive practical guide. 1st ed. Hoboken: Wiley; 2016. 167-232 p.

[26] Jain S. Quality by design (QBD): A comprehensive understanding of implementation and challenges in pharmaceuticals development. Int J Pharm Pharm Sci. 2014;6:29-35.

[27] Osborne DW. Impact of quality by design on topical product excipient suppliers, Part I: A drug manufacturer's perspective. Pharm Technol. 2016;40: 38-43.

[28] Santos P, Watkinson AC, Hadgraft J, Lane ME. Oxybutynin permeation in skin: The influence of drug and solvent activity. Int J Pharm. 2010;384:67-72.

[29] Hadgraft J, Whitefield M, Rosher PH. Skin penetration of topical formulations of ibuprofen 5%: An in vitro comparative study. Skin Pharmacol Physiol. 2003;16:137-142.

[30] Dave V S, Saoji SD, Raut NA, Haware RV. Excipient variability and its impact on dosage form functionality. J Pharm Sci. 2015;104:906-915.

[31] Lewis GA, Mathieu D, Phan-Tan-Lu R . Pharmaceutical Experimental Design. 2nd ed. New York: Marcel Dekker; 1999. 498 p. DOI: https://doi.org/10.1002/(SICI)1099-128X(200003/04)14:2<93::AID-CEM574>3.0.CO;2-F.

[32] International conference on harmonization (ICH). The international conference on harmonization of technical requirements for registration of pharmaceuticals for human use, quality guideline Q8(R2) pharmaceutical development [Internet]. 2009. Available from: http://www.ich.org/fileadmin/Public_Web_Site/ICH_Products/Guidelines/Quality/Q8R1/Step4/Q8_R2_Guideline.pdf. [Accessed: 2021-01-30].

[33] NIST/SEMATECH. e-Handbook of Statistical Methods [Internet]. 2012. Available from: http://www.itl.nist.gov/div898/handbook/. [Accessed: 2021-02-17].

[34] Bezerra MA, Santelli RE, Oliveira EP, Villar LS, Escaleira LA. Response surface methodology (RSM) as a tool for optimization in analytical chemistry. Talanta. 2008;76(5):965-977.

[35] Candioti LV, De-Zan MM, Camara MS, Goichoechea HC. Experimental design and multiple response optimization: Using the desirability function in analytical methods development. Talanta. 2014; 124:123-138.

[36] Politis SN, Colombo P, Colombo G, Rekkas DM. Design of experiments (DoE) in pharmaceutical development. Drug Develop Ind Pharm. 2017;43(6): 889-901.

[37] Singh B, Bhatowa R, Tripathi CB, Kapil R. International journal of pharmaceutical investigation. 2011;1(2): 75-87.

[38] Collins LM, Dziak JJ, Kugler KC, Trail JB. Factorial experiments efficient tools for evaluation of intervention components. Am J Prev Med. 2014; 47(4):498-504.

[39] Baker TB, Smith SS, Bolt DM, Loh WY, Mermelstein R, Fiore MC, Piper ME, Collins LM. Implementing clinical research using factorial designs: A primer. Behav Ther. 2017;48(4):567-580.

[40] Dziak JJ, Nahum-Shani I, Collins LM. Multilevel factorial experiments for developing behavioral interventions: Power, sample size, and resource considerations. Psychol Methods. 2012;17(2):153-175.

[41] Chakraborty B, Collins LM, Strecher VJ, Murphy SA. Developing multicomponent interventions using fractional factorial designs. Stat Med. 2009;28(21):2687-2708.

[42] Collins LM, Dziak JJ, Li RZ. Design of experiments with multiple independent variables: A resource management perspective on complete and reduced factorial designs. Psychol Methods, 2009;14(3):202-24.

[43] Vaddemukkala Y, Syed M, Srinivasarao. A research article on optimization of olmesartan tablet formulation by 2^3 factorial design. Int J Res Pharm Nano Sci. 2015;4:188-95.

[44] Barhatei S, Husain M. Development of hydrophilic matrix tablet of carbamazepine using 3^3 full factorial experimental designs. Int J Pharm Sci. 2015;7:369-375.

[45] Sharma P, Tailang M. Design, optimization, and evaluation of hydrogel of primaquine loaded nanoemulsion for malaria therapy. Futur J Pharm Sci. 2020; 6:26.

[46] Kumar RG, Sanghvi I. Optimization techniques: an overview for formulation development. Asian J Pharm Res. 2015;5: 217-221.

[47] Bolton S. Optimization techniques in pharmaceutical statistics; Practical and clinical applications. 3rd ed. New York: Marcel Dekker; 1997. 435 p.

[48] Nekkanti V, Muniyappan T, Karatgi P. Spray-drying process optimization for the manufacture of drug-cyclodextrin complex powder using the design of experiments. Drug Dev Ind Pharm. 2009;35:9-29.

[49] Rosas JG, Blanco M, Gonzalez JM, Alcala M. Quality by design approach of a pharmaceutical gel manufacturing process, part 1: determination of the design space. J Pharm Sci. 2011;100(10): 4432-4441.

[50] Xie L, Wu H, Shen M, Augsburger LL, Lyon RC, Khan MA,

Hussain AS, Hoag SW. Quality-by-design (QbD): effects of testing parameters and formulation variables on the segregation tendency of pharmaceutical powder measured by the ASTM D 6940-04 segregation tester. J Pharm Sci. 2008;97(10):4485-4497.

[51] Dash RN, Habibuddin M, Touseef H, Ramesh D. Design, optimization and evaluation of glipizide solid self-nano emulsifying drug delivery for enhanced solubility and dissolution. Saudi Pharm J. 2015;23:528-540.

[52] Central Composite Design [Internet]. 2020. Available from: https://en.wikipedia.org/wiki/Central_composite_design. [Accessed: 2020-02-17].

[53] Pramod K, Tahir MA, Charoo NA, Ansari SH, Ali J. Pharmaceutical product development: A quality by design approach. Int J Pharma Investig. 2016;6:129-138.

[54] Westerhuis JA, Coenegracht PMJ. Multivariate modelling of the pharmaceutical two-step process of wet granulation and tabletting with multiblock partial least squares. Chemometrics. 1997;11:372-392.

[55] Schneider A, Hommel G, Blettner M. Linear regression analysis. Dtsch Arztebl Int. 2010;107(44):776-782.

Index